Textbook of Medicine for Nurses

Textbook of Medicine for Nurses

Winifred Hector MPhil

Senior Lecturer in Education to the Course for Sister Tutor's Diploma,
Queen Elizabeth College, University of London

in association with

J. S. Malpas DPhil FRCP

Director of the Imperial Cancer Research Fund Unit of Medical Oncology,
St. Bartholomew's Hospital

Third Edition

William Heinemann Medical Books Ltd London

First Published 1967
Reprinted 1969
Second Edition 1973
Reprinted 1974
Third Edition 1977
Reprinted 1979

By the Same Author

Modern Nursing: Theory and Practice   *Sixth Edition*

Modern Gynaecology with Obstetrics for Nurses   *Fifth Edition* with Gordon Bourne

ISBN 0 433 14214 6

Printed in Great Britain by The Whitefriars Press Ltd., London and Tonbridge

Contents

Preface to the First Edition

In order to understand why symptoms arise in medical illnesses, and the reasons for a particular method of treatment, it is often necessary to recall some basic facts of structure and of physiology, and it is with this in mind that this book has been written.

It is felt that the student nurse who reads a medical text has had an introductory course of anatomy and physiology, but will want to be reminded of those facts that will widen understanding of medical diseases and how they are treated.

Although the actual writing of the text was done by a nurse, the project was the result of collaboration between a tutor and a physician. Dr. Hamilton Fairley read each chapter, offered suggestions and emendations, and taught his colleague a great deal. Without his knowledge the book could not have been written.

With such a large subject, there will inevitably be disagreement among nurse-tutors as to what conditions should be described, and the writer must sometimes make an arbitrary decision on which subjects to include, and whether to treat them in depth.

Best thanks are due to Professor Linford Rees for his chapter on psychiatry, and to Mrs. Besterman for her illustrations. She is not only an accomplished artist, but can offer intelligent suggestions on visual interpretations of the text. Mr. Owen R. Evans of Heinemann Medical Books Ltd. has worked very hard at all stages of production, and gratitude is owed to him for support when the going was difficult.

Mr. David Tredinnick of the Department of Medical Illustration, St. Bartholomew's Hospital, took most of the photographs, and is thanked not only for his professional skill, but for the helpful interest he and his staff have always shown in the School of Nursing.

Winifred Hector

September 1967

Preface to the Third Edition

Since the last edition of this book, Professor Gordon Hamilton Fairley's tragic death has saddened not only doctors and nurses but the many patients to whom he devoted his brilliant talents. It has been a pleasure to receive the assistance in Gordon's place of his friend Dr. J. S. Malpas.

Two new chapters have been added, one on SI units, and the other on elementary statistics. This is a subject which touches the nurse's work at so many points that it seems desirable to introduce some of the terms and concepts in common use. Developments in drugs have necessitated revision in all sections. Anticoagulant therapy, iron metabolism, hay fever, asbestosis, idiopathic steatorrhoea, Parkinson's disease, hypertension, anaemia, coronary artery disease and its treatment in the intensive care unit have been revised or extended.

Professor Linford Rees is thanked for his attention to the psychiatric chapter, and Dr. R. N. T. Thin, M.D. (Edinburgh), F.R.C.P. (Edinburgh) Physician in Charge of the Venereal Diseases Department, St Bartholomew's Hospital, for his detailed advice on his special subject. Dr. Peter Baillie, Queen Elizabeth College, University of London, gave valuable advice on statistics. David Tredinnick of the Medical Illustration Department of St. Bartholomew's Hospital is responsible for all the photographs in this book, and is especially thanked for his continuing interest as well as his professional skill. Mrs. Audrey Besterman has revised and augmented the illustrations, and I am grateful for her help and friendship. Owen Evans of Heinemann Medical Books has seen this edition into print with his usual efficiency and kindness.

Winifred Hector

Chapter 1

The Nature of Disease

Disease means the impairment of health, either mental or physical, and it is easier to recognize than it is to define. Many people who have a disease know that something is wrong with them; they have complaints, or **symptoms,** which they can relate to their doctor or nurse. They have a pain, or feel depressed, or cannot move some part. There are others who are not conscious of illness, but in whom the doctor on examination detects **signs** of disease. He finds the blood pressure is raised, or that there is albumin in the urine. By considering these signs and symptoms, and by referring to his past experience and knowledge, the doctor makes his **diagnosis** of what is wrong. This may be easy, as when the ends of a broken bone protrude through the skin, or so difficult that in spite of exhaustive tests and examinations, no definite diagnosis is reached. On the basis of his knowledge of the patient and his illness, the doctor may make a **prognosis,** or a surmise about the likely outcome.

These are points that nurses want to know about their patients. They ask, what is the matter with him? What worries him? Is he going to get better? And they also ask, what **treatment** should he have? And in particular, what can I as a nurse do for him? There may be some drug that will cure him; this is a **specific** treatment, and is a logical and satisfactory one that pleases everyone. Often, however, there is no such specific cure, and the physician may choose some **empirical** treatment, which is observed sometimes to be effective, but for which there is no known reason. Sometimes the physician can do nothing that will affect the course of the disease, but he can usually relieve the symptoms, such as pain, or nausea. The nurse is always able to do something for her patient; she can always promote his comfort in a dozen ways.

Disease is said to be **acute** when it arises suddenly; a man sets out for work apparently healthy, begins to shiver at lunch time, and before the evening has pneumonia. **Chronic** disease is usually insidious in onset and may last for years, as in the case of untreated pulmonary tuberculosis. Often the body adjusts to the effects of chronic disease in a remarkable way. A woman who becomes acutely anaemic by suddenly losing a litre of blood may be white, fainting and pulseless; a woman who develops anaemia slowly by losing blood gradually over a year may still continue with her housework, although wearily.

A word of some importance and interest used in describing diseases is
aetiology. This means the study of causes. The cause of tuberculosis is the
tubercle bacillus and yet, although almost everyone is exposed at some time to
this bacillus, comparatively few people get the disease. This leads doctors to a
belief in **multiple aetiology;** questions of sex, age, temperament, diet, physical
build and many others may decide if a person will get a disease and why at one
time rather than at another. Some of these are fairly easy to understand; for
instance, anyone who has no immunity to smallpox and comes into contact

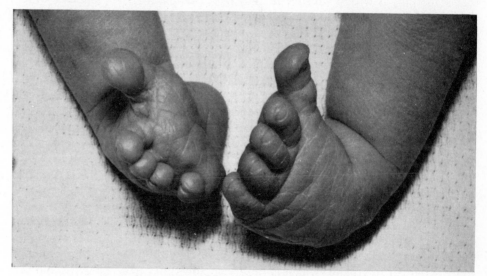

Fig. 1. A congenital condition. Bilateral club foot, or talipes equino-varus.

with an infected person will almost certainly get smallpox. Most people who
have strokes are elderly, most patients with chickenpox are children. This is
because strokes are commonly associated with ageing of the arteries, while
most people with chickenpox are children because most adults have already
had the disease. But often aetiology is puzzling; among duodenal ulcer patients
men predominate, while more women than men have toxic thyroid glands.

Diseases may be classified into types according to their causes. These vary
in importance from one country to another, and from one time to another. The
simple classification offered here will show the variety of illness the nurse may
meet, and the lines on which it is treated.

CONGENITAL

A baby may be born with a disease. This may be a basic abnormality in its cells, as in the case of the **mongol** baby, who has an unusual number of chromosomes. He may be diagnosed at birth by his appearance, and will prove mentally retarded. The baby may have been damaged in the uterus by some hostile factor. A mother who has German measles (rubella) about the third month of pregnancy may have a baby with a congenital heart defect, or cataract, or

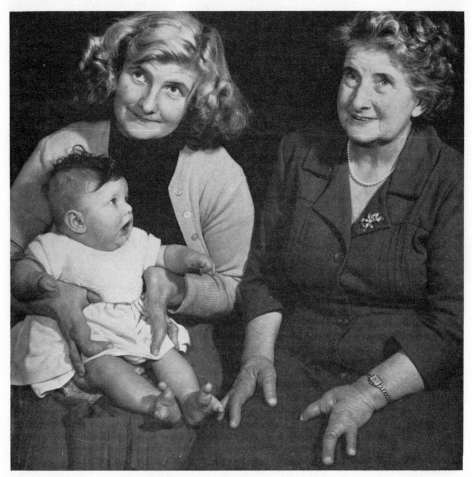

Fig. 2. A congenital condition that is also hereditary. This cheerful family group have made a good social adjustment.

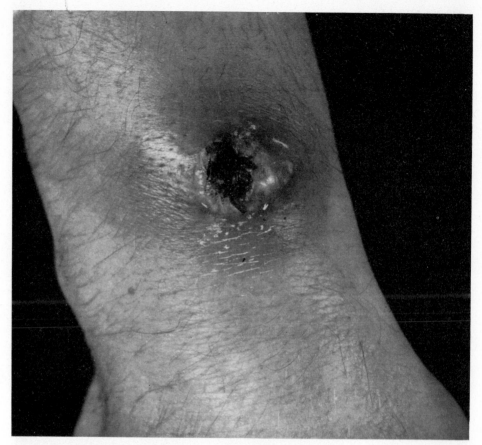

Fig. 3. Inflammation.

deafness. In the early 60's many women in all parts of the world received a drug, thalidomide, as a sedative "anti-emetic" during early pregnancy, and had limb-less children as a result. Such tragedies we ought to be able to prevent. Some malformations are severe, such as communication between the trachea and the oesophagus, some are slight, such as webbing of fingers.

With the improvement in infant welfare more babies with congenital defects are likely to survive. Anatomical defects are usually the province of the surgeon. Biologists are concerned in the advice to be given to parents in whom the possibility of having handicapped children is a high one. Nurses and physicians may have to help in the long-term and often painful adjustment that a congenitally affected child and his parents may have to make.

All disease that is not congenital is **acquired,** and some of the more important groups are as follows.

A. INFLAMMATORY

These are conditions in which the body reacts to injury by micro-organisms or chemicals, or heat or cold. It is the injury by micro-organisms, or **infective** conditions, that form the biggest section of this group. This will be considered at length in chapter 5, but we may notice here that it is in the control of infectious disease that some of the greatest medical victories have been won. It is in the interests of all countries to co-operate in the international control of infection, and the exchange of information at this level may lead to better understanding in other relations.

B. TRAUMATIC OR CAUSED BY INJURY

Injuries are common in modern life. The speed at which machines of all kinds move ensures a high rate of accidents to the people using them. It is hoped that improvements in safety design in cars and roads may reduce the hazards of traffic accident, but nurses should recall that most injuries take place in the home, where burns, scalds, falls and electrocution occur with distressing frequency, especially among children and the old. This is a field in which by advice and teaching nurses may help to reduce pain and illness. Another place is in factories and workshops, where the occupational health nurse is active in trying to prevent industrial injury.

C. NEOPLASTIC OR CAUSED BY NEW GROWTH

To patients the word "growth" means cancer, and nurses should avoid using both words which are open to misunderstanding.

Not all growths are "cancers". Some are not dangerous unless their size or position makes them so. An innocent glandular growth of the thyroid, an adenoma, may look ugly, and if it compresses the trachea may be dangerous, but will not otherwise endanger life. Innocent or benign tumours

1. tend to grow more slowly than malignant ones,
2. resemble in structure the tissue from which they sprang,
3. often have a capsule surrounding them,
4. do not invade neighbouring structures,
5. do not spread to distant parts of the body.

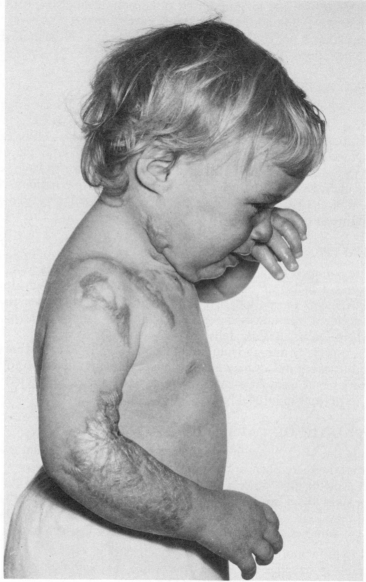

Fig. 4. Trauma. This little girl has suffered burns that have injured her not only physically but also mentally.

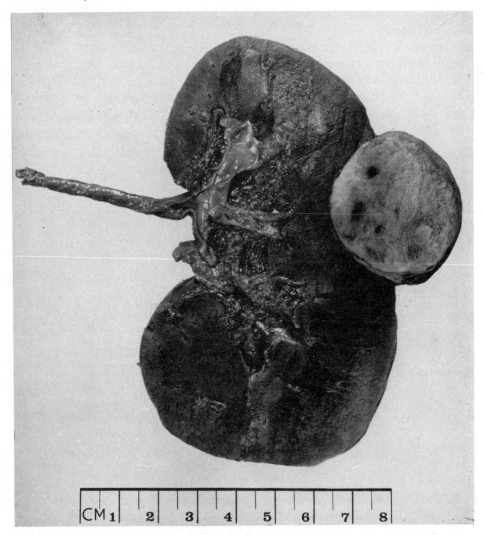

Fig. 5. Neoplasm. An innocent growth, enclosed in a capsule and not invading the kidney in which it originated.

In general, these are removed by the surgeon. Usually they are quite easily shelled out and the patient is relieved. No other treatment is effective.

Malignant tumours
1. often grow rapidly,
2. are often primitive in cell-structure,
3. do not have a capsule defining them,
4. invade and destroy neighbouring tissue,
5. spread by means of detached cells into the bloodstream and the lymphatic system.

In addition, patients with malignant growth often have anaemia and wasting.

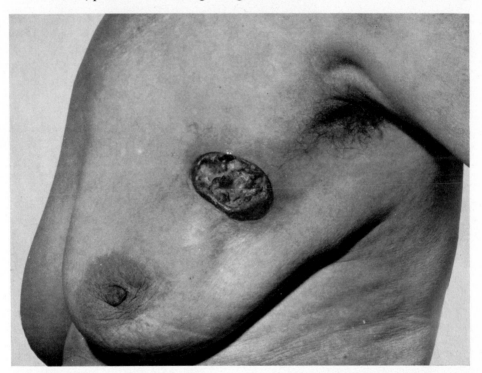

Fig. 6. Neoplasm. A malignant growth of the breast that has ulcerated through the skin.

The treatment of malignant growths has been primarily the province of the surgeon, and since we do not understand the cause of these growths, their removal at any early stage, perhaps with the lymphatic glands into which they drain is logical and may be curative. The surgeon is also concerned in one big advance in the prevention of malignant disease. Cancer of the cervix can be detected before any symptoms appear by examining cells scraped from the surface of the cervix or deposited in the posterior fornix. If 1000 well women of 40 or over are examined in this way, three will be found about to develop cancer of cervix, and they can be cured by simple removal of the uterus.

Radiotherapy from various sources has proved successful in many forms of cancer treatment, and in some (for example, skin cancers) may be the treatment of choice. Most people would probably now believe that the answer to malignant growth will be provided by the biochemist. Cancers originate at cell level, with a pattern of disorganized growth, and hopes of specific cure presumably depend on our ability to reverse or inhibit this process. The cytotoxic drugs (page 176) are a first step in this direction.

D. NUTRITIONAL DISEASES

In large parts of the world, people do not get enough food to eat. In under-developed countries where poverty and lack of knowledge limits food production, natural calamities like drought and floods are bigger hazards than else-where, and bring acute exacerbations of a chronic situation of want. In slightly less hard situations there may be enough food, but not of the right kind. Protein is often in short supply, since it is everywhere expensive, and mal-nutrition from protein lack is common, especially among children, who cannot grow without it. Vitamin deficiencies of many kinds exist. Subnutrition can still be seen in some groups, such as the old and solitary who lack interest or money for adequate food, and other underprivileged people.

In Western Europe and North America, the biggest nutritional problem today is obesity, as a walk down the street of most cities will confirm. Many overweight children are seen, who consume large quantities of sweets and ice-cream. Obesity makes many conditions worse—arthritis and heart disease are examples.

E. METABOLIC DISORDERS

Inability to deal in the normal way with certain elements of the diet may result in accumulation of unwanted chemicals that may lead to troublesome or even disastrous consequences. Though gout (page 343) seems to be primarily a condition of joints, the underlying cause is a metabolic one, uric acid. Children with phenylketonuria are unable to metabolize an amino-acid, alanine, and unless they can be restricted to food low in this particular amino-acid, will be mentally retarded. In these, as in many other conditions, the **diet** may be of prime importance.

A subdivision of this section are the **endocrine** disorders, in which as a result of over- or under-secretion of a ductless gland, upsets in the balance of such substances as sodium, calcium or sugar may occur.

F. ALLERGIC DISORDERS

Allergy means "altered reaction", and a person with an allergic disease reacts with physical symptoms to substances which other people ignore. Some substances are more common than others as allergens, though there is nothing to which someone cannot become sensitized. Allergens may be animal (bacteria; dust from the skin of horses, dogs and cats; shell fish); vegetable (grass pollen; strawberries and blackcurrants; primulas, lily bulbs and many varieties of plant) or chemical, a group increasing in importance with the creation of new industrial substances. These substances can be eaten; inhaled; come into contact with the skin; or be injected into the tissues by a hypodermic needle or an insect bite.

There are many tissues that can be involved in an allergic reaction. They include:

 a) the skin (eczema, contact dermatitis),
 b) the respiratory system (hay fever, asthma),
 c) the digestive system (food allergies),
 d) the joints (bacterial allergy).

The reactions involved may be very slight; many people notice a mild skin reaction after a meal of lobster, or the first season's strawberries. But occasionally a very severe effect, occasionally fatal may ensue. This is **anaphylactic shock.** It most frequently occurs in people who have received an injection of a foreign serum, such as anti-tetanus serum, which is the serum from a horse immunized against tetanus. This dose sensitizes the recipient to the protein in about 10 days and afterwards he remains in an acutely sensitive state for about six months. If during this phase he receives a second injection of the allergen, he experiences a profound and severe reaction that may result in death. Cardiac arrest may occur at once, or tachycardia, dyspnoea, bronchospasms, swelling of the face, and acute anxiety and restlessness may occur. Injection of adrenaline will usually relieve the symptoms, but anaphylactic shock may usually be avoided by taking precautions. Before giving an injection of serum, a test dose of 0·1 ml. should be given into the skin, and the patient observed for 10 minutes for swelling around the injection site or a rise of pulse rate.

Allergic reactions form the basis of some medical tests. For instance, the positive Mantoux test is an allergic reaction to tuberculin displayed by those who have encountered the tubercle bacillus. The word has come into general

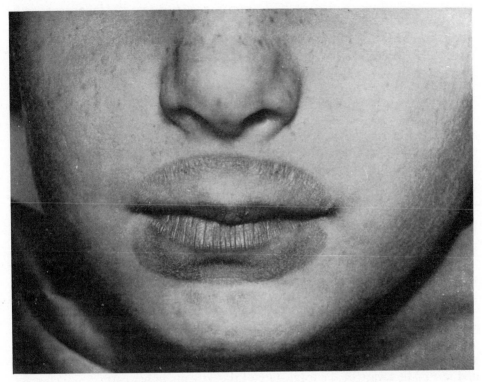

Fig. 7. Allergy. This boy has become sensitive to the dye in iced lollies.

use, and many who have no idea of its medical meaning speak of being "allergic" to something they dislike.

G. DEGENERATIVE DISEASE

The ageing process falls most heavily on three areas. The weight-bearing **joints** such as those of spine, hip and knee are affected, and their articular surfaces abraded by wear. This condition, **osteoarthritis** (page 340) affects most old people to a certain extent. The cells of the **brain** tend to diminish in number with the accidents of life, and since these do not regenerate, loss of mental power and memory is noticed. Most important of all, because it affects all systems, the **blood vessels** harden and degenerate, decreasing the supply of blood to vital organs, and by the narrowing of the interior of the arteries predisposing to clotting. The coronary arteries to the heart may be occluded, clotting or rupture of the cerebral arteries give rise to a "stroke", while the blood supply to the leg may be insufficient, and gangrene results.

Whether it is possible to delay or reverse this ageing process remains to be seen. It has been felt that these are diseases of civilization, and that therefore some cause must be found in the diet, or the tension of modern life. Over-eating and muscular inactivity may load the circulation unduly, while smoking, which is certainly associated with cancer of the bronchus, may, because of the vaso-constrictor action of nicotine, predispose to coronary disease. Apart from this, no conclusive evidence emerges, in spite of long research into dietetic factors. We are often told that primitive peoples do not get these degenerative diseases, but in fact primitive people less often reach the age at which they occur.

H. IATROGENIC EFFECTS

This word means "caused by treatment or therapy", and implies that the patient has signs and symptoms due to the treatment given for another illness. It is something of great importance to the nurse, who is constantly with the patient, and on whom the physician must rely for information about undesirable reactions to drugs or treatment. We now have at our disposal many powerful drugs, and the dividing line between the dose that will give the maximum effect, and the one that will cause serious side effects may be a very narrow one. Steroids (page 322), hypotensive drugs (page 113), cytotoxic drugs (page 176) and many others are potentially dangerous as well as beneficial. The nurse should try to be familiar with the toxic effects of the drugs she is asked to give, and should be aware of the total state of the patients in her care. Small changes in temperature or pulse, variations in the fluid output, rashes, vomiting, head noises, depression, complaints of sore throat or cramp may all be important. "How are you?" is the traditional greeting of the nurse to the patient; she should not omit it, and should listen carefully to the reply.

I. IDIOPATHIC DISEASE

This word refers to diseases whose cause is unknown and there are of course many of these, though the number is decreasing. They are a challenge to the research worker, since while we may control the effects of idiopathic disease, as in epilepsy, we cannot hope to find a specific cure.

J. MENTAL ILLNESS

This is one of the commonest kinds; nearly half the hospital beds in Great Britain are for patients with psychiatric disorders, and there are many more people with mental illness who do not require hospital treatment.

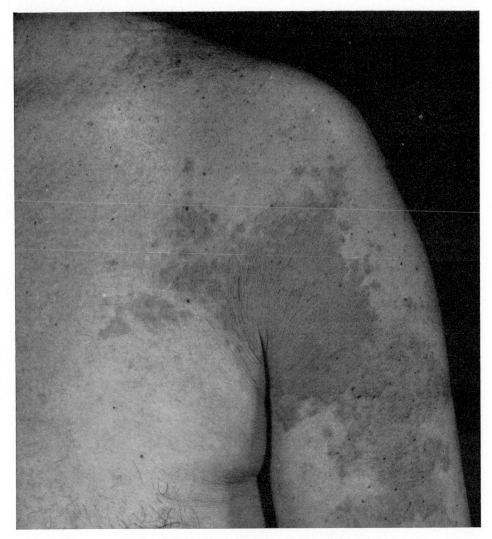

Fig. 8. An iatrogenic eruption, due to ampicillin.

   Since it is through the mind that one thinks and feels, mental disorders are characterized by upset thought and emotion, and because one can only express thought and feeling through the body, actions may become bizarre or even violent.

Many factors are concerned in mental illness, and may decide whether some-one breaks down at a particular time, and with a particular disorder. Mental illness is more commonly diagnosed in urban and highly developed com-munities than in rural and undeveloped ones. People live so closely together in cities, and sophisticated lives and manners are so easily upset by unusual behaviour that patients with mental symptoms are poorly tolerated, and there is pressure to keep people with such symptoms confined to institutions. In country areas there may be a more permissive attitude.

Some of the circumstances that precipitate mental illness are infections; vitamin deficiencies; endocrine imbalance; the personality pattern of the patient; inherited factors; lack of a stable family life in early childhood; sexual maladjustment; financial anxiety, and grief over personal tragedies. Others, such as changes in the chemistry of the nervous system, are doubtless involved, and the progress made today in the diagnosis of mental illness and control of its symptoms has been a feature of medicine in the second half of the twentieth century.

Chapter 2

Some Medical Measures

RELIEF OF PAIN

Pain is one of the most common and most urgent of the symptoms from which people seek relief, and in most cases this relief can be given by a suitable régime. There are three components to severe pain:

1. That of the cause, which must be identified and if possible relieved. Various causes are considered below.
2. Autonomic reactions. Severe pain is accompanied by sweating, vomiting, tachycardia and fainting due to a fall in the blood pressure.
3. Emotional reactions. Some people have a lower pain threshold than others, and are acutely distressed by pain which others may bear with composure. Fear that pain may presage the need for surgery, or portend serious illness or death, fear that relief will not be forthcoming, anxiety about strange surroundings in hospital or separation from families—all these may affect the way in which the patient reacts to pain. The role of the nurse in identifying these feelings and alleviating such fears is of great importance in the control of pain.

These are some of the commoner varieties of pain.

A. COLIC

This is pain caused by violent muscular contraction of a hollow organ, often in an attempt to overcome an obstruction. Colic is felt in the intestine in intestinal obstruction; in the common bile duct and ureter when stones are formed in them; in the uterus in the course of labour. Since these structures are supplied by the autonomic nervous system, vomiting and sweating are frequent accompaniments.

The pain comes in waves with the violent peristalsis that causes it, and while it is at its height the patient is restless, rolling about and groaning, then relaxing as it dies away. The cause of colic can usually be successfully treated. The pains of labour cease after delivery, intestinal obstruction can be relieved surgically. Colic in the ureter or common bile duct may be helped not only by analgesics (pain relieving drugs), but by plain muscle relaxants such as atropine or hyoscine.

B. INFLAMMATION

Inflammation in the superficial tissues is accompanied by swelling, heat and redness, as well as pain, which tends to be throbbing in nature. The pain is due to irritation of the nerve endings by toxic products and by pressure from the local oedema. Rest, elevation and warmth are soothing to pain of this nature, and if the inflammation is infective, the administration of the appropriate antibiotic by curing the inflammation will remove the pain.

The peritoneum is a very large membrane, and if it is inflamed (for instance, following the perforation of a hollow organ) pain is intense. The patient typically lies on his back with knees flexed, moving little; the abdomen is rigid, and respiration is shallow in order to avoid increasing the pain by movement.

C. ISCHAEMIA

If the blood supply to a muscle is interrupted, intense and cramping pain is felt. The most striking example is angina pectoris, when the blood supply to the heart muscle becomes inadequate. The patient stops motionless, thus reducing the work of the heart to a minimum, and his physician will endeavour to prevent such attacks of pain by prescribing a drug that will dilate the arteries, e.g. glyceryl trinitrate.

D. TRAUMA

Injuries cause pain by exposing nerve endings, and by allowing extravasation of blood or other body fluids into serous cavities. Extensive superficial burns are among the most painful of injuries. It is in pain of this kind that the prompt use of analgesics in adequate dosage is outstandingly successful.

E. NERVE INVOLVEMENT

Most people have had toothache, and so have minor experience of this type of pain, which is sharp and darting in character and can be triggered off by small stimuli. Trigeminal neuralgia (page 368) is pain in the distribution of the fifth cranial nerve, which supplies sensation to the skin of the face, and the pain from this condition is so severe that it has caused suicide. The pain of malignant disease (page 19) is often due to involvement of the nervous system.

F. RAISED INTRACRANIAL TENSION

The skull cannot expand, so that the occurrence in it of anything that takes up space—oedema, haemorrhage, or new growth—must result in compression of the brain. This causes severe headache and patients with pain of this type are seen in both medical and surgical wards.

G. POSTURAL CAUSES

Poor posture stretches ligaments and causes pain in the back, legs and feet. Many of the complaints of backache and footstrain come into this category, and pain can be lessened by exercises and re-education.

H. PSYCHOGENIC CAUSES

Many people with anxiety complain not directly of their fears, but of headache, stomach pain and other physical symptoms. They commonly describe these pains in vivid terms—they are excruciating, terrible, unbearable. Some nurses and even doctors find it less easy to sympathize with these feelings, when they know they have no discoverable physical cause. There is no justification for such a feeling; patients really feel pain, and their complaints are a plea for help. On the other hand, the fact that they describe their pain as unbearable does not mean that it will need unusual amounts of analgesic to relieve it. These people are by temperament liable to the risk of drug addiction, unless their analgesics are carefully prescribed, and the underlying psychological condition treated.

ANALGESICS

The physician who treats a patient in pain asks himself, what is the cause, and how may this be relieved? What is the most suitable analgesic to prescribe, having regard to the patient's age and temperament, and whether the pain is acute or chronic? Are any other drugs being taken, the action of which may be affected? Is there liver or kidney disease or respiratory difficulty? The answer is likely to be one of the drugs described here.

Opium derivatives. The most important of these are morphine, diamorphine (heroin) and codeine. Morphine (10–20 mg by subcutaneous or intramuscular injection) is an excellent analgesic, not only relieving pain but calming fear and anxiety. Its drawbacks are that it often causes vomiting, that it depresses the respiratory centre, and is a drug of addiction. It is most useful for acute pain and anxiety which is not likely to be recurrent (e.g. coronary thrombosis, post-operative wound pain) or in inoperable malignant disease where the problem of addiction is not important.

Diamorphine (heroin; 5–10 mg by injection) is banned from use in some countries because of its addictive tendencies. Its action is shorter than that of morphine, it is less liable to cause nausea, but equally depressing to the respiratory centre. Both morphine and diamorphine are controlled under the Misuse of Drugs Act, and all nurses must be aware of their responsibilities under this Act. Although the prescription of drugs for individual patients is done by the doctor, the nurse in hospital is responsible for the ordering and custody of stock supplies, and the key of the cupboard in which Controlled Drugs are locked is kept on the person of the nurse in charge of the ward. In addition to the legal requirements, each hospital has its rules on the checking of individual injections, and of the stock remaining after each dose is given. Addicts sometimes seek employment in hospital in the hope of gaining access to such drugs, and any discrepancy in stock balances or suspicious incidents must be reported at once.

Morphine and diamorphine are sometimes constituents of elixirs which can be used for patients with terminal illness; these people are often better treated with medicines by mouth rather than by injections repeated over a long period. Papaveretum and proprietary drugs such as omnopon are mixtures of opium alkaloids, and have the same drawbacks as morphine, which is the principal ingredient.

Codeine is an opium alkaloid with no addictive tendencies, but is much weaker than morphine. Codeine is an ingredient of several compound tablets along with such drugs as aspirin and paracetamol. Their use is not encouraged, because such mixtures may contain phenacetin, a substance once widely used as a pain-reliever, until the damage that it inflicts on the kidneys of the regular user became known.

Dihydrocodeine (DF118) is an analgesic of moderate strength which can be used for patients who are up and about. It is not wise to prescibe it for long continued use.

Aspirin (acetosalicylic acid) 300 mg per tablet is the most widely used drug for pain, and is especially effective for pain in joints and muscles, and for headaches, but is less so for pain in internal organs. It is not given to people with peptic ulcer, in whom it may cause haemorrhage, and even apparently normal people who use aspirin regularly may get slow oozing of blood from the gastro-intestinal tract which may lead to iron deficiency anaemia. Asthmatics, who are often sensitive to it, should not receive aspirin. Aspirin reacts with certain other drugs, most importantly perhaps with the anticoagulant Warfarin.

Paracetamol (500 mg per tablet) is a mild analgesic with no tendency to cause gastric bleeding. If taken in massive dosage it will damage the liver.

Pethidine (50–100 mg by mouth or intramuscular injection) is a synthetic drug similar in action to morphine but not as powerful. It has a relaxing effect on plain muscle, and so is useful in midwifery and in gallstone or renal colic. It is a controlled Drug, and the risk of addiction is high, so it is not prescribed for regular use. It is less depressing to respiration than morphine, and so is useful for people with head injury in whom brain damage has possibly occurred.

Pentazocine (*Fortral*) is prescribed in 30 or 60 mg ampoules for injection, and in 25 mg tablets, and it is less powerful than morphine but stronger than codeine. It is not addictive, but does not have the calming effect of morphine which is so valuable for patients with myocardial infarction or internal bleeding.

Methadone is a synthetic drug similar in strength to morphine, but without its tranquillizing effects. An advantage is that it is active by mouth, and it is sometimes useful when it is desired to relieve pain without clouding the consciousness. It frequently induces drug-dependence.

PAIN IN MALIGNANT DISEASE

A malignant growth erodes the normal tissue around it, and also metastasizes to lymph glands, bone, lung and brain. The pain of inoperable or extensive disease may be severe, but can always be relieved if suitable measures are taken. A plan should be made to prevent pain, rather than to wait until pain is severe and then attempt to relieve it. It is usually wise to prescribe an analgesic in medium quantities at four- or six-hourly intervals, not "as required". This may be quite a simple remedy at first, like codeine or dihydrocodeine. The amount can be increased, and the interval between doses decreased as time goes on. Eventually morphine or heroin will be required to control pain, and these drugs too must finally be given in increasing quantities, but since the outcome in such cases must be fatal, the fear of addiction need not arise. If morphine is given regularly in small doses, the total needed may be less than if one waits until the patient is in severe need. It should not occasion surprise or alarm, however, if doses above the normal range have finally to be given. The comfort of these patients is the paramount consideration.

Pain in bones or due to brain secondaries is often effectively controlled by adequate doses of aspirin. Where anxiety, or fear of pain returning is high, a tranquillizer such as chlorpromazine may reduce the need for high doses of analgesics. At night a hypnotic should be given, so that further doses of analgesic in the night may be avoided. Alcohol (e.g. brandy) may also promote sleep and relaxation if given at bedtime.

SLEEP

Average people sleep soundly at night because they are comfortable physically and at peace in their minds. People who are ill may fail to sleep because they are disturbed by such symptoms as pain, cough or breathlessness. They may be anxious about forthcoming operations, or the outcome of their illness for themselves or their families. If they are in hospital, they may be disturbed by a strange bed, the presence of others, unusual noises, and light.

Some of these barriers to sleep may be removed by the nurse or physician. Pain may be relieved and in suitable cases cough can be suppressed. Cold feet, a full bladder or thirst can easily be relieved. Wards should be kept as quiet as circumstances permit, and patients should be shielded from light. Co-operation between nurses and social workers may help to relieve anxieties where these are capable of solution.

In a proportion of cases, a hypnotic must be prescribed, either as an emergency measure or as part of a longer-term programme. The physician prescribing a sleeping drug considers what is the cause of the sleeplessness; is the patient accustomed to any particular drug; what is the age and weight. The drug is often prescribed to be given if necessary, and then it is the nurse's discretion to decide if it is to be given and at what time, or perhaps which of two alternatives is to be chosen.

In general, the dosage should be one adequate to ensure its purpose; if the patient fails to sleep after the first dose, he may lose confidence in it. It should be administered in good time, so that the patient does not have to be awakened before he has finished his sleep.

A hypnotic is a drug that produces sleep. A sedative will calm a patient without causing sleepiness, and a small dose of a hypnotic will often have a sedative effect. A tranquillizer will relieve tension and anxiety without affecting consciousness. Since people sometimes complain of sleeplessness because of anxiety, and if this is helped by a sedative or tranquillizer the insomnia may disappear. It will be seen that the boundaries between these types of drug are not clear-cut.

Large quantities of sedatives are consumed, and many people are dependent on repeated prescriptions to get sleep. Women form the larger part of the group Some of these patients were first introduced to hypnotics or sedatives while in hospital, and this indicates the care that doctors and nurses should exercise over the use of these drugs. The tranquillizers used in psychiatry are described in chapter 15; the drugs used to produce sleep and treat minor tensions are discussed below.

The **benzodiazepines** are a group of drugs important for both these effects. Nitrazepam (Mogadon) is a good hypnotic; it acts rapidly, and its effects lasts about eight hours, so that if it is given early the patient will awaken with no hangover. Accidental or intentional overdose is not usually dangerous, and this is a vauloble point. Nausea and rashes are occasionally caused.

Diazepam (Valium) and chlordiazepoxide (Librium) are other widely prescribed members of the group. When used as mild tranquillizers they may by relieving tension improve the sleep pattern. A more rational approach to the problem might be to uncover and hope to remove the cause of the anxiety, and thus avoid the necessity for such prescriptions, but this is a counsel of perfection in modern living conditions.

Choral hydrate is a safe effective hypnotic, but is a liquid with an unpleasant taste and is an irritant to the stomach, so it is not suitable for people with peptic ulcer.

The **barbiturates** are a large group of drugs, formerly widely used, but now fast losing popularity because of the dependence they cause, their danger when taken in large doses, and their abuse by addicts. They tend to cause confusion in elderly patients, and should not be prescribed for those who are depressed, since, they are often used in suicide attempts. Barbiturates increase the rate of destruction of anticoagulant drugs like warfarin. Phenobarbitone 30 to 60 mg or amylobarbitone 50 to 60 mg may still sometimes be used as a sedative, and thiopentone is very widely used as an intravenous anaesthetic.

DRUG OVERDOSE

Drug poisoning, either as a suicide attempt or as an attention-seeking device, is one of the commonest medical emergencies in casualty departments. Barbiturates are still prescribed, and are very dangerous in overdose; the newer hypnotics and tranquillizers are less, so, but patients frequently take them in excess, often with other drugs and alcohol as well. The most acute dangers are respiratory depression; circulatory and kidney failure; and disturbance of fluid and electrolyte balance. Pneumonia is a later and important complication.

The unconscious patient is laid on the side with the head low to facilitate the flow of blood towards the brain. If breathing is shallow, a cuffed endotracheal tube is passed so that intermittent positive pressure respiration, oxygen administration and tracheal suction can be performed. Aspiration of the stomach contents is usually done if the drug was taken less than four hours previously, and is always used if aspirin is known to be the cause, since aspirin may remain in the stomach for many hours. A stomach tube should not be passed on an unconscious patient until the endotracheal tube has been inserted, because of the danger of aspiration of the stomach contents into the respiratory tract. Penicillin is often given to protect the patient from pneumonia. Admission to an intensive care unit is desirable for all unconscious patients, since important decisions about management will depend on monitoring of the heart, the urine output, and the electrolyte levels. Aspirin and phenobarbitone are excreted in the urine, and for people with severe poisoning from these drugs forced diuresis with mannitol or frusemide may be used to hasten this excretion.

Aspirin poisoning has some distinctive features. The patients are often young people in emotional turmoil who do not have access to more sophisticated drugs. Consciousness is usually retained, and this must not mislead nurses or doctors into thinking the condition is not serious. Sweating and rapid breathing are important signs; the hyperpnoea is due to upset of the acid/base equilibrium by the salicylic acid swallowed. The stomach should always be washed out, and the amount of salicylate in the blood estimated.

Drug overdose is not an illness in itself; it is an episode which once it is surmounted indicates a need of help in other directions. It may be part of a psychiatric illness that needs treatment, or of social problems. Even apparently trivial incidents merit careful and considerate investigation, since people who eventually commit suicide may have made unsuccessful attempts previously.

REST

Before one gets up in the morning, metabolic activity is at its lowest level. Energy is being used only to sustain the circulation and the breathing. After rising, calories must be expended and oxygen supplied for muscular activity and the processes of digestion, so cardiac and respiratory effort must be increased greatly. People with impaired hearts or respiratory infections will therefore benefit from being kept at rest in bed, and those with acute cardiac conditions (e.g. coronary thrombosis) may be ordered "absolute" rest—the nurse performs the patient's toilet and feeds him, so that muscular activity is reduced to the minimum possible. Joints which are acutely inflamed will heal more quickly if they are kept still at this stage, and the patient with acute arthritis is often treated by supporting the joints in light splints.

Confinement to bed also provides mental rest, since the patient no longer has to make the decisions and meet the stresses of working life. If the patient is in hospital rather than in bed at home, he is still further protected from anxiety. Peptic ulcers will heal more rapidly if the patient rests in bed in hospital rather than undertakes the same dietetic and drug treatment while ambulant.

EXERCISE

Although rest is of inestimable value in selected cases, there are drawbacks to complete inactivity. If breathing is shallow during bedrest, and the patient moves little, fluid may accumulate at the bases of the lungs, and hypostatic pneumonia develops. Shallow movement of the diaphragm fails to exert the normal pumping action on the inferior vena cava, and venous blood tends to stagnate in the lower limbs. If the movement of the legs is minimal, the muscular contractions that normally assist the upward flow of venous blood no longer help the circulation, and because of these two factors clotting may occur in the deep veins. Portions of this clot may detach, and pass upwards through the inferior vena cava to the right heart, and thence to the lungs as a pulmonary embolus. Constipation is common in bedfast patients, and retention of urine may occur in elderly men with enlargement of the prostate gland.

Exercise is therefore the counterpart of rest, and is used in connection with it. Deep breathing exercises are given even those at absolute rest, and passive movements of the legs are undertaken by the physiotherapist. Elderly patients are not kept entirely at rest in bed if hypostatic pneumonia is feared, and in some cases it may be better not to confine them to bed at all.

Patients who have been kept at rest need graduated exercise to restore their muscle tone and self-confidence. They need precise instructions on discharge as to the amount of activity they should undertake. Vague instructions to "take things easy", or "go slow", may result in undue invalidism.

Chapter 3

Nutrition

Physicians and nurses are deeply concerned in the prevention of disease, as well as in its detection and cure, and the field of nutrition is one in which there are wide opportunities for such work. Very large differences in food intake in quality and quantity are seen, depending on income, social class, habits, race, religion and climate, but whatever these differences, everyone requires for health certain basic necessities in the diet. In addition, some groups, e.g. children and adolescents, pregnant and lactating women and those doing very heavy manual work have special needs. In large areas of the world, the average diet is grossly deficient in many respects, while in others over-eating is prevalent.

The items in respect of which the intake should approach optimum levels are these.

1. Calorie (kilojoule) value.
2. Protein.
3. Fat.
4. Carbohydrate.
5. Vitamins.
6. Mineral salts.
7. Water.

CALORIE (KILOJOULE) VALUE

The nutrient value of food has for long been measured in Calories (with a capital C = kilocalorie). A Calorie is the amount of heat required to raise the temperature of 1000 grams of water through 1°C. 1 Calorie (kilocalorie) = 4.186 kilojoules (kJ) in SI units).

A basic quantity of energy is always expended in maintaining the body temperature, the circulation and respiration. In an adult man, this is about 1500 C (63000 kJ). In addition, enough calories must be taken to provide for muscular activity, and in children and pregnant women, for growth. If intake is in excess of the amount required for these needs, food is converted into fat, and if such excess is habitually taken, obesity results. If food is below the required level, body fat is oxidized to provide the necessary calories, and eventually muscle is also sacrificed and wasting ensues. People who have a diet which is chronically short of calories usually lack essential nutritional as well, and mal-nutrition may be more usefully considered later, in connection with multiple deficiencies.

OBESITY

Overweight due to accumulation of excess fat in the storage depots of the body is a common disorder in prosperous Western societies. While it is commonest among the middle-aged, no age is immune, and in Britain today the variety of malnutrition most often found in schoolchildren is obesity.

The cause of obesity is a calorie intake in excess of calorie output. It is true that many obese people do not appear to eat largely, but this is because when overweight is established, it only takes a moderate diet to keep a fat person fat. Pathological causes of overweight are not common. They are
   a) Cushing's disease (p. 321).
   b) Myxoedema (p. 306). The deposits in these cases are not fat.
   c) Lesions of the hypothalamus in the brain, where the appetite centre is
      situated.

Obesity is often thought to be hereditary, but it appears more likely that eating habits tend to be learnt by children from parents, so that the condition is really environmental.

Overeating may be only the result of habit. With the onset of middle age, physical activities become less vigorous, and if the usual diet is taken the weight will begin to rise. This in turn restricts exercise, and a vicious circle is set up. Eating may also be a solace in times of depression or deprivation of esteem or affection, and such episodes are again more likely in middle age. The ill effects of obesity fall into four categories.
   a) *Cosmetic.* Consciousness of public notice and difficulty in buying clothes
      are painful.
   b) *Locomotor.* The obese person strains the joints of the hips and knees with
      the excess weight and may suffer from osteoarthritis, or painful feet.
   c) *Cardiovascular.* The effort of respiration when the rib cage is handicapped
      by obesity may lead to heart failure, and difficulty in removing carbon
      dioxide from the blood may cause sleepiness (Pickwick syndrome). Hyper-tension is a common complication of obesity.
   d) *Metabolic.* Diabetes mellitus (p. 310) is in middle age most common in
      the obese, and if the weight of these people can be reduced to normal, the
      glycosuria may disappear.

The treatment of obesity is not outstandingly successful; many of those who express a desire to lose weight are unable to persevere with the dietetic restric-

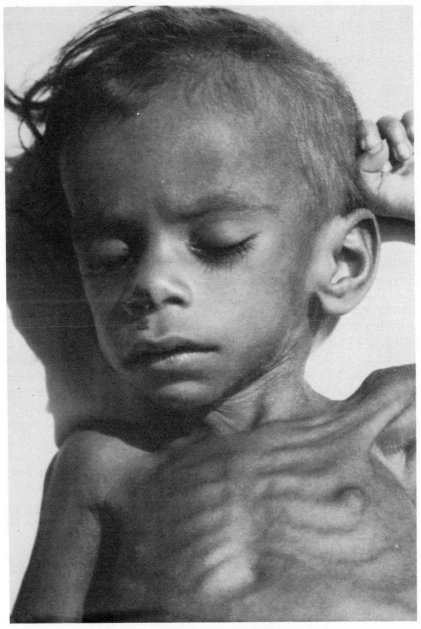

Fig. 9. Chronic sub-nutrition.

(Reproduced by courtesy of the Wellcome Trustees)

tions required. The co-operation of the patient is essential, and the best results are obtained if the patient is seen regularly to be weighed and encouraged.

There are many diets that are effective in weight control; they all have in common that they are low in calorie value. Complete starvation is possible for weeks or months, if fluids and vitamins are given, and after the first day or two hunger is not felt. Spectacular weight loss may be obtained, but close medical supervision must be given.

"Slimming" foods mostly contain methyl cellulose, which provides bulk but not calories; they have no power in themselves to cause weight reduction. "Slimming" drugs, such as fenfluramine, merely serve to suppress the appetite and thus make it easier to follow the diet. This must be one suited to the patient's personal circumstances, and must be fully explained. One that is popular currently is the low carbohydrate diet, which has the advantage that the patient can be allowed a variety of attractive and satisfying food. Meat, fish, eggs, cheese, butter, cream and green vegetables can be taken freely. Carbohydrate is severely restricted, and the total intake of calories is thus reduced. It is a diet that can be followed indefinitely without deprivation.

The diet given below has been well-tried and if strictly followed will permit steady weight loss.

REDUCING DIET OF 1000 CALORIES (4200 kJ)

BREAKFAST
Tea or coffee with milk from allowance—no sugar. Egg or grilled bacon, or lean ham or fish. Grapefruit (no sugar); tomatoes or mushrooms if desired. 1 slice brown or white bread—toasted if liked. Scraping of butter or margarine from allowance.

MID-MORNING
Coffee or tea with milk from allowance or fruit drink (no sugar); or meat or vegetable extract.

DINNER
Midday or evening
Clear soup, tomato juice, melon or grapefruit—no sugar. Meat—fresh or tinned, unthickened gravy. Fish—grilled, baked, steamed or boiled, or liver, ham or cheese. Green vegetables as desired—see list. Root vegetables—1 tablespoon. Fruit—fresh or stewed—no sugar.

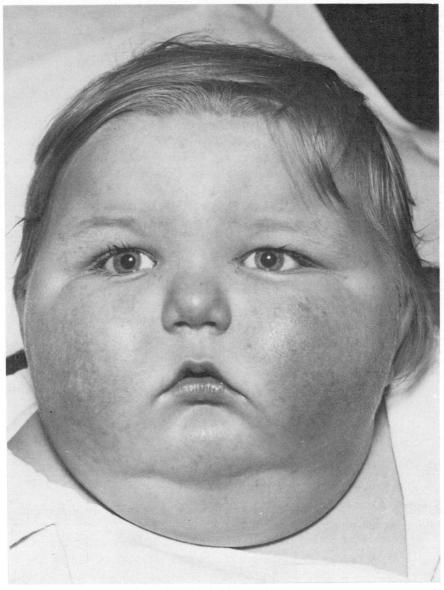

Fig. 10. Obesity in a child.

TEA OR BEDTIME	Tea with milk from allowance—no sugar. 1 slice bread or 2 plain biscuits. Scraping of butter or margarine from allowance. Tomato, lettuce, cucumber, cress, meat or fish paste, or meat or vegetable extract as desired.
SUPPER OR MIDDAY	Meat, egg, cheese or fish—no thick sauce. Salad or green vegetables as desired. Fruit—fresh or stewed—no sugar. Tea or coffee with milk from allowance—no sugar.
BEDTIME OR AFTERNOON	Remainder of milk from allowance. Tea or coffee if liked. No sugar.
DAILY ALLOWANCE	$\frac{1}{2}$ pint (8 dl) of milk. $\frac{1}{4}$ oz. butter or margarine (2oz (60 g) to last 8 days). 2 slices (2 oz.) (60 g) of a large thin cut loaf of bread *or* 3 slices of a small cut loaf. *or* 4 plain biscuits (cream crackers, Ryvita, Vita-wheat, RyKing, Marie, Osborne, Petit Beurre) or 1 square Matzoz. To increase to **1200 Calories** (54000 kJ) add 2 slices of bread and $\frac{1}{4}$ oz. (7 g) butter daily.

THE PATIENT MAY EAT—Average helpings of the following:

Lean meat
Beef, veal, corned beef, lamb, mutton, liver, poultry, rabbit, ham and grilled bacon.

Fish
White fish, herrings, kippers, smoked haddock, salmon—not fried.

Eggs
Boiled or poached.

Cheese
Not more than 2 oz. a day. No cream cheese.

Green vegetables and salads
Brussels sprouts, cabbage, cauliflower, celery, cucumber, marrow, mustard and cress, onions, radishes, runner beans, spinach, tomatoes, watercress—a large helping.

Other vegetables
Carrots, parsnips, peas, swedes, turnips—not more than one tablespoon a day.
NO potatoes or beetroot.

Fruit
Fresh or stewed (no sugar). Not more than 3 portions daily.

Saccharin or other sweetening tablets
May be used for sweetening if desired.

Miscellaneous
Tea, ground or instant coffee, water, soda water. Low Calorie (kJ) drinks, dietetic squash.

Condiments
Pickles in vinegar, Worcestershire sauce, vinegar, lemon juice, pepper, mustard, salt, herbs, gelatine, rennet, spices.

Soup
Clear soup, meat or vegetable extracts or green vegetable water with vegetable extract.

THE PATIENT MUST AVOID:
Fried foods, dripping, oil, cream. Salad cream and mayonnaise.
Thickened soups, sauces, gravies. Tinned or packet soups.
Sugar, glucose, sorbitol.
Jam, marmalade, honey, syrup.
Sweets, chocolates, peppermints, ice cream, iced lollies.
Cocoa, malted milk drinks, tinned milk, yoghourt.
Bottled drinks sweetened with sugar or glucose. Packet jellies.
Cakes, pastries, puddings, pies.
Breakfast cereals, barley, lentils, macaroni, rice, sago or semolina.
Potatoes, dried peas, beans, baked beans.
Grapes, bananas, tinned fruit in syrup, dried fruit. Nuts.
Extra bread, toast or biscuits.

PROTEINS
Proteins form part of all living cells, and so are an essential part of the diet, since without them growth and tissue repair cannot take place. Proteins differ from all other foodstuffs in containing nitrogen. Chemically they are highly

complex substances formed of chains of amino-acids, and before they can be absorbed from the intestine they must be broken down to their constituent amino-acids. They are subsequently re-synthesized in the tissues. Twenty-two amino-acids are important in nutrition, and eight are thought to be essential: phenylalanine, lysine, leucine, tryptophan, methionine, valine, threonine and isoleucine. Those protein foods from animal sources usually contain all eight, while vegetable proteins do not, so that vegetarians must take a varied diet if they are to obtain all the necessary amino-acids.

Sources of animal protein are:

Meat	Milk
Fish	Eggs

Vegetable sources:

Peas and beans

Nuts

Cereals

Protein is not stored in the body, if it is taken in excess of requirements, the nitrogen containing part is split off in the liver and excreted as urea by the kidneys, while the rest of the molecule is oxidized to produce energy. Protein used as fuel yields 4 calories (17 kJ) per gram. Since protein foods are more expensive than any others, it is extravagant to take a diet which contains an excess of it.

In many parts of the world, protein shortage is grave because of the economic difficulties. Such deficiency is felt most severely by children, who need protein in order to grow. **Kwashiorkor** is a protein deficiency disorder from which thousands of young children suffer in Africa, South America and the Far East. The child is usually between six months and four years old, and is undersized, apathetic and miserable. Wasting may not be obvious because of oedema, and the abdomen is distended by ascites. The skin is dry and scaly ("crazy pavement") and the hair often changes colour, a change particularly striking in negro children, whose hair may be red or grey. Diarrhoea and anaemia are common, and fatty degeneration of the liver always exists. Vitamin deficiencies and parasitic infections often require treatment as well.

Mortality is high without treatment, but adjustment of the diet with protein supplements is highly successful. Dried skim milk is very useful, as such children are intolerant of fat. UNICEF, the United Nations Children's Fund, distributes skim milk powder in under-privileged countries, and instruction on dietetic principles and agricultural advice on producing protein foods is given.

Protein deficiency is not often encountered in Great Britain, though there may be old people whose health would benefit from an increased protein intake.

They are often indifferent to their own needs, and short of money for the more expensive foods. In hospital practice, many patients require extra protein if they have suffered loss from haemorrhage, exudate from burns, or purulent discharge from infected wounds, or in ulcerative colitis. For such people, proprietary protein supplements may be added to the diet, e.g. Casilan or Complan.

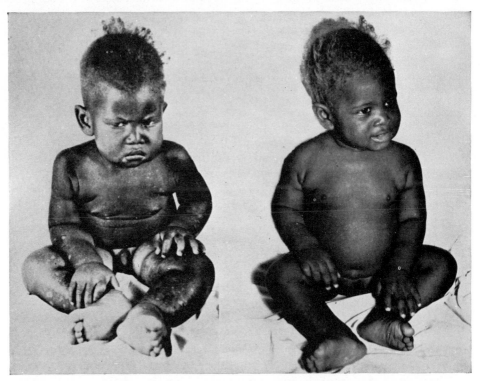

Fig. 11. Kwashiorkor before and after dietetic treatment. The child has been transformed mentally as well as physically.

(Reproduced by courtesy of the Wellcome Trustees)

FAT

Fat is a fuel food, and provides twice as many calories weight-for-weight as protein or carbohydrate. It is the storage substance of the body: any food taken in excess of energy requirements is converted to fat, and deposited under the skin, in the great omentum, or around the kidneys.

Animal sources:

Butter, cheese, cream, fat meat, fat fish such as herring and salmon, whale oil.

Vegetable sources:

Olive oil, corn oil, nut oil, margarine manufactured from vegetable oils.

Fat adds palatibity to the diet, and is also important because the fat-soluble vitamins A, D and K are found in it. In countries were dairy herds can be kept, butter is the most popular fat in the diet, while in hotter climates vegetable oil takes its place. Margarine fortified with vitamins A and D is an efficient substitute in food value for butter, and its flavour has been greatly improved by manufacturers.

Fat is composed of glycerol combined with a variety of fatty acids, with different properties. Those fats like butter which are solid at medium temperatures contain a high proportion of saturated fatty acids, while those like olive oil and corn oil which are liquids contain unsaturated fatty acids. The importance of the distinction is that a connection between coronary thrombosis and a diet high in saturated fats has been suggested. This condition is more common in countries where the diet contains a high proportion of animal fats than in those where vegetable oils are used in cooking. Some physicians prescribe for coronary patients diets containing these unsaturated fats instead of butter, while others believe there is no firm evidence that such restrictions are useful. It is of course important that no patient with heart disease receives enough fat in the diet to cause overweight.

CARBOHYDRATES

Carbohydrates are made of carbon, hydrogen and oxygen, and they range in chemical structure from the simple to the complex. Considered in this order, they include:

Sugars. The simplest sugars are glucose and fructose; slightly more complex are sucrose (cane sugar) and lactose (milk sugar). Honey and sweet fruits are natural sources of sugar.

Starches. These are insoluble carbohydrates, found in all cereals such as wheat and rice, and in root vegetables like potatoes and carrots.

Cellulose is the fibrous framework found in many vegetables (such as cabbage and celery). It is not digestible in the human alimentary canal, but provides bulk which helps to satisfy appetite and promote peristalsis.

Starches form a large part of the diet in most parts of the world, since they are bulky, and usually less expensive than protein or fat. In Great Britain bread and potatoes are the common starch foods, in Mediterranean countries pasta made from wheat flour is eaten and in the East rice is the staple diet.

The consumption of sugar in the form of candy and chocolates has increased enormously in the West in the last quarter of a century. Nutrition experts do not view this trend with satisfaction, it is partly responsible for the number of obese children, and for the incidence of dental decay.

VITAMINS

Vitamins are substances with no calorie value. They are only required in minute amounts in the diet, but unless these amounts are forthcoming, ill health and even death may result. When the vitamins were first described they were given letters to distinguish them and, although their chemical construction is now known, they are often alluded to by their letters, and will be described in alphabetical order.

Vitamin A is a fat soluble vitamin found in liver, dairy produce and cod liver oil. A coloured substance, carotene, found in red and orange fruits and vegetables is converted to vitamin A in the body, so tomatoes, carrots, swedes and apricots are sources of vitamin A.

Vitamin A maintains the health of mucous membranes, e.g. the conjunctiva, and in combination with a protein forms visual purple (rhodopsin), a pigment in the retina which is necessary for sight in dim light.

Dietetic deficiency first causes difficulty in seeing in poor light (night blindness) and eventually thickening and opacity of the conjunctiva may lead to blindness. Fat soluble vitamins can be stored in the body, so excess vitamin A in concentrate form, such as fish liver oils, should not be given to children except on medical advice.

Vitamin B complex. The vitamin B group contains many related substances, all water soluble. The following are the more important ones.

B1 (thiamin) is found in meat, whole grain cereals and wholemeal bread. Prolonged lack causes **beri-beri,** a disease causing polyneuritis, oedema and heart failure. It is not often seen outside the tropics, but chronic alcoholics in any country may suffer from neuritis, since alcohol interferes with the appetite, and hence with the supply of B1.

Nicotinic acid (niacin) is found in liver, yeast and in all whole cereals except maize. Deficiency causes **pellagra** with dermatitis, diarrhoea and mental changes. It used to be common in South America, in areas where maize was the staple article of diet, but as rising economic levels permit a more varied diet, the incidence is falling.

Vitamin B$_{12}$ (cyanocobalamin) is found in high quantities in liver, and if it is not absorbed in adequate amounts, pernicious anaemia (page 158) results.

Folic acid is present in many foods and is also made in the intestine by the colon bacteria. It is necessary for normal blood formation, and if it is lacking anaemia of a large-celled type develops. Deficiency is common if absorption from the intestine is interfered with. Folic acid is often given with iron to prevent anaemia in pregnancy.

Vitamin C (ascorbic acid) is water soluble, found in citrus fruits, blackcurrants, rose hips, tomatoes, green vegetables. It is necessary for the formation of fibrous tissue and for the health of the capillaries.

The deficiency state that results from lack of this vitamin, **scurvy,** has been known for centuries, from the experience of sailors on long voyages without fresh food. Adults suffer from haemorrhages into the gums, skin and joints, anaemia and failure to heal wounds. Infants also suffer from scurvy if they are fed on boiled milk without supplements. The outstanding symptom is pain and tenderness in the bones and joints, especially of the legs, so that the child is apprehensive at being handled, and screams when it fears that it is going to be moved.

Scurvy responds readily to the administration of ascorbic acid or fresh orange juice. While severe scurvy is rare in Great Britain, mild forms may be seen in elderly people living alone, and in people who have "indigestion", and live on restricted diets without fresh food. Patients with cancer of the stomach may lack ascorbic acid because of anorexia, and need the vitamin to promote wound healing if operation is undertaken.

Vitamin D is fat soluble and is found in fat fish, fish liver, butter, cheese and fortified margarine. It is made in the skin by the action of sunlight on the sterol it contains, and since vitamin D is not found in a wide range of foods, this method of vitamin manufacture is important.

Vitamin D is necessary for the absorption of calcium, and without it changes take place in the skeleton. Children develop **rickets,** and this disease was prevalent in the industrial towns of nineteenth-century England, before its cause and method of prevention was discovered. Calcification of bones and appearance of teeth is delayed and leads to many deformities. The epiphyses of bones enlarge and those of the ribs may be prominent ("rickety rosary"). The arm bones may bend when the child sits up and begins to support its weight on them, and when

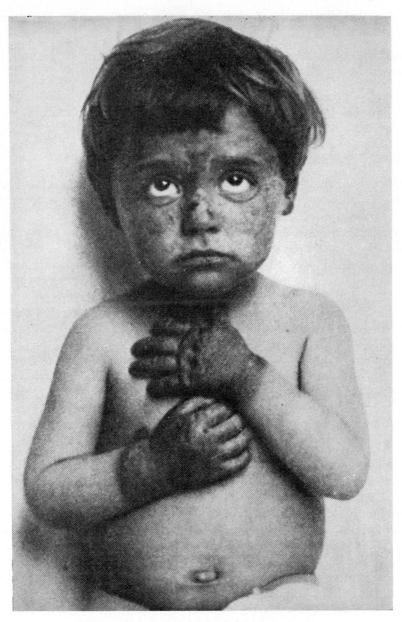

Fig. 12. Vitamin deficiency. Child with pellagra.

(Reproduced by courtesy of the Wellcome Trustees)

it stands up the leg bones bend, producing bow legs. The skull is enlarged, with bossing of the forehead and parietal eminences. The spine curves and all muscles are weak. Anaemia is common and the child gets frequent infections.

Adults who are deficient in vitamin D may suffer from osteomalacia. It is especially a disease of women whose calcium reserves are depleted by pregnancy. Fatigue, stiffness and pain in bones appear early, and as the disease progresses pathological fractures and deformity of the pelvis may follow.

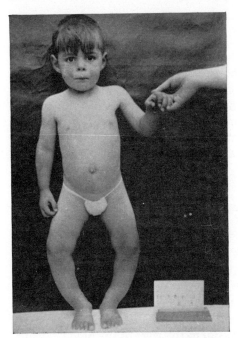 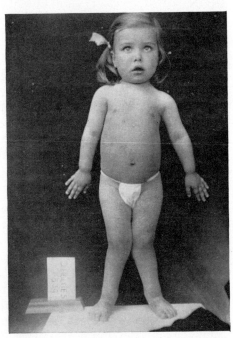

Fig. 12a. Vitamin deficiency. Children with rickets.
(*Reproduced by permission of F. Wilson Harlow, FRCS Eng.*)

These deficiency diseases are preventible, and with effective health teaching, welfare service to the elderly and other vulnerable groups and improved economic conditions it is hoped that they will become rare all over the world.

MINERALS

IODINE

Iodine is required in very small amounts in the diet for the health of the thyroid gland. It forms part of thyroxine, the thyroid hormone, and in its absence the gland enlarges to form a swelling in the neck called a goitre. Iodine is found in sea fish, and in vegetables grown near the sea, so that places far removed from the sea, e.g. Switzerland are the areas in which goitre is most common. It is less frequently encountered now that the cause is known, and in many countries potassium iodide is added to table salt, and this supplies the small amount of iodine required to prevent goitre.

IRON

Iron is a constituent of haemoglobin, the pigment which carries oxygen to the tissues. Without it red cells cannot be made in adequate numbers and anaemia results.

When red cells break up, the iron in the haemoglobin is not excreted, but is used in the formation of new molecules of haemoglobin. Adults therefore need only a very small intake of iron to maintain satisfactory blood levels, unless iron is lost in haemorrhage. Women are more vulnerable in this way than men, because of the natural losses of menstruation and childbirth. The best natural sources of iron are meat, liver, egg yolk and green vegetables.

CALCIUM

Calcium phosphate forms the mineral part of bones and teeth, and is present in the blood at a level of 2.1 to 2.6 mmol/l. It is necessary for muscle contraction and for the clotting of blood.

The best natural source of calcium is milk and milk products. In Britain white flour is fortified with calcium chloride, and this provides a valuable source of the mineral. Calcium is absorbed from the small intestine in the presence of vitamin D, so that for normal calcium metabolism, an adequate intake and sufficient vitamin D must both be present. If either is in chronically short supply, infants develop rickets (page 35). A fall in the level of the blood calcium causes tetany (page 308). Excess calcium in the blood can cause cardiac arrest, and injections of calcium chloride can be used by the cardiac surgeon to stop the heart during operations on it.

FLUORINE

In areas where fluorine is absent from the drinking water, dental decay is more common in children than it is in places where fluorine is present in small amounts. Health authorities advocate the addition of minute amounts of fluorine to the water in such districts, but there is opposition in some quarters to the "adulteration" of water, and it has been suggested that fluoride tooth paste for children is preferable to administering it to everyone. No other function has been attributed to fluorine in human nutrition.

WATER AND SALT METABOLISM

All the physiological processes take place through the medium of water. Foods are digested, nutriments absorbed and distributed, and waste products excreted in watery solutions. Body temperature is largely regulated by evaporation of water from the skin. Plasma, urine, tears, sweat and cerebrospinal fluid consist largely of water.

Water constitutes about 70 per cent of body weight, and this quantity remains remarkably constant in health. About 260 dl. is lost every day in the urine, sweat, stools and by respiration. For convenience in arithmetic, this will be considered as 300 dl. Unless this amount is replaced, life cannot be sustained for more than a few days. Fluid (1) is drunk as such, (2) is also a constituent of all foods, and (3) is derived in the tissues from oxidation of foods. The intake is regulated by thirst; if an undue amount of water is lost (e.g. by sweating in hot weather) more is drunk, and so the fluid balance is maintained. If more fluid than usual is drunk, an increased quantity of dilute urine is passed.

Nurses make use of this balancing action when they ask a patient with a urinary infection to increase his fluid intake, which will increase the output and so dilute the infected urine. A patient who is unable to take food must drink an increased amount of fluid, to make up for the water content of normal food. Feverish patients lose an abnormal amount of water through the skin, and through the lungs because of the increased respiration rate.

Loss may occur in abnormal ways in many surgical and medical patients. Fluid may be vomited, or aspirated from the stomach; diarrhoea, haemorrhage, loss of plasma from burns, and excessive sweating are possible causes of fluid loss. If this cannot be made good by drinking, the patient is said to be in negative fluid balance, and suffers from **dehydration.**

Of the 45 or so litres of water in the body of an adult, 30 litres is contained within the cells, and is termed **intracellular.** The rest of the body fluid is **extracellular,** and is found either within the blood vessels as plasma, or in the tissue spaces between the cells. Movement of fluid containing oxygen, nutrients and waste products is constant and rapid.

Water metabolism is intimately connected with the mineral salts that are dissolved in it. Of these the most important is common salt, or **sodium chloride.** Salt is constantly lost in the sweat, and no difficulty is encountered in temperate climates in replacing it from the food. Usually more is consumed than is required, and this excess is regularly excreted in the urine, which usually contains

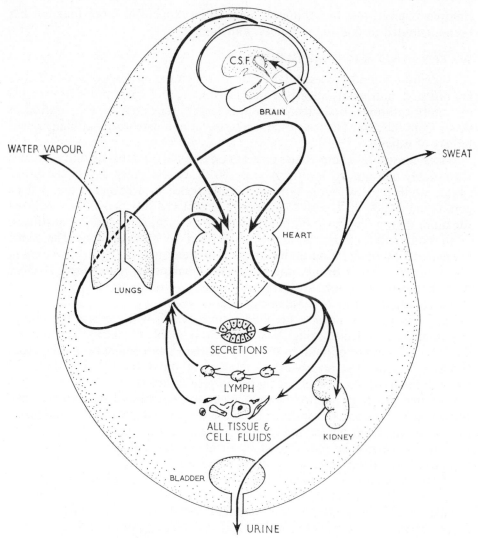

Fig. 13. Some of the fluid elements of the body.

5 g. of sodium chloride per litre. Excessive sweating causes loss of abnormal quantities of salt, and athletes often take salt tablets, especially in hot weather, to guard against salt lack.

The amount of sodium chloride in the plasma is 0·9 per cent, and this quantity

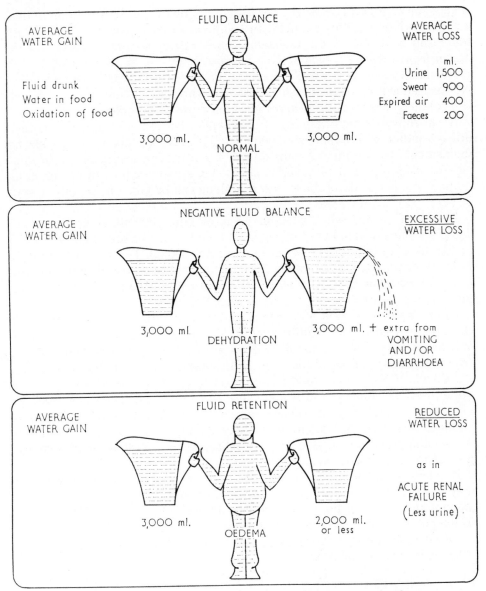

Fig. 14. Normally the fluid taken and excreted balance each other.

If extra fluid is lost, and is not balanced by increased intake, the patient passes into negative fluid balance, or dehydration.

If the intake is normal but excretion is reduced oedema develops.

is kept constant because the red blood cells are unable to withstand more than a slight variation in this strength. In solutions weaker than this, they absorb water and finally break up, or haemolyse. In strong solutions, water is withdrawn from the cells which shrivel and are destroyed. A solution of 0·9 per cent sodium chloride is therefore spoken of as physiological or **normal saline.** Normal saline is equal in strength or **isotonic** with the salt content of the blood, and solutions used for intravenous injection must be isotonic.

It was shown at the beginning of the chapter that in a person with a normal urinary output, a fluid intake of 3000 ml. a day must be maintained to make up the amount lost. To this we must now add that the salt lost in the sweat must also be made up, and that this is about 5 g. Anyone who can eat or drink normally finds this no problem, but if nothing can be taken by mouth, it must be supplied in another way.

100 ml. of normal saline contains 0·9 g. of salt; 1000 ml. (1 litre) contains 9 g. If we want to supply 5 g. of salt in 24 hours, it will be found in $1000 \times 5/9 = 555$ ml. of normal saline, or in round figures 600 ml. To this must be added 2400 ml. of water to make up the 3000 ml. of fluid to which we have alluded. It will be seen that the total is made 1/5 of normal saline and 4/5 water. This is fifth-strength normal saline, usually written N/5 saline.

N/5 saline is quite well absorbed if given rectally, and it is possible over a short period to maintain fluid balance in this way. It is not, however, a comfortable method, and patients too ill to drink are unlikely to be able to absorb the required amount. The usual route for fluid administration is the **intravenous** one.

3000 ml. of N/5 saline could not however be given intravenously, since it is not an isotonic solution and would cause haemolysis. Neither would 3000 ml. of normal saline be given (unless salt was being lost in other ways) since although this would be isotonic, it would contain too much salt ($3 \times 9 = 27$ g.). A common practice is to give **dextrose saline,** which is N/5 saline plus enough glucose to make it isotonic.

Problems of intravenous therapy are rarely as simple as this. The patient may have suffered blood loss, or be vomiting and thus losing chloride. The amount and choice of fluid will then depend not only on clinical observations of the pulse and skin, and consideration of the fluid balance chart, but also on chemical estimation of the mineral salt content of the plasma, and sodium chloride is only one of these.

ELECTROLYTES

The electric cell that one puts into a transistor set has two poles, marked $+$ and $-$, that are connected to the appropriate terminals. The positive ($+$) pole is called the anode, the negative (−) one is the cathode. If the two poles of a battery are connected to rods which are put into a dilute mineral salt solution, and the current switched on, the salt breaks up in the form of charged particles, called **ions.** The positively charged particles are attracted to the negative pole (cathode) and are called **cations;** the negatively charged ones go to the anode, and are called **anions.** Mineral salts which will in dilute solution break up into these electrically charged ions are called **electrolytes.** The most important ones in the blood are sodium chloride, sodium bicarbonate, potassium bicarbonate, potassium chloride and calcium chloride and calcium phosphate. These dissociate into these ions.

Cations (+)	*Anions* (−)
Potassium (K+)	Bicarbonate (HCO_3−)
Sodium (Na$^+$)	Chloride (Cl−)
Calcium (Ca^{++})	Phosphate (PO_4−−−)

Estimation of the blood electrolytes is necessary in many diseases. Potassium is of special importance because it is found chiefly inside the cells. If salt loss from the body is prolonged, as in intractable vomiting, potassium is withdrawn from the cells in an attempt to maintain the potassium level in the blood. This fall in potassium levels should be foreseen, and potassium supplied, or the patient will become weak, drowsy and confused, and may suffer cardiac arrest.

The infusion fluid that a patient receives is determined by his needs. If he has suffered a haemorrhage, he will require transfusion of whole blood. If he is grossly anaemic, i.e. severely lacking in red cells, giving whole blood in quantities sufficient to relieve the anaemia may overload the circulation with fluid, so packed cell transfusion may be given. If extensive burns or superficial injuries have caused loss of serum, plasma is given. If water and electrolytes have been lost by vomiting or diarrhoea, then water and the appropriate salts must be given intravenously in an isotonic solution.

ACID-BASE BALANCE

The maintenance of stable conditions within the body is essential for life, and there are many mechanisms constantly at work to keep the temperature, the metabolic rate and the electrolyte content of the blood steady. The nervous system, the endocrine glands and the kidneys are among the more important agents involved.

One of the constants that must be maintained within narrow limits is the amount of acid in the tissues. The acidity of a solution is measured by the quantity of hydrogen (H) ions it contains. Water, which is neutral in reaction, contains 1/10,000,000 of a gramme of hydrogen ions in every litre. This can be written as $1/10^7$, or 10^{-7}. Water is said to have a hydrogen ion concentration (pH) of 7. Acids have a pH of less than 7, and the lower the figure the stronger the acid. Alkalis or bases have a pH of more than 7.

The pH of the plasma is 7·4, that is, it is slightly alkaline. Acid is constantly being produced in the body by oxidation of carbon to produce carbon dioxide, and by metabolic processes. This must be constantly excreted or neutralized if the pH of the blood is to be kept up, and it is done in three ways.

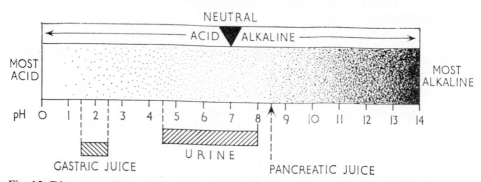

Fig. 15. Diagram to illustrate the pH of body fluids. The pH of water, which is neutral, is 7. Fluids with a higher pH than 7 (e.g. pancreatic juice) are alkaline. Gastric juice (pH 1·5 to 2·3) is strongly acid.

1. By use of salts as buffering agents. Students who would like to know more of the chemistry involved should consult a larger book, e.g. *A Short Textbook of Medicine* by Houston, Joiner & Trounce, chapter 12.
2. By respiration. Carbonic acid (H_2CO_3) consists of carbon-dioxide (CO_2) and water (H_2O). Carbon dioxide is exhaled from the lungs and so the amount of carbonic acid in the blood is reduced. The respiratory centre in the medulla is sensitive to CO_2, and if the level rises, respiration increases in rate and depth to wash out the acid.
3. By urinary excretion. The kidney is exceedingly sensitive to the pH of the blood, and if this tends to fall, the urine becomes more acid.

These mechanisms are efficient in ordinary circumstances to keep the pH constant, but in pathological conditions they may fail to maintain the balance, and acid or alkali may predominate in the blood.

Acidaemia. Acid may accumulate in the blood for two main reasons.

1. Respiration is inadequate to eliminate acid, e.g. in chronic bronchitis with

emphysema. The most extreme example is seen in cardiac arrest, when cessation of respiration leads to accumulation of acid in the blood, which must be corrected by administration of sodium bicarbonate if recovery is to be achieved.

2. Abnormal acids are produced, often by upsets of fat metabolism. In diabetic coma, the acids produced are keto-acids or ketones. The deep breathing so characteristic of this condition is due to an effort to increase acid excretion by over-breathing.

ALKALAEMIA

Alkalaemia may, like acidaemia arise from metabolic or respiratory causes. It may result because acid is lost through excessive vomiting, or because excess alkali has been taken, perhaps in the treatment of gastric ulcer. In such patients, the respiratory movement is decreased, in an effort to conserve acid and so restore balance.

Acid may also be lost through over-breathing which may occur in anxiety states. An example of the link between breathing and the pH of the blood is seen in Cheyne-Stokes respiration (page 183). Increasingly deep breathing washes acid from the blood until it falls below the level at which it stimulates the respiratory centre. Breathing ceases for a time, during which acid accumulates in the blood, and eventually the medulla is stimulated to start the cycle again.

The treatment of upsets of acid-base balance depends on the cause. Abnormal production of acids must be prevented, lung disease must be treated, drug treatment must be reviewed, the electrolyte balance must be frequently estimated, and the body mechanisms for regulating the acid-base balance given an opportunity to restore the equilibrium.

Chapter 4

Immune Reactions

There are several ways in which the body can respond to invasion by foreign substances.

a) **Phagocytosis.** This is the primitive method of defence adopted by the amoeba, which deals with suitably sized particles by engulfing and digesting them, thus combining self-defence and nutrition. The polymorphs are the most important and numerous phagocytes in the body, and are the first line of defence, migrating to sites of infection very quickly, and eating up bacteria.

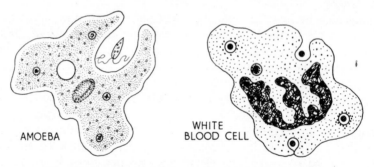

AMOEBA

WHITE
BLOOD CELL

Fig. 16. Amoeba and polymorphs are similar in action.

b) **Formation** of **non-specific anti-bacterial substances.** An example of such substances with a general action against all types of organism is lysozyme. This is a digestive enzyme that can kill bacteria. It is found in many body fluids, such as tears.

c) **Antibody formation.** Antibodies are produced in response to the introduction into the tissues of an antigen. The first antibodies that interested doctors were those made against bacteria, but the events connected with allergy (page 10), graft rejection (page 51), anaphylactic shock (page 10), and autoimmunity (page 51) showed that the immune reaction was not confined to bacteria. Antigens are usually proteins, but some carbohydrates can excite antibody formation. All antigens have one or more places in their molecules, called antigen combining sites, onto which the antibody locks, rendering the antigen inert and harmless. The fit between the two is specific, e.g. the measles antibody cannot combine with the virus of mumps. Although food contains many antigens, these do not usually excite antibody formation because they are broken down in the intestine before being absorbed into the portal vein.

It has been known for centuries that someone who survived an attack of an infectious disease like smallpox was in some way protected against a second attack, and in 1798 Jenner demonstrated that inoculation with material from cowpox lesions could produce immunity to smallpox. In the second half of the nineteenth century the organisms causing infectious disease were identified, and doctors became concerned with practical problems of immunization against these organisms. It was recognized that the lymphatic system was intimately connected with the phenomena of resistance to infection. In the middle of this century there was an upsurge of interest in this subject, when we became aware that immunity was not merely a matter of resisting bacterial attack, but was concerned in defence against cancer, in the rapid destruction of grafted organs, in allergy, and in a whole group of diseases in which the tissues mounted an attack, not against invading bacteria, but against proteins from its own cells. Some of the facts about the structure of the lymphatic system should be recalled before describing its part in immune reactions.

The organs of the digestive and respiratory systems are grouped together, and are easily recognized as serving a common function.

The **reticulo-endothelial system,** however, consists of tissues rather than organs, and these are scattered widely through the body, and are concerned especially with blood formation and destruction, and with the establishment of immunity. These cells line the liver, spleen, thymus gland, bone marrow, and the lymphatic system.

The **lymphatic system.** Fluid escapes from the blood capillaries, carrying dissolved foodstuffs and other necessities to the tissues. These do not become waterlogged because this fluid is collected by the lymphatic capillaries. These vessels are at their origin open-ended, and drain the spaces between the cells.

At intervals along the lymphatic vessels are lymphatic glands, and all tissue fluid passes through one or more of these glands before returning to the blood stream. These glands act like a series of filters, and diagram 17 shows the complicated interior of a gland and some of its functions, to be described later. The thymus gland (page 48) and the spleen are seen by their structure to be part of the lymphatic system. The spleen is richly supplied with blood from the portal circulation, but it is made of lymphoid tissue, which can make lymphocytes.

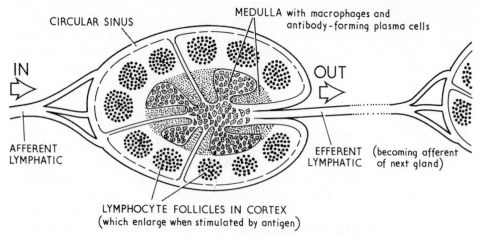

CIRCULAR SINUS

MEDULLA with macrophages and
antibody-forming plasma cells

IN

OUT

AFFERENT
LYMPHATIC

EFFERENT (becoming afferent
LYMPHATIC   of next gland)

LYMPHOCYTE FOLLICLES IN CORTEX
(which enlarge when stimulated by antigen)

Fig. 17. A diagram of the structure of a lymph gland.

During foetal life it makes red blood cells, and can resume this function in adult life in times of stress. The spleen destroys aged red blood cells, but it seems to have no function that cannot be taken up by other organs, and no ill effects follow its removal.

Collections of lymphoid tissue occur in the nasopharynx and fauces (adenoids and tonsils) and in the intestinal tract (Peyer's patches; the appendix) to deal with the high risk of infection in these sites. The lymphatic capillaries join to become larger vessels, and eventually these empty into one of two ducts that drain into the innominate veins in the chest. The pressure is low in the great veins here, and the lymph is sucked out of the ducts into the blood circulation. The larger is the thoracic duct, which drains the body below the waist, and the left side of the body above it.

THE THYMUS GLAND

This gland lies in the chest, just beneath the sternum, and it can be seen from its structure that it is related to the lymphatic system. The central medulla of the gland contains many lymphocytes, and the outer cortex is packed with them. The thymus is quite large at birth, attains its maximum size at puberty, and then slowly shrinks until it is very small in old age. The cortex decreases very markedly during the course of long illnesses.

At birth, the function of the thymus is to make lymphocytes, which travel to the peripheral glands and populate them, and it is known from animal

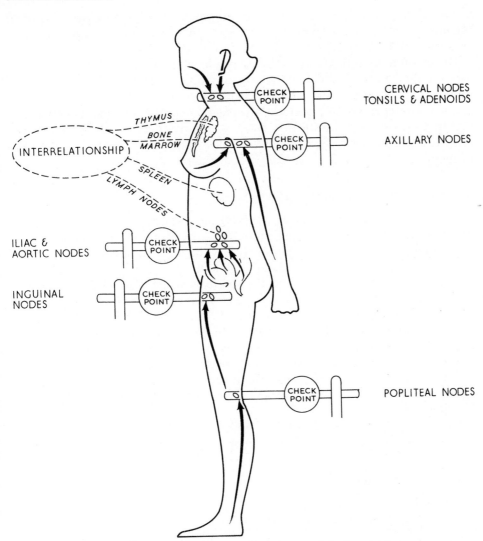

CERVICAL NODES
TONSILS & ADENOIDS

AXILLARY NODES

ILIAC &
AORTIC NODES

INGUINAL
NODES

POPLITEAL NODES

THYMUS
BONE MARROW
INTERRELATIONSHIP
SPLEEN
LYMPH NODES

CHECK POINT

Fig. 18. A diagram of the functions and relations of the lymphatic system.

experiments that, without the thymus, the lymph glands and Peyer's patches in the intestine do not develop properly, so that resistance to infection is absent. The thymus makes a hormone which enables primitive cells in the bone marrow to develop into lymphocytes capable of undertaking their work for immunity.

In the adult, the thymus maintains the supply of such lymphocytes, though it becomes of decreasing importance with age, when immunity to most common organisms is most likely to have been established.

The amount of antibody in the blood can be measured; for instance, one can measure the ability of serum containing antibodies to form a precipitate with a solution containing antigen. Antibody can be seen with the electron microscope, and if the antigen is whole bacteria, the reaction consists of such large particles that they can be seen with the naked eye. Antibodies against foreign blood cells can cause visible clumping or agglutination of these cells, and this is the basis of the well known test for the ABO blood groups.

STRUCTURE OF ANTIBODY

There are five different types of antibody in man, and most antigens cause production of all types. They are globulins, a kind of protein, and used to be classed together as immunoglobulins. IgG is the most common in humans and animals. It was formerly called gamma globulin, and this rather vague term is still used to describe the substances derived from blood that are used to provide temporary protection against certain diseases (e.g. measles) or to treat them. It is very effective in neutralizing toxins such as those of diphtheria. IgA has the special ability to cross cell membranes, so tears, saliva and mucus contain quite a lot of this antibody. It protects the body tissues from the bacteria inside the intestine, and its presence in sweat helps to deal with bacteria on the skin.

IgM has a bigger molecule than the others, and seems more primitive. It is the first antibody to appear in response to an antigen, and is particularly effective in killing bacteria.

IgE is responsible for the allergic reaction. It must have some other useful function, but this has not yet been discovered.

MODE OF ACTION

Antibodies work in various ways:

a) By uniting with antigen and immobilizing it.

b) By coating bacteria in a way that makes them easier for phagocytes to devour. An example of this was seen in lobar pneumonia before the use of antibiotics. The patient was gravely ill for a week or ten days, although the lung was crowded with phagocytes. Then antibody production began, and if he survived to this stage there was a dramatic change for the better in his condition as the phagocytes were enabled to engulf the pneumococci.

c) Another way involves a set of blood proteins called the complement system. The antigen-antibody complex attracts and fixes complement, which facilitates the breakdown or lysis of bacteria. IgM is especially effective in complement fixation.

d) By covering vital structures of organisms, especially viruses, which cannot grow until they have penetrated host cells. If their surface structures are covered, they cannot do this.

FORMATION OF ANTIBODIES

When an antigen enters the tissues, it is drained with the tissue fluid into a lymphatic capillary to the nearest lymphatic gland. Once the antigen has been processed by the big cells in the medulla, lymphocytes begin to multiply rapidly, and eventually their mature descendants begin to manufacture antibody. It seems likely that individual lymphocytes only make one kind of antibody, and some of these lymphocytes are "memory cells", which respond rapidly if a second dose of antigen is introduced.

CELLULAR IMMUNITY

Antibodies are carried in the lymph and blood stream to meet with antigen, but there is another way in which antigens can be attacked. This is by means of lymphocytes which can make direct contact with foreign cells and mount a local attack. This is the mechanism by which skin grafts or kidney grafts from another incompatible individual are rejected. The grafts are invaded by large numbers of the host's lymphocytes, which destroy them. The physician looking after the patient who has received an organ transplant has to find a way of controlling this cellular immune response.

AUTO-IMMUNITY

The immunity systems that protect the tissues from foreign invasion are so complex that it need not be surprising that anomalies and failures can occur at times. For instance, the allergic reaction (page 10) is often highly inconvenient if no worse. Cases in which the body fails to recognize and display tolerance to parts of itself, and makes antibodies to these constituents, are attracting increasing attention. Some human diseases are known to be caused by attack on its own tissues by auto-antibodies, and many more diseases of which the cause has long been obscure are now suspected of falling within this group of auto-immune diseases.

A recognized example of such a condition is auto-immune haemolytic anaemia, in which the patient forms antibodies to his own red blood cells, breaking them up and inducing a severe and even fatal anaemia. Since the spleen is largely responsible for haemolysis or red cell breakdown, it becomes greatly enlarged, the patient's skin is jaundiced because of the presence of more blood pigments from the broken down red blood cells than can be excreted in the bile. Laboratory tests on the red cells show that they are coated with anti-body, and this confirms the diagnosis of auto-immune disease. The treatment of this condition is described on page 164.

Known types of auto-immune disease fall into two groups. In the first, one organ is the main target of attack; in the second, the effects of the condition is felt in many different systems. An example of the first group is **Hashimoto's disease** of the thyroid gland. The patient, most commonly an adult woman, has an enlarged thyroid gland, and signs of thyroid insufficiency. Blood examination shows the presence of antibodies to thyroglobulin, and the condition will continue until the gland has been converted to fibrous tissue. The symptoms of thyroid deficiency can be controlled by giving thyroxine on a maintenance basis.

An example of a condition in which many organs appear to be attacked is **systemic lupus erythematosus** (SLE). Symptoms occur in connection with the kidneys, skin, joints, lymphatic system, liver, lungs, and the gastrointestinal tract, so that such diverse symptoms as renal failure, rashes, arthritis, pleurisy pericarditis and hepatitis may occur. Antibodies are formed to the proteins in the patient's own cell nuclei though whether this antibody formation is a cause or an effect of the illness is not yet clear. Life can now be prolonged for years by treatment with corticosteroids, and immuno suppressive drugs such as azathio-prine; renal failure is usually the terminal event. Other diseases which may eventually prove to be auto-immune are rheumatic fever, rheumatoid arthritis, nephritis and myasthenia gravis. Diabetes mellitus is another possibility, and even mental illness such as schizophrenia has received consideration from this aspect.

Chapter 5

Infectious Diseases and Allied Conditions

Many diseases in men, animals and plants are caused by infection from micro-organisms. These are found on the surface of the body and in its digestive canal, in the air and in the soil. Many of these are harmless; others are normal inhabitants of such organs as the colon, but if they gain entry to sterile organs, such as the kidney, will set up an infection. A few are disease-producers, or **pathogens.**

The fall in the amount of infectious disease in the world is due to a combination of causes—identification of organisms, and their means of transmission; improvements in hygiene, especially of food and water; vaccination against specific disease; discovery of potent drugs to prevent or cure infectious disease; better nutrition; eradication of breeding grounds of micro-organisms. The number of beds in Western Europe and North America reserved for infectious diseases has dwindled away to a very low number, and developing countries show the same general trend, though at a slower speed.

Some diseases caused by micro-organisms are infections, but are not "catching", or infectious to others. Pneumonia and pyelitis are examples. Others, such as smallpox or measles, are readily transmitted, producing in all those affected a disease running a similar course. These are spoken of as the *specific fevers*, and once a patient has acquired one of these, the possible course of the disease can be forecast with reasonable accuracy.

Specific fevers often occur in *epidemics;* that is, a number of cases closely related in time and place appear. Sometimes they appear in *sporadic* episodes, few in number, scattered, and not obviously connected with each other. Some are *endemic;* i.e. a small number of cases are usually present in certain areas of the world, as rabies is in India. From such reservoirs of infection epidemics are always threatening to arise. Occasionally waves of infection may sweep large areas of the world in the form of *pandemics*; in the middle ages it was plague that claimed so many victims; in modern times influenza is one of the commonest diseases to occur as a pandemic.

SOURCES OF INFECTION

The sources from which infection can arise are as follows:

1. PATIENTS

People already suffering from a disease can transmit it to others. This was the way in which the great pandemics of the past arose. Today it is of less importance, since methods of isolation, knowledge of routes of transmission, and ways of protecting staff are all so much improved. The greatest danger comes from the mild unsuspected or undiagnosed case.

2. CARRIERS

Convalescent carriers are those who have had the disease and recovered, but still continue to harbour the organism. Typhoid fever is an important example, and a dangerous one, since the typhoid bacilli may be excreted in the urine or faeces for years, and a carrier may be the source of a big epidemic if his excreta contaminate milk, or water, or a supply of food.

Healthy carriers who are not susceptible themselves to an infection may harbour micro-organisms and pass them on to others.

3. ANIMALS

Some diseases of animals can be transmitted to man, and these will be described in the text. The best known to the layman is rabies, which can be transferred to a man who is bitten by an infected dog.

4. INSECTS

Some of the most important diseases that affect man and his domestic animals are insect-borne. The mosquito, which is concerned in the transmission of yellow fever and malaria, is undoubtedly the most important of these, since these two diseases, though reduced in power, are still formidable. Below are some of the diseases so transmitted, and their insect vector.

DISEASE	INSECT VECTOR
Yellow fever	Mosquito
Malaria	Mosquito
Plague	Rat flea
African sleeping sickness	Tsetse fly
Epidemic typhus	Louse
Endemic typhus	Rat flea
Scrub typhus	Mite larva
Q fever	Tick
Rocky Mountain spotted fever	Tick

Among the methods of combating such diseases, destruction of the insect carrier and its breeding places must obviously be important.

5. SOIL

The organisms found in soil are of more interest to the surgeon than the physician since they are mostly anaerobic ones (growing in the absence of oxygen), and causing such wound infections as gas gangrene and tetanus.

METHODS OF INFECTION

1. BY INHALATION

(Usually derived from man). Many infectious diseases have inflammation of the naso-pharynx (respiratory tract) as a prominent symptom (scarlet fever, diphtheria, measles), and patients who cough or sneeze may expel infected drops of moisture into the air, whence they may be inhaled by others.

This is known as droplet infection, and is a traditional method of spread. Not all bacteriologists are convinced that droplet infection is quite as straight forward as this; they feel that organisms are deposited on articles, and think that contaminated fingers are an important method of transfer.

Whatever the facts, the nurse has an important role in preventing spread of such infection from her patients. Effective isolation; good ventilation; use of tissues that can be burnt for collection of respiratory discharge; damp dusting; and careful hand toilet after contact with the patient or his surroundings are all important.

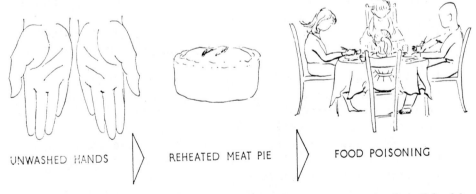

UNWASHED HANDS ▷ REHEATED MEAT PIE ▷ FOOD POISONING

Fig. 19. Intestinal infections are most commonly conveyed by contamination of food by faecal organisms.

2. BY INGESTION

(Most commonly from man). Organisms excreted in the urine or faeces may be transferred to food or drink and infect others. Food poisoning, typhoid, dysentery and poliomyelitis are examples. Sudden large outbreaks of illness with gastro-intestinal symptoms are usually due to contamination of water, or milk, or food in a shop or restaurant.

3. BY ENTRY THROUGH SKIN OR MUCOUS MEMBRANE

e.g. wound infections, syphilis. These infections may be contracted from man, or animals, or the soil.

DEFENCE AGAINST INFECTION

As long as the skin is whole, it is a powerful barrier to infection. Good general nutrition, and an adequate diet with sufficient protein and vitamins are helpful. The most important defence against any organism, however, is *specific immunity* to the organism concerned. Entry of infection into the body should provoke the production of *antibody* which neutralizes the effects of the organism.

Natural immunity is possessed by some animals to the diseases of others. Man does not normally contact foot and mouth disease, or distemper. Babies are usually immune to the same diseases as the mother for the first few months of life. The most important kind of immunity, however, is that made in the body in response to a stimulus; this is **active immunity**. The methods by which this is produced is as follows:—

1. By infection with the disease. The effect on immunity after some infections is enough to protect for life against a second attack. Measles, rubella and chickenpox are examples.
2. By subclinical infection, not severe enough to cause an acute attack, but sufficient to mobilize the body's defences. It is an important way of acquiring resistance to tuberculosis.
3. By artificial immunization. The importance of this method is that people may be protected against an attack by injecting a killed culture of the organism, or a preparation of its toxin, or a similar but weaker organism, causing production of antibody. Smallpox, diphtheria, whooping cough, poliomyelitis and tetanus can be prevented by active immunization in youth. Plague, cholera, yellow fever and typhoid are other diseases against which artificial immunity is possible.

Passive immunity is not made by the subject, but conferred on him by the injection of serum which contains an antibody. Passive immunity to tetanus can be established by giving injections of serum from a horse which has been actively immunized to tetanus. Serum from adults who have had measles contains antibody, and the gamma globulin portion in which it is concentrated can be given to children to establish passive immunity. This kind of immunity only lasts a few weeks, and so is only of minor importance, but the use of immune serum to modify the course of a disease may be useful as a method of treatment, or to enable a mild attack to occur and stimulate active immunity.

PREVENTION OF INFECTIOUS DISEASE

It is more important to be able to prevent disease than to cure it. Illness means loss of work, loss of money, and chronic disease. It entails the spending of capital on hospital buildings and equipment, and keeping a staff on twenty-four hour duty. Prevention is not only cheaper, but obviously preferable. The leading methods are:

1. Active immunization, to reduce the number of susceptible people. This has been successful in many diseases, including diphtheria. It entails convincing the public that it is worthwhile and without risk.

2. Recognition and isolation of cases. In many countries, the more important infectious diseases are *notifiable*, and the Medical Officer of Health sends figures of the fevers in his area to a central authority, so that country-wide trends may be watched.

3. Detection of carriers. Evidence of cure should be sought before a patient is discharged from hospital.

4. Safeguarding water supplies. Water is scarce in many parts of the world, and shallow wells may be used that are grossly polluted. In developed countries a very high standard of purity exists in water supplies, but if a breach in this standard of hygiene occurs, large outbreaks may occur.

5. Hygiene of food sources. Milk and meat are readily contaminated, and at all stages of producing and transporting such foods health regulations should be enforced. Food handlers in stores should be given instruction on avoiding direct handling of unwrapped food.

6. Destruction of insect vectors. Flies contaminate food, and other insects may carry specific diseases, as mentioned earlier.

7. International pooling of information. Travel is now so fast that a patient in the first stages of an infection may be thousands of miles away from the place

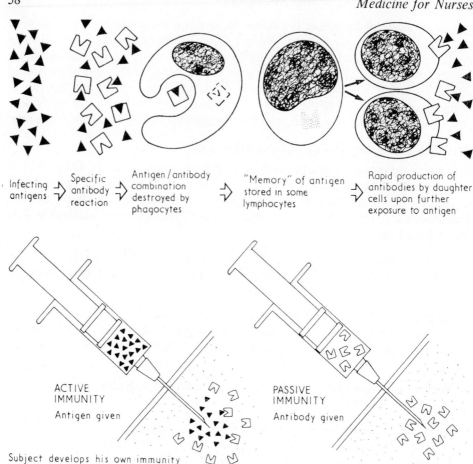

Fig. 20. The upper line of pictures describes the way in which active immunity develops in response to a specific infection. The two lower sketches show the difference between active and passive immunization.

of origin when his condition is first diagnosed. Warnings of the approach of an influenza epidemic may be possible months ahead of its arrival. Great population shifts are taking place all over the world, bringing diseases into areas where they were previously unknown. The work of the World Health Organization in disseminating information and promoting health education is increasingly important.

THE COURSE OF A SPECIFIC FEVER

There is a basic similarity in the course run by all the specific fevers, since in all there is bacterial invasion, a struggle between the organism and the infection-resisting powers of the body, and recovery (it is hoped) when these powers become strong enough to destroy the infecting organisms. The stages passed are as follows:

1. Incubation. This is the period that follows the entry of organisms into the system. Antibody is manufactured, often the white blood count rises, and all the mechanisms for defeating infection come into play. Often of course these are successful, as is seen by the number of people who have active immunity to diseases which they have never "had". But if there is no specific immunity, symptoms of infection appear, and these mark the end of the incubation period, and the beginning of the next phase.

Incubation periods may be as short as a day in scarlet fever, or as long as six months in rabies, but they are usually fairly constant in any one condition, and sometimes very markedly so. In smallpox, for instance, it is most usually 12 days.

2. Onset. The signs and symptoms which first appear are usually due to the general reactions to the infection. Fever, raised pulse rate, and increased respiration rate are usual. Headache, vague back ache and joint pains are common, and dry tongue, concentrated urine and constipation accompany almost all fevers. Those which enter via the nasopharynx may be accompanied by sore throat, watering of the eyes, running of the nose and swollen glands.

3. The height of the disease shows the fully-developed picture of the disease, and the symptoms depend on the system attacked. Those in which there is intestinal infection will be marked by diarrhoea, the respiratory ones with tracheitis.

The appearance of a rash is common to many fevers, and shows that the organism is one that produces a toxin that affects the skin blood vessels. Rashes are a great help in diagnosis; their colour, distribution, nature, intensity and date of appearance are all carefully noted.

4. Defervescence. The duration of the acute symptoms is again characteristic; it is only a day or two in rubella, and may be four weeks in untreated typhoid fever. A fall in temperature and pulse rate indicates that the body defences have the upper hand in the struggle with the infection.

5. Convalescence. After a feverish illness of any length, there is a period of sub-health. Muscles have become slack, weight may have been lost, and a period of convalescence with fresh air, sunlight, a judicious mixture of graded exercise and rest, and a diet with plenty of protein should be arranged if possible.

COMPLICATIONS OF SPECIFIC FEVERS

The course of the specific fevers is often made more severe by extension of infection to neighbouring organs, or by the effects of the infection on distant structures. One important group will be better understood after looking at Fig. 21.

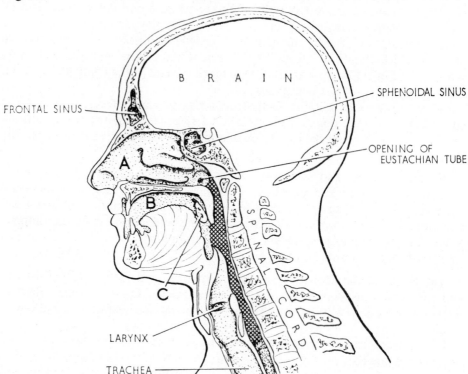

Fig. 21. A sagittal section of the head and neck, to show the structures to which infection may spread by direct extension.

A. DIRECT EXTENSION

The hatched portion is the pharynx; in front of this area is A, the nose; B, the mouth; and C, the tonsils. This is the area attacked in such infections as measles and scarlet fever, and from it spread can occur in several directions.

Laryngitis can give rise to *tracheitis*, whence infection can descend to cause *bronchitis* and *pneumonia*. On the side wall of the pharynx behind the nose can be seen the orifice of the Eustachian tube, leading to the middle ear; up this duct can pass organisms from the pharynx to cause inflammation, i.e. *otitis media*. From the tonsils, infection can pass along the lymphatics to the glands in the neck, causing cervical *lymphadenitis* (Fig. 22).

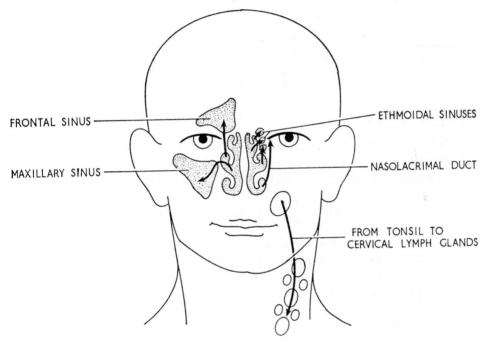

FRONTAL SINUS

ETHMOIDAL SINUSES

MAXILLARY SINUS

NASOLACRIMAL DUCT

FROM TONSIL TO
CERVICAL LYMPH GLANDS

Fig. 22. Infection may spread from the mouth and pharynx to the sinuses, the conjunctival sac and the cervical lymph glands.

Opening into the nose on each side is the maxillary *antrum*. The lining of this hollow in the upper jaw is continuous with that of the nose, and since its connection with the nose is half-way up the antrum if infection enters here, it may be difficult to clear, and maxillary *sinusitis* can be troublesome. Other sinuses in the frontal, ethmoid and sphenoid bones are less often involved.

The same diagram (Fig. 22) shows on the left side the lacrimal duct, by which the tears drain from the conjunctival sac of the eye into the nose. *Conjunctivitis* of some degree is common in measles.

B. NERVOUS

In conditions like tetanus and poliomyelitis the main brunt of the attack falls on the nervous system, but in others, of which diphtheria is an example, the nervous system may be affected by toxins, and paralyses of various muscles may result, and will be described in the appropriate section.

C. CARDIAC

Like all other tissues, heart muscle depends on its blood supply for its efficient performance, and in diseases in which general toxaemia is a feature, myocardial failure may occur. A pulse rising in rate and diminishing in volume, especially if the temperature is falling, is a danger sign.

D. RESPIRATORY

There are three reasons why pneumonia is a common complication of severe infectious disease.

1. There may be direct extension of the infection from the nasopharynx, as described above.
2. There may be secondary invasion of the inflamed tissues by another pathogen.
3. Unless medical and nursing care is effective, weakness may mean that the patient spends long periods without moving, and may be too feeble to cough. Congestion of the lung bases results, and causes hypostatic pneumonia (page 194).

E. DIGESTIVE

In the enteric fevers, of which typhoid is the chief, the inflammation of the lymphatic patches in the small intestine may be severe enough to perforate the gut wall, and allow the escape of intestinal contents into the peritoneal cavity, or there may be erosion of a blood vessel, causing haemorrhage.

NURSING PRECAUTIONS

The precautions necessary to prevent spread of an infectious disease depend on the nature of the disease and the route by which infection occurs.

This list is intended as a guide. Each patient will of course need to be considered individually by the physician in charge.

KEY TO SYMBOLS

Isolation
0 = no action
1 = barrier nurse in open ward
2 = barrier nurse in side room or cubicle
3 = remove to isolation ward or hospital

Faeces and Urine
0 = no special action
1 = add Sudol (1 per cent) leave 1 hour

Terminal Disinfection
0 = no action required
1 = wash floors, walls and furniture with a detergent + hypochlorite
2 = treat with gaseous formalin

BARRIER NURSING

Barrier nursing includes the following precautions:

Wearing of gowns. Gowns should be worn for all procedures involving disturbance of the bedclothes and personal attention to the patient. They are not necessary for serving meals.

Masks. Should be worn in the same circumstances as gowns, on the instructions of the physician or surgeon in charge of the patient.

China. Feeding utensils should be washed and kept for the patient alone and terminally disinfected by autoclaving. They should be washed in a special bowl or sink reserved for their use. Where all ward china is washed in a heated washing-up machine no precautions are needed.

Linen. Bed linen should be put into an "infected" laundry sack for disinfection by formalin before being sent to the laundry. Disposable sheets may be available.

Mattresses. Mattresses enclosed in a plastic cover should be swabbed with hypochlorite solution containing 1 per cent of available chlorine on discharge of the patient. Foam-rubber mattresses and pillows should be dealt within the same way. Other mattresses and pillows should be sent for disinfection by formalin.

DISEASE	ISOLATION	FAECES and URINE	DISINFECTION
Anthrax	2–0	0	2
Ascariasis	0	1	0
Brucellosis	0	0	0
Chicken pox	3	0	1

DISEASE	ISOLATION	FAECES and URINE	DISINFECTION
Cholera*	3	1	1
Diphtheria*	3	0	1
Dysentery*			
amoebic	1	1	0
bacillary	2/3	1	1
infantile	2/3	1	1
Gas gangrene	0	0	0
Glandular fever	0	0	0
Gonorrhoea	1–0	0	0
Hepatitis, infectious	2	1	0
Herpes simplex			
adult	0	0	0
infants	2	0	0
Herpes zoster	3	0	1
Histoplasmosis	2	0	0
Influenza	0	0	0
Leprosy	2	0	0
Malaria	0	0	0
Measles*	3	0	0
Meningitis			
aseptic	2	1	1
meningococcal*	2–0	0	0
pneumococcal	0	0	0
tuberculous	2/3	0	1
Meningo-encephalitis*	2	1	1
Mumps	3	0	0
Ophthalmia neonatorum*	1–0	0	0
Paratyphoid fever*	2/3	1	1
Pneumonia*			
atypical	0	0	0
pneumococcal	0	0	0
Poliomyelitis*	3	1	1
Psittacosis	2/3	0	0
Rheumatic fever	0	0	0

* Notification required by law.

DISEASE	ISOLATION	FAECES and URINE	DISINFECTION
Rubella	3	0	0
Salmonella infection	2/3	1	1
Smallpox*	3	1	2
Staphylococcal infection		Follow local rules	
Known streptococcal infection			
erysipelas*	2–0	0	1
scarlet fever*	2–0	0	1
sore throat	2–0	0	1
puerperal fever*	2–0	0	1
Syphilis, infectious	1–0	0	0
Tapeworm infestation	0	1	0
Tetanus	0	0	0
Tuberculosis			
pulmonary*	2/3	0	1
extra-pulmonary infectious*	2/3	0/1	1
non-infectious*	0	0	0
Typhoid*	2/3	1	1
Whooping cough	3	0	0

No special precautions are required for Actinomycosis, Aspergillosis, Ancylostomiasis, Candidiasis, Catscratch disease, Leptospirosis, Q fever or Toxoplasmosis.

* Notification required by law.

1 or 2–0 = transfer to open ward after 48 hours treatment with adequate doses of penicillin—then patient will no longer be infectious.

GENERAL NURSING PRINCIPLES

Prevention. The public health nurse who runs immunity clinics and is concerned with infant welfare has an obvious role in the prevention of infectious disease. So does every nurse in hospital, in the community and her own family, where hygiene should be thought about and promoted.

ISOLATION TECHNIQUES

Many people are concerned with patients besides nurses and doctors, and these must understand the precautions used and observe them. Medical students, radiographers, physiotherapists, visitors, other patients and domestic staff must be taught the rules and helped to observe them. Patients greatly dislike barrier techniques even when they realize the necessity for them, and nurses must try to see that they do not feel outcast.

During this illness there will be articles taken out of the cubicle which must be made safe. This practice is *current disinfection*. When the illness is over, all the contents of the cubicle must be dealt with by *terminal disinfection*. It is obvious that the amount of current disinfection should be kept to a minimum, so that articles like thermometers, bowls, and books, should be kept in the unit and only dealt with once after the disease is over. The patient's notes, charts and X-rays should be kept outside, so that they may be freely consulted.

Of all techniques used, scrupulous hand-washing after attention has been given is the most important. Some points that apply to nursing many patients with specific fevers are given below.

1. *Ventilation.* A good supply of fresh air will reduce the number of airborne bacteria, and lessen the risk of infection by such organisms to other patients and staff. An extractor system which withdraws air to the exterior, instead of allowing it to circulate to other parts of the ward, is an advantage. A buoyant atmosphere is refreshing to a feverish patient.

2. *Bed.* The mattress should be completely enclosed in a plastic cover, which can be sterilized as indicated in the disinfection chart, and avoids the difficulty of disinfecting the mattress itself. If a mackintosh is needed below the draw sheet, disposable plastic sheeting should be used. Blankets should be of cellular cotton, or disposable ones used. Overheating of a feverish patient will cause sweating and fluid loss, but the patient's impression about the best number of blankets should be considered. If the illness is likely to be lengthy, a bed cradle should be used and a support to prevent foot drop.

3. *Food.* When the temperature is raised, so also is the basal metabolic rate, so that fluid loss from the body by the skin and expiration is increased, and the rate of oxidation of foodstuffs rises. Since the appetite is usually reduced in such illnesses, the patient may be reluctant to take food, and too apathetic to increase the fluid intake.

It is important that the patient drinks plenty, in order to dilute the circulating toxins, keep up the urinary output, and ensure a fresh moist tongue. It may be necessary to consider the energy content of drinks if the illness is a long or severe one, but usually the patient may have what he prefers. A jug of water on the locker is a convenience to the nurse, but daunting to the patient, and a glass of water or fruit juice with ice, replenished when necessary is more likely to be drunk. Small children are often difficult over drinks, and should be given a small cup or mug, and encouraged to drink a few mouthfuls at frequent intervals.

If it is required to raise the energy value of drinks, milk, beaten eggs, sugar, casilan, malted milk extracts or brandy may be used to fortify drinks, in accordance with the patient's tastes and age.

There is no need to press a reluctant patient to eat if the illness is only likely to last a day or two, but in more severe or protracted illness, a high protein diet is given, to prevent wasting, and low residue foods should be selected in order to keep the calorie intake high. Ice-cream, fruit purees, jellies, thickened soups, eggs, minced meat and fish are examples. Low residue foods are especially important in the intestinal infections, such as typhoid, but in general there is no need to prohibit foods which the patient feels he can eat.

4. *Skin toilet.* A daily bed bath is welcome to the feverish patient, and it is a pleasure to the nurse who finds a patient hot and uncomfortable in a tousled bed, to leave him cool, clean and comfortable. It is also an opportunity to examine the skin for rashes, assess the muscle tone, look at and treat the pressure areas, and to listen to the patient. Regular turning helps to keep the skin over the pressure areas healthy, and to prevent hypostatic pneumonia.

5. *Mouth care.* Patients with pyrexia often breathe through the mouth, so that the tongue and lips become dry. Eating and brushing the teeth suffice to keep the mouth fresh in ordinary life, but the feverish patient may not be eating and may be too ill to care about dental hygiene. The nurse must clean the tongue and the inner surfaces of the cheeks frequently with a refreshing lotion and should encourage the patient to clean his teeth or rinse his mouth if he is able. A good fluid intake will help to keep the mouth moist and a film of petroleum jelly applied to the lips will prevent cracking.

6. *Eyes.* Conjunctivitis is seldom well marked, but some reddening of the eyes, and complaints that the light hurts are not uncommon. If possible the bed should be placed so that light is not an inconvenience, but drawing the blind should be avoided if possible, since a dark room is depressing and sunlight a good antiseptic. Sore eyes can be bathed with boracic, and if the lids of a semi-conscious patient do not completely close, a drop of paroleine should be instilled into the conjunctival sac to prevent ulceration of the cornea.

7. *Discharges.* Paper handkerchiefs should be used for running noses or watery eyes, and these should be put in a paper bag and burnt.

8. *Excreta.* Measurements of the fluid intake and output are often indicated, and tests of the urine for albumin and blood may be required every few days, especially if nephritis is a complication that may occur.

A daily bowel action is hardly to be expected if the diet is a fluid one, and aperients are not generally indicated. A suppository may sometimes be required.

SCARLET FEVER

Organism. A haemolytic streptococcus, which produces a skin toxin, which causes the rash that gives the disease its name.

Method of spread. Airborne, or spread by contaminated hands to the mouth and thence to the pharynx.

Incubation period. Less than a week; (2–4 days).

Course. It is mostly a disease of children, and used to be a severe and often fatal disease. There is at first sore throat, with shivering, fever, nausea and lack of appetite. The rash appears on the next day, a widespread bright red one, usually starting behind the ears, and worst in the bends of the elbows, hips and knees. The face is flushed, but a pale area around the mouth gives a characteristic appearance. The tongue is coated with a white fur through which the red papillae show. The symptoms abate and the rash fades in about a week, usually to be followed by peeling of the skin.

Complications. Early treatment will usually avert these, but otitis media (middle ear infection), inflammation of the cervical lymph glands and pneumonia are not unknown. Rheumatic fever and acute nephritis occasionally follow, and are manifestations of sensitization to the streptococcus.

Treatment. Nursing care as above. An oral penicillin will quickly bring the infection under control. The child should be kept in bed till the rash has gone and the temperature is normal. The urine should be examined for blood and/or albumin after a fortnight.

Prevention. Neither active nor passive immunity is useful clinically.

MEASLES
(Morbilli)

Organism. A virus.

Method of spread. Respiratory.

Incubation period. 1–2 weeks; average 10 days.

Course. Most adults are immune to measles, since they had this highly infectious disease as children. Babies under six months old usually derive natural immunity from their mother.

Measles in the early stages resembles a severe cold, though experienced observers usually diagnose it early. There is fever, running nose, sneezing, reddened and watering eyes and a characteristic loud brassy cough. Koplik's spots are tiny white points with surrounding inflammation, which are found on the insides of the cheeks near the opening of the duct from the parotid gland.

On the third day the fever often subsides, to rise again on the fourth day as the rash appears. It is a blotchy red rash, most profuse on the face but usually covering the whole body. The child is wretched and irritable now, hot and with an irritating skin, disturbing cough and painful eyes. Gradually the fever abates and the rash fades.

Complications. The nurse must be alert to detect the early signs of *otitis media* (pain, fever, rolling the head, screaming) and *bronchopneumonia*. Careful eye toilet should avert *corneal ulceration*, but if the child has severe photophobia this condition should be suspected and the doctor informed. *Encephalitis* is rare.

Treatment. No drug is effective against the virus, but a sulphonamide or oral penicillin is often given to avert the complications referred to. The nursing aims to relieve the symptoms, as described above. After a severe attack the child is often pale and tired, and convalescence in fresh air and sunshine is beneficial.

Prevention. Passive immunity can be conferred by injections of gamma globulin prepared from the pooled blood plasma of adults who have had the disease. It may be used to protect infants or unwell children from the disease. A vaccine exists to confer active immunity, and is widely used in the United States. The acceptance rate in the United Kingdom is not high.

GERMAN MEASLES
(Rubella)

Organism. A virus.

Method of spread. Respiratory.

Incubation period. Over 2 weeks; (about 18 days).

Course. It is less a disease of small children than some others, e.g. teenagers and young adults. An attack, even if mild, confers life-long immunity. Often it is a very mild affair, with headache, stiff neck, running nose and a rash of pink spots behind the ears and on the forehead. Enlargement of the occipital lymph glands is quite common, but usually the whole episode is over in three or four days.

Complications. The only serious one occurs in women who develop the disease in the first twelve weeks of pregnancy, since the baby may be born with congenital malformations such as cataract, deafness or heart abnormalities.

Prevention. Vaccination against rubella is offered to girls between 11 and 14 years old. Four weeks should separate the giving of this vaccine and any other. Exposure of children to infection should not be avoided, especially of girls who should preferably contract the disease early. Pregnant women should be protected from exposure, and if infection is feared should be given an intramuscular injection of gamma globulin.

WHOOPING COUGH
(Pertussis)

Organism. A bacillus, *Haemophilus pertussis.*

Method of spread. Respiratory.

Incubation period. 1–2 weeks.

Course. Almost all the patients are under five years old, and in the early stages, which are highly infectious, the illness is indistinguishable from the common cold, with a harsh cough. The coughing increases in frequency, until the typical pattern that gives the disease its name is manifest. The paroxysm begins with a series of short hard coughs, ending in a deep inspiration through the half-shut glottis which causes the "whoop". These attacks may be frequent and tiring. The child may sit up as the coughing begins, holding the side of its cot, and becomes first red and then cyanosed. Fluid runs from the nose and eyes; the tongue is protruded and the lower surface is often abraded by friction against the teeth. The coughing ends with the production of thick mucus, and often vomiting. Mother and child may both be exhausted by these attacks, and the vomiting may cause weight loss. Coughing may continue for several weeks.

Complications. Bronchopneumonia is the most common serious one. Sometimes collapse of a lobe of a lung leads to bronchiectasis (page 199) in later life. Fits may appear, and are a serious sign.

Treatment. Tetracycline is often prescribed, and helps to prevent complications in the chest. Linctus to allay the cough is useful. The child is kept warm, and moist inhalations may help to loosen thick sputum.

Children should be supported and comforted during the paroxysms, which they find very frightening. If vomiting is frequent, a feed should be given immediately the attack is over, in the hope that it will be retained and absorbed before the next fit of coughing.

A pertussis vaccine is available but some public anxiety is felt about its use, since a small proportion of children suffer brain damage following its use. It must be remembered that such damage may also be caused by whooping cough itself. The vaccine should not be used for infants less than six months old, or those with asthma or eczema.

DIPHTHERIA

Organism. A bacillus, *Corynebacterium diphtheriae*.

Method of spread. Respiratory, from cases or from carriers.

Incubation period. Under a week (1–6 days).

Course. The infection is usually of the tonsils and fauces, but sometimes affects the anterior part of the nose. Where diphtheria bacillus is widespread infection of wounds may occur, but this is now virtually unknown in England. The usual first symptoms are sore throat, headache and general feverish symptoms. The temperature is often only slightly raised, while the pulse rate is markedly raised and the blood pressure low. Over the tonsils and fauces appears a dirty greyish membrane closely adherent, and with an inflamed area around it. From this area toxins are absorbed into the bloodstream, and cause symptoms throughout the body. The condition can be diagnosed at this stage from a throat swab and from the clinical picture. If the disease is suspected, treatment on the lines given below is begun at once, since delay may lessen the chances of recovery from this disease, which has serious complications and, though easily prevented, is dangerous when it occurs.

The dangerous complications are:

a) *respiratory obstruction from spread of the membrane into the larynx.* This danger is greatest in young patients whose small airway is easily occluded. In severe infections, tracheostomy may be life saving.

b) *Heart failure.* The soft rapid pulse indicates that the heart muscle is always affected by the toxins, and the danger of sudden death from myocardial failure is a serious one.

c) *Involvement of the nervous system.* The muscles most commonly affected are those of the soft palate, which shut off the nasopharynx during swallowing. Paralysis allows fluids to regurgitate through the nose when attempts are made to drink, and a nasal tone of voice develops. Other muscles may be involved later, occasionally including those of respiration, but recovery from diphtheritic paralysis is always complete.

Treatment. Nursing care is directed to keeping the patient lying down at complete rest to avert the risk of heart failure. Cyanosis, respiratory difficulty, or a pulse rising in rate and diminishing in volume are signs that must be immediately reported to the physician. Fluid intake must be kept high.

Anti-diphtheritic serum is given as soon as the diagnosis is made, and to avoid anaphylactic shock (page 10) a test dose is given by subcutaneous injection. The diphtheria bacillus is sensitive to penicillin, and this is also given.

As the condition improves, extra pillows are added and more activity allowed. It will be some weeks before the patient is ready to leave hospital even in a mild case, while if paralysis has occurred it will be some months before recovery is complete.

Prevention. Diphtheria can be prevented by active immunization, and outbreaks in the western world are small and infrequent. It is still a dangerous disease in parts of the Far East, and could be so again in the west if the level of immunization were allowed to fall. Epidemics are usually caused by a carrier, and if a case occurs, contacts should have the throat and nose swabbed, and a Schi test will detect those who are unprotected and need immunization.

ENTERIC FEVER
(Typhoid and Paratyphoid)

Organisms. These are bacilli of the Salmonella group.

Method of spread. The organisms are swallowed in food or water contaminated by sewage or excreta, and the source of an epidemic is usually a carrier. Large epidemics are uncommon in countries where sanitation is good, but the Salmonella is still responsible for a great deal of illness in many parts of the world.

The biggest epidemics are caused when water supplies are affected, but in developed countries outbreaks are usually caused by a carrier who is also a food-handler, or by shell fish affected by sewage. The last outbreak in Great Britain was due to corned beef, tins of which had been cooled in water con-containing sewage.

Course. Paratyphoid and typhoid are similar in their course, but paratyphoid is usually a less severe disease. The description given here is of typhoid, which if diagnosed and treated early will not run the protracted course which used to be seen before the introduction of chloramphenicol.

The onset is gradual, with malaise and a little fever which tends slowly to get worse, falling in the morning and rising at night. Headache and constipation are usual, and sometimes there are nose-bleeds. The rise of temperature is proportionately greater than the increase in the pulse rate. At this stage the typhoid bacillus is in the bloodstream, and may be discovered if blood is taken for culture. On the eighth day a rash may appear, not often profuse, of rose-red spots on the abdomen and back. In the second week fever may be continuous and diarrhoea usually occurs, with loose offensive stools. During this week and the next the patient is profoundly ill; the temperature swings markedly and this is the time of most risk of the complications given below. The bacillus is present in large numbers in the stools, and often in the urine. During the fourth week the temperature gradually falls and the symptoms abate.

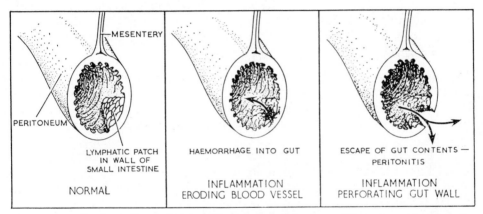

Fig. 23. Complications of typhoid fever. Haemorrhage into the small intestine and perforation into the peritoneal cavity.

Complications. These are many and serious. As in all severe fevers, heart failure and bronchopneumonia are to be feared. Ulceration of Peyer's patches, the lymphoid areas of the small intestine, may cause haemorrhage, or perforation into the peritoneal cavity. These complications are commonest in the third week, when sudden falls in temperature or blood pressure, sweating, fainting or abdominal pain must be instantly reported. Perforation must be repaired surgically, and blood transfusion will be needed if there is bleeding.

Some people recover from typhoid, but continue to excrete the bacillus and become carriers. Occasionally the gall bladder is the source of infection, and cholecystectomy may cure it. Carriers must understand that they are a potential source of infection to others and that scrupulous hand toilet after defaecation is essential.

Treatment. Chloramphenicol is the specific cure, and once the diagnosis has been made and the drug begun, improvement is seen within 48 hours. The lengthy disease described above is thus not now seen in its classic form.

The patient is nursed at complete rest to avert the risk of heart failure, and the strictest barrier technique is necessary to prevent the infection of others. Dehydration will readily occur if there is diarrhoea, and a high fluid intake is vital. The pressure areas and the mouth must be given intensive care. Regular accurate observations of the temperature, pulse and respiration, and of any complaints of abdominal pain, may give early warning of the onset of complications.

As the condition improves, a high calorie, low-residue diet is given to build up the patient's depleted strength. The stools are regularly examined for the presence of typhoid bacilli, and the patient can be considered no longer infectious when six consecutive stools are negative.

Prevention. Effective sewage disposal and safeguarding of water supplies is the cause of the decrease in typhoid in the countries where the disease is now uncommon. Washing the hands after using the w.c. would prevent many outbreaks of "food poisoning", and must be urged in plain terms on all food handlers.

T.A.B. is a vaccine made from the bacilli of typhoid, and of paratyphoid A and B, and it will provide immunity for a year or two. Those going to areas where typhoid is present should be immunized by two subcutaneous injections at 10-day intervals. Local and general reactions following the injection are common, though generally mild.

CEREBRO-SPINAL MENINGITIS

Organism. The meningococcus.

Method of spread. From the nasopharynx to the blood stream and the meninges. Carriers are often responsible for epidemics, which are usually associated with overcrowding. It has been uncommon in Britain since the last war.

Incubation period. Less than a week.

Course. The onset is usually sudden, often with a rigor, or convulsions in children, and severe pain in the head and back, and vomiting. The neck feels stiff, and attempts to flex it are resisted. The patient shows the attitude typical of meningeal irritation from any cause; he lies on his side with his head buried under the bedclothes since dislike of light (photophobia) is often present, and brusquely resists any effort to examine or treat him. Lumbar puncture produces cerebro-spinal fluid which is cloudy, and in which meningococci can usually be found, and this will distinguish this form of meningitis from the others. Small haemorrhagic spots (petechiae) appear on the second or third day, and confusion and coma will follow unless the disease is successfully treated.

Treatment. Penicillin by injection is usually given, since strains of meningococcus are now frequent which are resistant to the sulpha drugs which were once effective.

The patient should be nursed in a quiet room, and shaded from direct light. If he is confused or drowsy incontinence of urine must be expected, and measurement of the intake is important, since if the patient cannot be induced to take enough by mouth, intravenous fluids may be necessary. The pressure areas must be treated, and headache relieved by use of the analgesics that will be ordered.

Prevention. Vaccines are available against meningococcus meningitis, and are useful in those parts of the world (e.g. The Sudan and Brazil) where the disease is common and drug resistant. Vaccination is not widely used in this country, since the sporadic case can be quite successfully treated. Small epidemics occasionally occur.

MUMPS
(Epidemic parotitis)

Organism. A virus.

Method of spread. Respiratory.

Incubation period. Over 2 weeks (18 days).

Course. There may be mild general malaise, but often there are no symptoms until one or both glands begin to swell, and there is painful spasm of the jaws. In a few days the swellings subside.

Complications. The virus may affect not only the salivary glands, but also the pancreas, ovaries or testis. Very occasionally orchitis may be bilateral, and cause subsequent sterility.

Treatment. No drug is effective. Keeping the mouth clean and moist is obviously important, and plenty of bland fluids should be given, if necessary through a straw.

Prevention. A vaccine exists but is not available through the National Health Service, since the disease is thought too mild for this to be necessary.

CHICKENPOX
(Varicella)

Cause. A virus.

Method of spread. Respiratory, and by discharge from rupture of the skin lesions.

Incubation period. 14 days.

Course. This is a very infectious disease, so most people have it as children and do not usually feel very ill.

The rash is often the first symptom. It appears first on the trunk, then on the face, and finally the limbs. The lesions are little vesicles (blisters), small and surrounded by a ring of inflammation, and because they are so superficial they rupture easily. The contents of the vesicles soon become cloudy and purulent, and within a few days dry up to form scabs. Several crops may occur, so that vesicles, pustules and scabs may all be seen. Scarring is not usual, unless scratching and secondary infection have occurred.

Treatment. Children may be miserable for a day or so, and adults who contract chickenpox often feel quite ill, with severe headache, but on the whole, care of the skin with prevention of chafing, is the only problem. Calamine lotion can be dabbed on irritating areas.

Prevention. Chickenpox usually spreads from child to child, but the virus can, if transferred to an adult, cause herpes zoster or shingles (page 369). Occasionally an adult with shingles can cause chickenpox in a child by transfer of virus. Gamma globulin from convalescent patients can be used to confer passive immunity where necessary. For instance, in children with leukaemia, chickenpox is a very dangerous condition that can cause death. If such a child is exposed to infection the mother should consult the doctor and if the child develops chickenpox he must be admitted to hospital.

In regions where smallpox is endemic, or during epidemics in other countries, it is important that every case of chickenpox is carefully considered to ensure that it is not a mild case of smallpox. The differences between the two will be considered in the next section.

SMALLPOX
(Variola)

Cause. A virus, of which major and minor forms exist.

Method of spread. By the respiratory system, or by contamination from the skin lesions. It is highly infectious to the unprotected.

Incubation period. 1 to 2 weeks, usually 12 days.

Course. On the first day there is shivering, pain in the head and back, sore throat and laryngitis, and sometimes nettle rash (urticaria), which is distinct from the true rash that appears on the next day. This rash first consists of

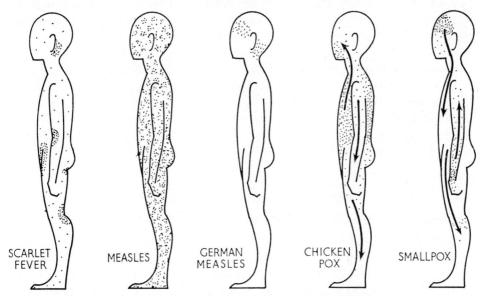

SCARLET FEVER   MEASLES   GERMAN MEASLES   CHICKEN POX   SMALLPOX

Fig. 24. The characteristic distribution of the rash in five infectious diseases.

macules (flat red areas) on the forehead and wrists, spreading to the arms, the trunk, and finally the legs. The rash is always thickest on the face and upper limbs, and where the skin is subject to pressure, as over bony prominences, or under wrist watches and shoulder straps. The macules soon develop into papules (raised red areas) and then into vesicles (blisters). These are deep set and hard unlike the flimsy superficial vesicles of chickenpox. The contents of the vesicles becomes cloudy and they turn to pustules. These gradually dry into hard scabs, which separate to leave deep scars or pock-marks.

The pustular stage is reached in about four days, and is marked by a deterioration in the patient's condition, and he may be extremely toxic. Secondary infection of the pustules may occur, and the throat and mouth may be ulcerated.

Complications. Heart failure and bronchopneumonia are the most common and the most serious. Corneal ulceration may threaten sight, and encephalitis (brain inflammation) can occur. Smallpox is frequently fatal.

Treatment. Nurses caring for smallpox patients should have been recently and successfully vaccinated. Care of the mouth and tongue is especially important, and a high calorie fluid diet is given. If swallowing is painful, aspirin mucilage may be helpful. Every effort must be made by aseptic nursing methods to protect the skin and respiratory system from bacterial infection. Prophylactic penicillin is often ordered with this aim in view.

Prevention. Though smallpox is still endemic in parts of the East, it has been eliminated from large areas of the world by vaccination, isolation of cases, and quarantine of suspects. Routine vaccination of all infants in Great Britain was discontinued in 1971, since the risk of a child contracting smallpox was even less than that of serious complications following vaccination. Medical and nursing staff will still need protection. Most countries require those entering from potentially infected areas to produce a certificate of vaccination.

RABIES

This condition is included as an example of a disease contracted from animals.

Organism. A virus, which affects the general nervous system.

Method of spread. Rabies virus is present in wild life in affected areas. In Western Europe foxes form the important reservoir, in the United States it is skunks, and in South America the vampire bat. In developed countries domestic animals form the link between wildlife and man in transmission of the disease. Dogs or cats which become infected can bite a human; there is virus in the saliva, which is injected into the wound.

Incubation period. This is from 10 days to a year, usually about 2 months.

Course. Depression, restlessness and sleeplessness occur. Spasm of the pharynx prevents drinking. Delirium, convulsions and paralysis follow. The disease is invariably fatal once symptoms appear.

Prevention. Rabies is unknown in England because there is no reservoir of infection in domestic dogs or wild animals, and dogs are not allowed into the country except after 6 months quarantine. From time to time there is agitation for relaxation of the quarantine rules, but the freedom of this country from rabies is a strong inducement to retain them. Some pessimism is felt about our ability to remain free, since rabies is steadily spreading towards the French coast.

A person who is bitten by an animal thought to have rabies is inoculated with attenuated virus, in order to produce immunity during the incubation period, often with success. If the animal responsible can be confined, the diagnosis can be confirmed by its death, or refuted if it survives for 10 days.

MALARIA

Malaria is included here because of its world-wide importance, although it does not now occur in Britain. It is a common disease of tropical and sub-tropical countries, caused by the injection into the host by an infected mosquito of the malaria parasite, which is a protozoon belonging to the genus Plasmodium. The disease is endemic in areas where there is enough warmth and moisture to maintain a breeding population of anopheles mosquitoes, and where there are people with malaria on whom the mosquito feeds. Malaria used to occur in marshy areas in the temperate zones from which it has now been banished, and in Britain it is now only seen in people who have returned from infected areas. These include tropical Africa, India, Pakistan, Ceylon, Indonesia, Northern Australia, Central and South America.

Several varieties of anopheles can transmit malaria, but in each case it is the female which is the blood-sucker. Mosquitoes are mainly nocturnal, avoiding bright light and flying in the evening. The eggs are laid on the surface of stagnant water, in which the larval stage is passed.

The malaria parasite belongs to the genus Plasmodium, and there are four varieties that affect man. These are:

1. **Plasmodium falciparum,** causing malignant tertian malaria. It is the most dangerous organism, with the most severe complications. Unlike the other three plasmodia, it does not persist in the liver. Malignant tertian malaria is the most common form throughout tropical Africa.

2. **Plasmodium vivax,** causing benign tertian malaria. It is the common parasite in India and South-east Asia.

3. **Plasmodium malariae,** causing quartan malaria.

4. **Plasmodium ovale,** causing benign tertian malaria. *P. malariae* and *P. ovale* are less common than the other two.

LIFE CYCLE OF THE MALARIA PARASITE

This takes place partly in the mosquito and partly in man.

Mosquito. 1. The female mosquito sucks infected blood, containing the sexual form (*gametocytes*) of the parasite.
   2. Male and female forms unite, and the egg cells become encysted in the stomach wall of the mosquito.
   3. In 1 to 3 weeks asexual forms (*sporozoites*) emerge, and reach the salivary glands.
   4. These sporozoites are injected into the next person bitten.

Man. 1. The sporozoites injected into the blood invade liver cells, where they develop.
   2. In about a week, the affected liver cells rupture, and release into the blood stream *merozoites*, which enter red blood cells.
   3. Asexual development occurs in the red blood cells.
   4. The affected red blood cells rupture, and release into the blood stream merozoites, a process accompanied by a rigor.
   5. These merozoites enter other cells. This process may be repeated several times before sexual forms (*gametocytes*) appear in the blood. The interval between rigors is 48 hours in tertian malaria, 72 hours in the quartan variety.
   6. In all except *P. falciparum* infections, sporozoites persist on the liver, and may reappear in the blood after considerable intervals, even years.

COURSE

The typical feature of malaria is the *rigor* that occurs when a new hatch of merozoites appears in the blood. Rigors are seen at the onset of several acute infections (e.g. pyelitis), and are a striking example of the power of the body to vary the temperature rapidly. The patient suddenly feels intensely cold, sometimes saying it is as if icy water were running down his back. He begins to shiver violently, and this muscular activity makes a large amount of heat. At the same time, heat loss is prevented because sweating ceases and the skin vessels constrict. The patient's distress is such that his attendants pile blankets on him, still further reducing heat loss. Headache is severe, and vomiting is a common symptom. This is called the "cold" stage of the rigor because of the patient's complaints, but in fact the temperature is climbing quickly. After 10 or 15 minutes the physical processes by which the temperature was raised are reversed. Shivering ceases, drenching perspiration starts, the skin vessels dilate, and the patient throws off his blankets. By these means the temperature is rapidly reduced to normal or subnormal, although the patient feels hot, and this is referred to as the hot stage of the rigor. The patient feels better now, and may be more normal until the next rigor occurs, either in two days (*tertian malaria*) or three (*quartan*). This regular periodicity may not be noticeable if the patient is infected by several batches of parasite, entering the blood stream at irregular intervals.

The spleen and liver gradually become enlarged, if the illness is not successfully treated. As blood cells are ruptured by the parasite, haemolytic anaemia is present in chronic malaria. In untreated ceases, the rigors will recur for about 6 weeks, then cease for long periods.

Children from the age of two or three are liable to contract malaria, and in remote under-developed areas the mortality in acute attacks is high. In chronic or relapsing malaria the child is listless from anaemia, wasted, with a distended abdomen due to enlargement of the spleen. The large spleen may rupture from quite minor injuries.

Diagnosis is made from examination of blood films.

COMPLICATIONS

Malaria often causes *abortion*, and since chronic malaria is often associated with anaemia, women may be badly affected by the normal blood loss of labour.

The worst complications are found only in malignant tertian malaria. In this condition the capillaries may be blocked by masses of affected red blood cells. If this occurs in the liver, there will be *jaundice;* if in the kidney, there may be acute *renal failure;* if in the intestine, there is severe diarrhoea with loss of fluids and electrolytes; if in the brain, the condition is named *cerebral malaria.* The symptoms are due to restriction of the oxygen supply to the brain through blocking of the vessels. The temperature is usually high, and there is drowsiness that may lead to coma, fits or hemiplegia. Sometimes the temperature is subnormal (*algid* form). Unless effective treatment is undertaken, the mortality rate is high.

Blackwater fever used to occur when malignant tertian malaria was treated with quinine, but it is now rarely seen since quinine has largely been superseded by newer drugs. Acute haemolysis caused release of haemoglobin in quantities too great to be metabolized normally, and it appeared in the urine, colouring it red or black.

PREVENTION OF MALARIA

1. Breeding places of mosquitoes may be drained, or the surfaces of stagnant water sprayed to lower the surface tension, and so prevent access of air to the larvae.

2. Places where adult mosquitoes rest by day (under eaves, in thatch or cellars) are sprayed with insecticide.

3. Wire mesh over windows prevents insects getting in at night, and mosquito nets can be used over beds.

4. Residents or visitors to affected areas should take a malaria suppressant, e.g. pyrimethamine (Daraprim) 50 mg (2 tablets) once a week. Proguanil, chloroquine and mepacrine are also used.

TREATMENT

Acute attacks. The aim of treatment is to eradicate the parasite by means of chemotherapy, and to treat other symptoms, such as anaemia or dehydration, that may be present. Chloroquine, mepacrine, proguanil, or pyrimethamine are all used, but resistance of the parasite to any or all of these may arise, and in this case quinine may have to be used. Gastrointestinal upsets may attend the use of the newer drugs, and giddiness or deafness is sometimes caused by quinine.

During a rigor the appropriate nursing care is given. In the cold phase, blankets are given, and after sweating the patient is bathed, dried and the clothes changed. Plenty of fluid must be given.

In cerebral malaria, hyperpyrexia is treated with sponging, or the use of fans and wet sheets. Chloroquine may be given by intravenous injection, and corticosteroids may be required. Patients with blackwater fever usually require transfusion, and are treated along the lines suggested for acute nephritis until symptoms diminish. Quinine must not be given.

STREPTOCOCCAL INFECTIONS

Pathogenic varieties of the streptococcus can produce a wide range of infections, which include tonsillitis, erysipelas (a skin inflammation), scarlet fever, and puerperal fever. The last three were at one time dangerous diseases with a high mortality, but since the introduction of antibacterial drugs these conditions have become less frequent, and can be efficiently treated in the very early stages.

The streptococcus is unique among disease-producing organisms in that sensitization to its toxins may cause two important diseases one to three weeks after the original infection. These are acute nephritis (page 223), and rheumatic fever, which is included in this chapter because of its link with streptococcal infections, though it is not a disease which is "catching" as are the other conditions described here.

RHEUMATIC FEVER
(Acute rheumatism)

Rheumatic fever is characterized in its acute stage by fever, joint inflammation and a tendency to affect the heart. The most important complication is chronic disease of the heart valves, which often causes heart failure later.

Aetiology. The connection with streptococcal infection has already been mentioned. It is usually a disease of children and young people, and is commoner among the underprivileged than among those in good economic circumstances.

Course. The onset is usually acute. Pain is felt in one or more of the big joints (knees, hips, elbows, ankles), which becomes red, hot, swollen and tender. The temperature is elevated, and the pulse rate raised out of proportion to the increase in temperature. Anaemia and a rise in the blood sedimentation rate are usually found. In a typical case, the joints originally inflamed improve, and others become affected. Sweating is marked, and fibrous (rheumatic) nodules may appear in the skin over bony prominences. If no complications arise, the symptoms subside in two or three weeks, though much longer periods are not uncommon.

Treatment. Skilled nursing and careful observation for complications is required, so the patient should be admitted to hospital, especially if home circumstances are unfavourable.

A bed cradle is supplied to prevent pressure on inflamed joints, and in view of the fever and sweating a draw macintosh should be omitted. A flannelette sheet next to the patient may be more comfortable than a linen one, which does not absorb perspiration. Absolute rest will be ordered in order to avoid any extra work for the heart, so one pillow will be used for a child, while an adult will be more comfortable with two or three.

Temperature, pulse and respiration should be estimated four hourly; a rising pulse rate indicates heart involvement, and must be reported. Intake and output are recorded, and a liberal fluid intake encouraged. A feeding cup must be used, to avoid making the patient sit up, or an angled plastic straw may be more acceptable to a child.

A daily warm bed bath, regular change of night clothes and pulling through the draw sheet will prevent discomfort from the sweating. Gentle handling will avoid causing pain to inflamed joints, which may be wrapped in gamgee, or allowed to rest on small pillows.

A course of penicillin is often prescribed at the outset, in case streptococci are still present in the throat. Sodium salicylate is prescribed to lower the temperature and relieve the joint pain, but it has no action that will prevent heart damage. Sodium salicylate may be given two hourly by day, four hourly by night, and an adult should have 8 to 12 g in twenty-four hours. Since it is a gastric irritant, it is usually prescribed in a mixture with sodium bicarbonate, and a good fluid intake will help prevent stomach upsets, as well as making good the fluid lost in sweat. Nausea, vomiting, ringing in the ears (tinnitus) and deafness are toxic signs, and it may be necessary to use calcium aspirin instead, since it is less irritating and better tolerated by children.

In a favourable case, when the temperature and especially the pulse rate fall and the joints become normal, activity may be gradually resumed. The patient may have another pillow, and feed himself, and if this has no adverse effect on the pulse, cautious return to normal may be begun.

Convalescence must be long and leisurely, and the parents of a child patient must be told that second attacks are not uncommon, and symptoms must be reported to the doctor at once. Sore throats are dangerous, and exposure to infection must be avoided. Phenoxymethicillin daily by mouth reduces to about one twentieth the onset of recurrent attacks. Prophylactic treatment of children is recommended to continue until the age of 20.

Complications. The heart muscle (myocardium) and the heart lining (endocardium) which also forms the valves are commonly affected. A rapid pulse of diminished volume is noticed by the nurse, and the doctor examining the heart hears abnormal sounds. Inflammation of the pericardium that surrounds the heart is accompanied by pain in the chest, fever, restlessness and sometimes cyanosis.

Danger to life from acute rheumatic carditis is not great, but the inflamed valves (especially the mitral valve between the left atrium and ventricle), may gradually become distorted by scar tissue, and many deaths from chronic heart failure are due to former attacks of rheumatism. People with chronic valvular disease are also more prone to bacterial endocarditis (page 188) than others, since if organisms gain entry to the bloodstream, they may colonize the layers of fibrin that form on such diseased valves.

CHOREA

The association of this condition with rheumatic fever is well established, but the nature of the connection is not known. Chorea is a disease of children, who display involuntary restless movement, sometimes violent and exhausting. Rheumatic heart disease may be present, or may occur later.

Girls are more often affected than boys, and there is often a history of anxiety or stress (about school examinations, for instance). The child is first noticed to be restless and clumsy, dropping things and grimacing. Movements are absent during sleep, but while awake, movement may be almost incessant, interfering with feeding and threatening injury. Attempts at carrying out simple instructions cause associated movements that may involve the whole body.

Treatment. Rest in hospital is required for all severe cases. The child's bed should be in a quiet place, and padded bedsides are required to prevent injury. It may also be necessary to cover the bars of the bed-head by tying a pillow in place. Soluble aspirin is usually prescribed, and a sedative such as phenobarbitone or a tranquillizer.

It may be easier to put the child in warm nightclothes and cover her with a rug, rather than to try to keep sheet and blankets in place. A good quality diet with adequate fluid intake is essential. Loss of weight will soon occur unless the intake provides for the energy expended. Inadequate fluid intake may cause ketosis, with the appearance of acetone in the urine. In very severe cases, oesophageal tube feeds may be required.

Recovery from chorea is the rule, and the nursing of such patients to normal health again is most rewarding.

ANTIBACTERIAL DRUGS

An antibiotic is a substance derived from another organism which can destroy bacteria within the body. The first ones discovered were the natural products of moulds, which they made to protect themselves against bacteria in which were their competitors for food supplies. The formula of many of these is now known, and they can be produced synthetically. New antibiotics become available quite frequently, and their method of administration and their value depends on these circumstances.

A. The organisms against which they are active. This range of activity is known as the spectrum: a wide-spectrum antibiotic is one which will destroy a variety of bacteria.

B. The effect of the hydrochloric acid in the stomach on them. Those which are destroyed by acids cannot be taken by mouth, but must be given by intramuscular or intravenous injection.

C. The toxic effects. These are powerful drugs, and some may affect the bone marrow (preventing the formation of blood cells), or the apparatus of the inner ear, (causing giddiness or deafness). Such antibiotics are reserved for severe infections, and watch must be kept for the earliest signs of ill-effects. Nurses should be aware of the specific dangers of the drugs they are using and report any untoward signs.

D. The ability of organisms to become resistant to certain antibiotics. Bacteria may be destroyed by an antibiotic when it is first administered, but survivors may learn to tolerate the drug, and the numbers of these will increase until further treatment with this antibiotic is ineffective. This is a serious occurrence, since any other people who may contract an infection from this patient will also have a condition which is resistant to treatment with this antibiotic. Many strains of staphylocci occur, especially in hospitals, which are resistant to many antibiotics.

E. Sensitization effects. Patients may become sensitized to antibiotics, and display fever or rashes. Once a person has become allergic to a drug he usually remains so, and if it is given on a second occasion, especially by injection, the severe symptoms of anaphylactic shock (page 10) may follow. Application of antibiotics to the skin is particularly liable to lead to sensitization, and those used for skin diseases or as eyedrops are either rarely used for other purposes, or are not absorbed from the intestine, and so are unlikely to cause systemic effects.

F. The blood levels attained. The majority of those in common use are absorbed from the injection site or the intestine into the blood, and the concentration in the blood falls fairly quickly as the antibiotic is excreted by the kidneys into the urine. The drug must be given at the intervals prescribed, in order to maintain an adequate level in the blood. If this falls too low, it encourages the appearance of drug-resistant bacteria, described in section D.

Some antibiotics are insoluble, and if they are given by mouth they remain in the intestine and are excreted in the stools. These would be useless for treating urinary infections or pneumonia, but are valuable to the surgeon who wants to sterilize the gut before operating on the colon, and in the treatment of intestinal infections. They are also used to prevent or cure coma in people with hepatic failure by reducing protein formation by bacteria in the intestine.

G. Side-effects may occur. These are effects which are unwanted, though not necessarily dangerous. For instance, wide-spectrum antibiotics which are given by mouth to treat respiratory or urinary conditions will also destroy the normal bacterial habitants of the mouth, colon and vagina, and this may allow invasion by thrush (candidiasis), or by drug-resistant bacteria.

PRESCRIBING ANTIBIOTICS

It will be seen from the preceding section that there are dangers attached to the giving of antibiotics, and they are only prescribed when they are likely to be effective. They are not active against viruses, and so are of no use for the common cold or influenza. Neither are they prescribed as a precaution against infection, unless this is highly likely, as in the patient with heart disease who is to have a dental extraction (page 138). In any severe infection, the nature of the organism and the antibiotics to which it is sensitive should be discovered by sending to the bacteriologist a specimen containing the organism. If treatment is urgent, a wide-spectrum antibiotic is prescribed, and this can be changed if necessary when the bacteriologist's report returns.

SOME COMMON ANTIBIOTICS

PENICILLIN GROUP

Penicillin was the earliest, and is still one of the safest and most useful of the antibiotics. It has no toxic effects, but has been used so widely that many people are sensitized to it, and allergic reactions, sometimes severe, may follow its administration to such people. Enquiry should be made about sensitivity before it is prescribed. It is effective against the streptococcus, gonococcus and the spirochaete of syphilis; many strains of staphylococci are penicillin-resistant, and it has no action on colon bacilli.

Benzyl penicillin is a soluble form given by intramuscular injection four times a day, in doses of 250,000 to 1 million units. The larger dose is required where abscesses exist, or collections of pus which oppose penetration by the drug. A high level of antibiotic in the blood is attained by this treatment. **Procaine benzyl penicillin** is a relatively insoluble form, slowly absorbed when given by intramuscular injection, and so only necessitating one injection a day.

The chief drawbacks to these older forms of penicillin are that they cannot be given by mouth; that staphylococci (which cause so much sepsis) are often resistant to them; and that because they are not active against *Escherichia coli* they are useless for many cases of urinary infections. Research into the structure of the penicillin molecule has been directed to finding new forms which do not have these drawbacks, and the following groups have been introduced.

1. Penicillins active against staphylococci.

   Methicillin (Celbenin) **Flucloxacillin** (Floxapen) and **Cloxacillin** (Orbenin) are resistant to the penicillinase which some staphylococci can make in order to inactivate penicillin. Methicillin must be given by injection, Cloxacillin and flucloxacillin can be given by injection or by mouth, but high doses by injection are painful.

2. Penicillins that can be given by mouth.

   Phenoxymethyl penicillin (Penicillin V) is not destroyed by gastric acid, and is given orally, in doses of about 250 mg six-hourly. People who are taking oral penicillin at home must be told how important it is not to miss a dose, and parents with sick children must know that the child must be awakened if necessary when the penicillin is due.

   Other oral varieties are **Phenethicillin** (Broxil), **Propillicin** (Brocillin), and **Phenbencillin** (Panspek). Rashes are not uncommonly caused.

3. Penicillins with wide-spectrum activity.

   Ampicillin (Penbritin) is active against most colon bacilli, and a high concentration can be attained in the urine. It can be given by mouth (250–500 mg six-hourly) as well as by injection. It is one of the most widely used of the penicillins, but is of no avail against penicillin-resistant staphylococci.

   Penicillin easily produces sensitization if applied to the skin, and doctors and nurses who administer it must protect their fingers from contamination.

CEPHALOSPORINS

These substances resemble penicillin in action. When widely used strains of staphylococci arise which are resistant to cloxacillin and methicillin as well as the cephalosporins. Cephaloridine is given by injection, but other preparations can be given by mouth.

STREPTOMYCIN AND GENTAMYCIN

Streptomycin is active against many organisms which are resistant to penicillin, including *Bacterium coli*. It has three drawbacks: (1) it must be given by injection; (2) resistance to its action by bacteria occurs very readily; (3) it is liable to produce damage to the inner ear, leading to giddiness and to loss of hearing that may amount to permanent deafness.

For these reasons its greatest use is in tuberculosis (page 205). If it is used for urinary infections, the dose does not normally exceed 1 g a day, and the course does not exceed five days. Special vigilance is needed with patients who have impaired kidney function, and with children and old people, and any complaints of giddiness or difficulty in hearing must be reported at once.

Streptomycin is another drug which readily causes sensitization if applied to the skin. This is of great importance to those caring for tuberculous patients, who use streptomycin daily, and nurses should wear gloves while preparing and giving injections.

Gentamycin is widely used for Gram negative infections, it is safer than streptomycin, but none the less can damage the vestibular branch of the auditory nerve.

CHLORAMPHENICOL

Chloramphenicol is one of the older antibiotics, and has the great drawback that it affects the bone marrow, and deaths from aplastic anaemia have followed its use. Though effective against many organisms, it is reserved for severe infections caused by bacteria resistant to safer antibiotics, and for typhoid fever, for which it is the specific treatment.

Because chloramphenicol is little used by mouth, it is often prescribed as drops for eye infections.

ERYTHROMYCIN CLINDAMYCIN AND LINCOMYCIN

These are similar in range to penicillin, but may be effective against penicillin-resistant staphylococci. Organisms establish resistance to them fairly readily. Lincomycin is popular with paediatricians. Fusidic acid is another antibiotic to which organisms soon display resistance.

THE TETRACYCLINES

This important group includes tetracycline itself, oxytetracycline, and some newer ones which may be found to have advantages over the first two.

Tetracycline can be given by mouth, and is effective against a wide range of organisms, including colon bacilli, so is often given at the outset of a severe infection, until the bacteriologist's report is available. The chief drawback of this group is that the sterilizing effect on the intestinal tract may allow infection by yeasts and fungi of the mouth, anus and vagina. A more serious complication is enteritis due to resistant-strains of staphylococci, which may cause diarrhoea leading to dehydration. The tetracyclines can cause discoloration of teeth in children; they should not be given to pregnant women or to children under seven years old.

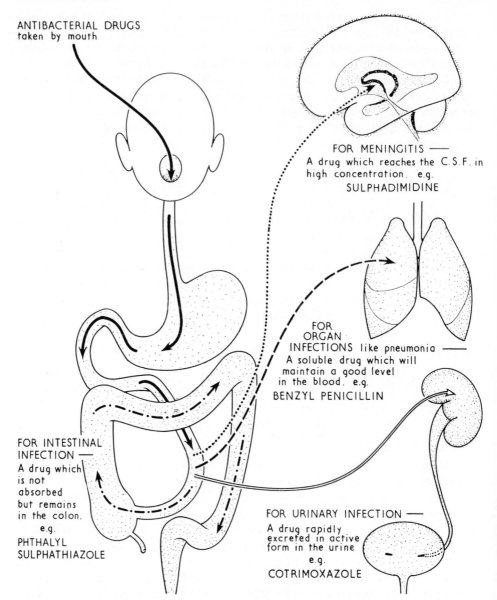

ANTIBACTERIAL DRUGS
taken by mouth

FOR MENINGITIS —
A drug which reaches the C.S.F. in
high concentration. e.g.
SULPHADIMIDINE

FOR
ORGAN
INFECTIONS like pneumonia —
A soluble drug which will
maintain a good level
in the blood. e.g.
BENZYL PENICILLIN

FOR INTESTINAL
INFECTION —
A drug which
is not
absorbed
but remains
in the colon.
       e.g.
PHTHALYL
SULPHATHIAZOLE

FOR URINARY INFECTION —
A drug rapidly
excreted in active
form in the urine
        e.g.
COTRIMOXAZOLE

Fig. 25. Some reasons for the choice of an antibacterial drug.

NEOMYCIN and KANAMYCIN

These are used for infections by *Bacterium coli, Bacillus proteus* and *Pseudomonas pyocyaneus*. Both are dangerous when given by injection, as they may injure the kidneys or cause deafness. Neomycin is not absorbed from the intestine, and so is useful in the treatment of dysentery, and in the preparation of patients for colonic operations, and in the treatment of hepatic pre-coma. Gentamycin has similar properties. *COLISTIN AND SULPHOMYXIN* are active against gram-negative infections, but readily produce toxic effects.

SULPHONAMIDES

This is a large group of antibacterial drugs with a broad spectrum of activity, some of which have fallen into disuse, because although effective they were toxic. Some are soluble, and are excreted by the kidneys, so that they are useful for urinary tract infections. Others are insoluble, so that they remain in the gut and exert their action there.

Sulphadimidine is the most useful sulphonamide. High levels can be maintained in the blood by six-hourly dosage by mouth, and it is relatively soluble in the urine. One of the drawbacks of this group is a tendency to come out of solution in the urine, especially when it is acid, and blockage of the ureters by crystals, or haematuria, may occur. Potassium citrate is often given at the same time, in an endeavour to make the urine alkaline, and the fluid intake must be high, in order to dilute the urine.

Sulphasalazine is of use in Crohn's disease and ulcerative colitis, in the prevention of recurrences of an attack rather than in the very acute stages.

Co-trimoxazole (Bactrim, Septrin) is a combination of sulphamethoxazole with trimethoprim. It has a wide range of uses in acute infections of the urinary and chest infections.

Phthalylsulphathiazole is scarcely absorbed at all from the alimentary canal, and so is used in preparing patients for operation on the large intestine, and in the treatment of bacillary dysentery.

VENEREAL DISEASES

The diseases grouped under this heading are acquired by sexual intercourse with an infected person. Although there are effective remedies for these diseases, unless treatment is begun early serious complications may occur, and infection of others is likely. The problems they present are social as well as medical, since incidence is high among the promiscuous, and promiscuity is an index of insecurity and disorganization in a community. Venereal disease figures rise in wartime, when large numbers of men and women are separated from their families, and in immigrant communities until these are stabilized.

When effective treatment became available for the venereal diseases, it was hoped that their incidence would fall rapidly and permanently, but this hope has not been realized, and there are few countries in the world where the number of new cases is not increasing annually. The incidence of syphilis is rising, and although the total number of cases may not be great, the late results of untreated syphilis are so serious that alarm must be felt. One of the most worrying facts about venereal disease is that the average age of patients is falling, and that many teenagers and even schoolchildren are infected.

It is usual to ascribe venereal disease to ignorance, but in spite of continual propaganda through all the mass-media, and considerable permissiveness in discussion of sexual affairs, there is as yet no sign that growth of knowledge about the transmission of venereal disease is likely to cause a fall in the number of people affected. Nurses and doctors concerned in this work must strive to ensure that treatment is readily available, and that contacts are traced and treated, so that the reservoir of infection in the community is kept at as low a level as possible. Censoriousness must be avoided, but it must always be remembered that venereal disease is largely preventible, since it mainly occurs among the sexually promiscuous. There is a mood of rebellion and restlessness among young people in many parts of the world, and they must be supported and helped with their problems, personal and social, in the hope that they may reach a more stable attitude, since these are the parents of tomorrow.

In the United Kingdom three conditions are defined as venereal diseases by law. These are syphilis, gonorrhoea and chancroid. Chancroid is rarely seen nowadays. In addition to these diseases it is now recognized that many other conditions are transmitted from person to person during the close bodily contact that occurs during sexual intercourse in its various forms. The more common diseases which are transmitted this way are non-specific genital infection in males and females, candidiasis and trichomoniasis in females more commonly than in males, and scabies, pediculosis, genital warts, genital herpes simplex, and genital molluscum contagiosum in both sexes.

In the United Kingdom most patients with one of these diseases are treated in a clinic for sexually transmitted diseases. Management in these clinics follows the usual lines. The patients are seen by a doctor who takes the full history with particular reference to his genital complaints but also covers his general health and past history. A full clinical examination is carried out with particular reference to the genitals but it must be remembered that these diseases can effect the rectum, the pharynx and occasionally every other part of the body. Appropriate specimens are taken for investigations some of which are done on the spot in the clinic. Blood is taken from every patient for examination for serum antibodies for syphilis. Once a diagnosis has been made appropriate treatment is given and the patient is advised about tracing his contacts; this is a most important part of the management of every patient with an infectious disease as this is one of the main ways of preventing the spread of infection. Patients with emotional and social problems will be seen by a social worker and patients with general medical complaints may be referred to their own practitioner or to the appropriate hospital department.

One of the most important aspects of the management of patients in a sexually transmitted diseases clinic is that treatment is confidential. This means that the patient's diagnosis is not told to anyone outside the clinic without his or her consent and certainly not to a partner. Many clinics keep their own notes which do not leave the department.

Nurses have a most important role in these clinics, helping the doctor to examine and investigate patients, and to help to comfort and soothe anxious patients.

SYPHILIS

Organism. A spirochaete, *Treponema pallidum*.

Method of spread. Syphilis is acquired by intercourse with an infected person, but may also be congenital in a baby born to an infected mother.

Incubation period. The average is 25 days, with a range from 9 to 90 days.

Course. The spirochaete enters the tissues through a small break in the skin or mucous membrane, and at the site of entry there appears a small raised lump which breaks down in the centre to form an ulcer which is known as the primary sore or chancre. The edges are well defined, there is no pus formation and the ulcer has a hard base with a zone of inflammation around it. The lesion is painless. The ulcer shows little tendency to heal, and within a few days the local lymph glands enlarge, and may reach a fair size.

The primary sore is usually on the penis in men, and in women may be on the labia minora or on the cervix. If in the latter situation there may be no symptoms at this stage. The diagnosis is confirmed when the spirochaete is found in the serum that oozes from the base of the ulcer. Without treatment the ulcer will take one or two months to heal.

Six or eight weeks after the primary infection the organism enters the blood stream and the secondary signs of syphilis appear. The patient feels ill, the temperature rises, there is anaemia and complaints of headache. The throat is sore, because of ulcers on the fauces. Skin rashes are very common, and may take many forms. Typically the lesions are papules, coppery or red in colour, and widely distributed over the body. Papules in moist areas coalesce to form masses called condylomata lata, in which spirochaetes are found.

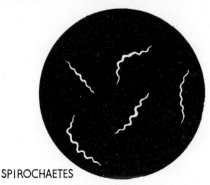

SPIROCHAETES

Fig. 26. Treponema pallidum. The causative organism of syphilis.

The moist lesions (e.g. faucial ulcers and condylomata) are all infectious. This secondary stage of infectious syphilis lasts in untreated patients up to 12 months, and then all signs disappear and the disease passes into the latent phase. Later there may follow one of the forms of tertiary syphilis, which principally affect the nervous system (p. 392) or the circulatory system, but may appear in many situations.

In the secondary stage of syphilis, spirochaetes may be found in the moist lesions, and since this is a stage of general invasion, blood tests now also become positive. The older ones are the Wassermann and Kahn reactions, and newer and more specific ones are the treponemal immobilization tests (T.P.I.) and the Reiter Protein Complement Fixation Test. These tests become positive during the infectious stage of syphilis, and will remain positive for years in the absence of treatment.

The typical lesion of late syphilis is the *gumma*, a mass of necrotic tissue, which if it is near the surface, ulcerates through the skin, forming an indolent sore, circular in shape, with sharply defined edges and a base which is often covered with a yellowish slough. Almost any organ can be affected, bones and the liver being among the more common.

The lesions in the circulatory system affect mainly the aorta. Inflammation weakens its walls, and the thinned portion may bulge out to form an *aneurysm*, which may eventually rupture. If the aorta is affected near its origin, the coronary arteries may be involved, and the aortic valves may become incompetent. Syphilis of the circulatory system is much less common than it once was, because it is now usually effectively treated at an earlier stage.

Congenital syphilis. A woman who has syphilis can pass it to her unborn child, even though she no longer has the moist lesions of early infectious syphilis. The spirochaete can pass through the placenta into the foetal circulation, so that the baby may be born with the general signs of syphilis, or may show them in the early weeks. Rashes are common, often papular and coppery red in colour, but sometimes large blisters or *bullae* are seen. The baby fails to thrive, and infection of the nasal mucous membranes causes discharge, and respiratory obstruction which makes sucking difficult because the baby has to stop frequently to breathe. Cracks at the angles of the mouth heal to form radiating scars or rhagades. Lymph glands are enlarged, and the bones are often tender because of periostitis.

Even without treatment, many children survive this acute infectious stage, and some time after the second year gummata begin to appear, often in the nose and mouth. The hard palate may be perforated, and the nasal bones may collapse, causing a saddle-shaped nose. The permanent teeth are affected, the central incisors being widely spaced and notched (*Hutchinson's teeth*). Inflammation of the cornea (*keratitis*) makes it hazy, and scars may be formed in it. Deafness due to involvement of the eighth nerve is common.

Treatment. The sooner treatment of syphilis is begun, the better the results, since in early cases complete cure can be obtained, while if destructive lesions are present, the disease can only be arrested. Penicillin is the drug of choice for the treatment of all forms of syphilis. The type and dose given depends on the stage of syphilis being treated. In the newborn babe with congenital syphilis the usual treatment is to give 200,000 units of procaine penicillin per pound and to divide the total into ten injections, thus a 4.5 kg baby requires 2,000,000 units of penicillin, i.e. 200,000 units of procaine penicillin once daily for ten days by injection. The older child with congenital syphilis will also require a 10 day course of penicillin the dose depending on the age and size of the child. In late congenital syphilis the dose will be similar to the dose used for acquired syphilis.

In primary acquired syphilis (in the earlier stage of this form of infection) it is still common practice to give 600,000 units of procaine penicillin daily for 10 to

12 days. In secondary acquired syphilis the same dose of penicillin is given for 14 or 15 days. This regime is used for early and late latent syphilis and for tertiary syphilis. In the various forms of neurosyphilis and cardiovascular syphilis this dose of penicillin may be continued for 21 days. In these last forms of syphilis other general medical measures may be required and in some forms of cardiovascular syphilis surgery may be indicated. Other forms of treatment are not usually necessary in the earlier stages. It may be difficult for a few patients to attend for daily injections, and these patients may be treated with longacting penicillin as Benzathine penicillin 2.4 mega units twice weekly for two or three weeks. Patients who are hypersensitive to penicillin may be given tetracycline 500 mg four times daily for 15 to 21 days. The disadvantage of this preparation is that it has to be taken orally and this requires on the patient's full co-operation. Alternatives to the tetracyclines are the erythromycins which can be given in the same dosage, and cephaloridine 2 g daily by intramuscular injection for 10 to 14 days. It must be remembered that with this last preparation some patients who are hypersensitive to penicillin are also hypersensitive to cephaloridine.

Careful follow up after the treatment of syphilis is most important and nurses have a role in helping to persuade the patients of the importance of their attendance for this follow up.

Prevention. Blood tests for syphilis should be made on all women attending antenatal clinics, and this should make congenital syphilis rare. Young people should be made aware of the dangers of promiscuity.

GONORRHOEA

Organism. A coccus discovered by Neisser in 1879. It is Gram negative, that is, it does not take up Gram's stain; and is often found in pairs inside pus cells, i.e. it is an intracellular diplococcus.

Method of spread. In adults, by sexual intercourse. The eyes of babies may be infected during birth if the mother has gonorrhoea. Accidental infection of small girls from towels or lavatory seats occasionally occurs.

Incubation period. Three to 10 days, the average being 5 days.

Course. In men, the infection is in the anterior urethra at first, and causes purulent discharge and pain on micturition. Unless this is treated, the inflammation spreads to the posterior urethra, when the local symptoms will be more severe, and general signs such as fever and headache usually appear. From the urethra the infection may spread to the bladder (cystitis), the seminal vesicles (vesiculitis), the prostate gland (prostatitis) and the epididymis and the testis

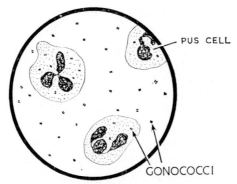

Fig. 27. Gonococci in smears are usually seen in pairs, often in pus cells.

(epididymo-orchitis). Infection of the rectum (proctitis) is sometimes found in homosexual men. Scarring and fibrous tissue formation after healing may cause urethral stricture, or may cause adhesions in the vas deferens which carries the semen from the epididymis to the ejaculatory duct, and so cause sterility.

In women, the cervix as well as the urethra is affected in acute gonorrhoea. Besides the urinary symptoms, there is profuse purulent discharge from the cervix via the vagina. Not infrequently, however, symptoms are slight and soon disappear. If spread occurs, it is usually to Bartholin's glands, where an abscess may form, or to the Fallopian tubes (salpingitis). Pus escaping from the tubes into the peritoneal cavity can give rise to gonococcal peritonitis. Even slight inflammation of the tubes may stick the delicate layers of the ciliated mucous membrane together and cause sterility.

A most important complication is gonococcal bacteraemia which is some times called disseminated gonococcal infection. This condition is commoner in females than in males and is characterized by fever, joint pains and a peripheral pustular rash. This is another emergency when the patient should be admitted to the hospital.

The diagnosis depends on finding the gonococcus in the discharges, or obtaining a culture from them. The gonococcus is very susceptible both to heat and drying, and if cultures cannot be made at once, the swab should be placed in Stuart's transport medium, in which the organism will survive for a few days. The gonococcal complement fixation test is a serum test, similar in principle to the Wassermann test for syphilis, but it is not specific, and is only really informative when it is negative.

Gonorrhoea is the most common infectious disease that responds to antibiotics, and it is one of the few infections which responds to a single dose of antibiotic provided an adequate dose of a suitable drug is given. Pencillin is usually the drug of choice for gonorrhoea, but the dose varies in different places. Some strains of gonococci are partially resistant to penicillin but no complete resistance has yet been reported. Partially resistant strains are particularly common in some parts of Africa and the Far East. In the U.K. uncomplicated gonorrhoea in a young adult can be treated with 1.2 to 2.4 mega units of procaine penicillin given in a single injection. Many clinics also give a gram of probenecid by mouth at the same time. Probenecid blocks the renal excretion of penicillin and so raises peak serum concentrations of the drug. In recent years many clinics have started to give oral treatment and 2 g of ampicillin plus 1 g of probenecid taken as a single oral dose under supervision in the clinic gives satisfactory results. For patients with uncomplicated gonorrhoea who are hypersensitive to penicillin, co-trimoxazole may be given. Unfortunately single doses of this drug involve taking many tablets and tend to cause vomiting. Multiple dose therapy is therefore recommended and a good regime is to give 4 tablets of co-trimoxazole twice daily for two days.

The most important local complication of gonorrhoea in the male is epididymitis. A patient with acute epididymitis should be advised to rest and to wear a suitable scrotal support. The usual standard dose of antibiotic should be given but it is advisable to continue with multiple dose therapy for several days. A suitable regime would be ampicillin 2 g and probenecid 1 g as a first dose, followed by ampicillin 500 g four times a day for 5 to 7 days. The most important local complication in the female is acute salpingitis or acute pelvic inflammatory disease as it is also called. This is one of the emergencies in venereology. The patient should be admitted to hospital for rest and for a few days she will require careful nursing with complete bed rest. Provided the diagnosis has been satisfactorily established by bacteriological investigations, treatment with penicillin by injection can be given. It is wise to start with a large loading dose such as crystalline penicillin 5 mega units in a single injection (given in 8 ml of 0.5% lignocaine) plus 1 g of probenecid. This should be followed by 1 mega unit of crystalline penicillin six hourly until all signs and symptoms have stopped. The patient can then be allowed out of bed and treatment can be continued with procaine penicillin 900,000 units once or twice daily to complete 10 days. An alternative is to give ampicillin by mouth. With a loading dose of 2 g plus 1 g of probenecid and continue with 0.5 to 1 g of ampicillin six hourly for 10 days. Another common local complication of gonorrhoea in the female is acute Bartholinitis. This usually responds to a single dose of antibiotic such as 2 g of ampicillin plus 1 g of probenecid and the abcess should be aspirated using a wide-borne needle inserted through the inner aspect of the labia minora after local anaesthesia with ethyl chloride spray. If this treatment is not followed by rapid resolution then the patient should be referred to a gynaecologist.

In all patients with gonorrhoea it is most important that their contacts be traced and they should all return for examination and bacteriological investigation after treatment. A common regime is to ask them to return three times in the 14 days after completing treatment.

Non-Specific Genital Infection

Non-specific genital infection in the male usually takes the form of non-specific urethritis. This condition has the same clinical features as gonococcal urethritis in the male, namely, urethral discharge and dysuria. However, although leucocytes are present in the discharge no organisms can be found. Experience has shown that although no organism can be found to cause this condition it responds to tetracycline. In some clinics the condition is still treated with Oxytetracycline 250 mg four times a day for 7 days. However, in others longer courses of treatment have been found necessary. Prolonged treatment is difficult for ambulant patients to remember and it is helpful to give them long-acting tetracycline which can be given twice a day. Detecto which is a mixture of Oxytetracycline, Chlortetracycline and demethylchlortetracycline, can be taken in a dose of one tablet, which is 300 mg twice daily, and courses of up to 21 days have been given. Many specialists believe that 21 day courses are to be recommended in this condition. No clinical equivalent of non-specific urethritis has been found in the female but is it becoming common practice to treat the regular female partners of men with non-specific urethritis using the same course of tetracycline.

Genital Herpes Simplex

The most common identifiable cause of genital ulceration is genital herpes simplex due to Herpes *Virus Type* II, as apposed to *Herpes Virus* Type I which causes labial herpes. Genital herpes is usually a recurrent condition which causes a cluster of vesicles on the genitals which rapidly break down to form erosions which may be painful and tender. Diagnosis is usually clinical but the virus can readily be cultured from vesicles and fresh erosions. Usually simple hygiene is all that is necessary for treatment. If secondary infection is present it can be treated with sulphadinidime 1 g t.i.d. for five to seven days or co-trimoxazole may be used as an alternative. The antiviral agent Idoxuridine has been used in the condition but so far there is no convincing evidence of its value.

Genital herpes may also affect the cervix but there is still no specific treatment for this condition. The most important aspect of it is that there is association between cervical herpes infection and subsequent carcinoma of the cervix but the nature of the association is not yet known. Women who have had herpetic cervicitis should be advised to have regular cervical cytology examinations.

Genital Warts

Warts may affect the penis and around the anus in the male, and on the female they affect the vulva, vagina, cervix, perineum and perianal region. The diagnosis is made from the appearance of the lesions and the treatment is Podophyllin which is a paint dissolved in spirit or Tinct. Benz. Co. It is made up in various strengths from 10 to 25%. It is painted on the warts. One usually starts with a dilute concentration such as 10% and leave it on for four hours. If this does not have a satisfactory result, 25% Podophyllin may be applied and left for fours hours too. A few patients need repeated application of Podophyllin and if so, the duration that it is left on should gradually be increased. After the appropriate interval the paint should be washed off with plenty of hot soapy water. Occasionally large or extensive warts require cauterization and this is best done under general anaesthesia.

An important part of the management of anyone with anogenital warts is to advise them about hygiene. They should keep the affected area as cool and as dry as possible.

Trichomoniasis

Trichomoniasis, which is due to the flagellate parasite *Trichomonas Vaginalis*, commonly causes vaginal discharge and discomfort although the organism may be present without there being any symptoms. The usual treatment for this condition is metronidazole. This can be given in 200 mg tablets taken three times daily for 7 days. A useful alternative in ambulant patients is to give them 400 mg tablets one twice a day for five days. An alternative is Nimorazole, a similar compound which can be given in a dose of 200 mg twice daily for 6 days, or 1 g every 12 hours for three doses. *Trichomonas vaginalis* is sexually transmitted and can cause balanitis, urethritis or prostatitis in the male, but the organism is often difficult to isolate from the male partner. It is considered good practice to examine the male and to treat him with a similar course of treatment.

Candidiasis

Vulvo-vaginal candidiasis or thrush is due to *Candida albicans* and is another common condition in women causing vaginal discharge and vulval itch. The usual treatment is Nystatin pessaries two at night for 14 nights plus Nystatin cream to the vulva twice daily. It is good practive to see any regular male partner who may have balanitis or may harbour candida under the prepuce without any symptoms. In both cases he should be treated with local Nystatin cream. Various alternatives to Nystatin are available and one suitable one is Canestin one pessary at night for six nights plus Canestin cream for the vulva. It is however more expensive than Nystatin and slightly less effective.

Chancroid, Granuloma Inguinale and Lymphogranuloma Venereum

Chancroid, granuloma inguinale and lymphogranuloma venereum are all basically tropical infections. They all produce a genital ulcer and swelling in the inguinal region. Chancroid, which is due to the bacillus *Haemophilis ducreyi*, produces a painful irregular genital ulcer and marked enlargement of the inguinal nodes which matt together and suppurate. The diagnosis is made by finding the causative organism in the ulcer and treatment is usually a sulphonamide such as sulphadimidine 2 to 4 g as a loading dose and 1 g four hourly until the healing is complete which may take some 10 to 14 days. Co-trimoxazole may also be used. An alternative is oxytetracycline 250 mg six hourly until healing is complete.

Granuloma inguinale is due to an organism called *Donovania granulomatis* or Donovan's body, a bacterium, which is now believed to be related to the *Klebsiella* group. It produces a comparatively large granulomatous ulcerated genital lesion and rounded swellings in the inguinal region which resemble enlarged lymph nodes but many of them are masses of granulomatous tissue. The diagnosis can only be made my biopsy of the lesions and identifying the causative organism in the biopsy. The treatment is tetracycline 500 mg six hourly for 10 to 20 days.

Lymphogranuloma venereum is due to one of the chlamydia organisms. There is often an insignificant genital lesion but suppurative enlargement of the lymph nodes occurs. There may also be quite marked constitutional symptoms and in the late stages there may be mild to moderate lumphatic oedema of the vulva and anal strictures may occur. Malignant changes have been described as squelae of genital elephantiasis and of anorectal stricture. The diagnosis can usually be suspected on clinical grounds but must be confirmed by isolating the organism or by serum antibody tests. The treatment consists of sulphadimidine 5 gm daily in divided doses for one to three weeks. Co-trimoxazole may also be used and the tetracyclines such as oxytetracycline 1 g six hourly for a week followed by 500 mg six hourly for 14 days are also effective.

In all these conditions it is important to exclude the presence of syphilis by the appropriate investigations.

Yaws, Endemic Syphilis and Pinta

Yaws, endemic syphilis and pinta are all childhood diseases due to treponema organisms which appear identical with *Treponema pallidum* of syphilis, They produce lesions of skin, subcutaneous tissues, mucosal and submucosal tissues and in the case of yaws and endemic syphilis, they also affect bones. The diagnosis is made in the same way as for syphilis for they affect the serum antibody tests in exactly the same manner. The treatment is penicillin and a single injection of 2·4 mega units of Benzathine penicillin is effective.

Other genital lesions

Patients may present at a clinic with many conditions such as psoriasis and even in alignant disease. Infestations like pediculosis pubis and scabies may also be acquired in the circumstances that give rise to sexually transmitted disease. It will be evident that those who arrive at clinics may have a very large range of medical, emotional and social needs to be considered.

Chapter 6

Diseases of the Circulatory System

If the front of the wrist or the back of the hand is examined, a network of blue vessels can be seen under the skin. These are superficial veins, carrying blood back towards the heart. At intervals, swellings can be seen which mark the site of the valves which direct the onward flow of blood. If a section of vein is emptied by pressure from two fingers, it will fill at once if the distal finger is taken away. If the proximal pressure is released, blood will only run back as far as the nearest valve.

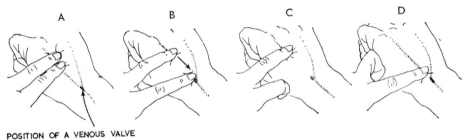

POSITION OF A VENOUS VALVE

Fig. 28.

A. Two fingers are placed on a vein distal to a valve.
B. The portion of vein is emptied by stroking it up to the valve.
C. The proximal finger is removed, but the valve prevents the vein filling from above.
D. The distal finger is removed, and the vein fills from below.

The deep veins, with which the superficial ones eventually join, lie between the muscles, whose tone and contractions help the onward movement of the blood. From the upper parts of the body, the return of venous blood to the right atrium is helped by gravity. The return of blood from the legs and abdomen via the inferior vena cava is assisted by the negative pressure in the chest, and by the movements of the diaphragm, through the central tendon of which the inferior vena cava passes to reach the heart.

Veins are thin walled, and are easily distended by increased pressure. Superficial ones are especially vulnerable because they are not supported by muscle, and if unduly stretched the valves may be damaged, blood begins to flow backwards along the veins, which become tortuous and dilated, or *varicose*. The legs and the anal canal are the most common site for varicose veins, which are treated, if severe, by the surgeon, either by injection or by operation.

The route taken by the blood is in effect a figure of eight, from the veins to the right heart, the heart to the lungs, back to the left side of the heart, out via the arteries to the capillaries which supply the tissues, and thence to the veins. Failure or obstruction at any point on this one-way system will cause congestion behind this point. For instance, failure of efficient action in the right ventricle

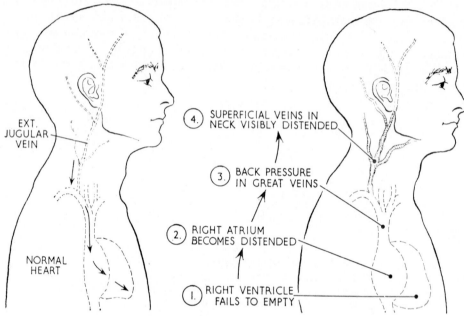

EXT. JUGULAR VEIN

NORMAL HEART

4. SUPERFICIAL VEINS IN NECK VISIBLY DISTENDED

3. BACK PRESSURE IN GREAT VEINS

2. RIGHT ATRIUM BECOMES DISTENDED

1. RIGHT VENTRICLE FAILS TO EMPTY

Fig. 29. The effect of right ventricular failure.

will cause engorgement of the veins which can be seen to be distended in the neck.

VENOUS THROMBOSIS

Clotting within the vessel is one of the most important pathological affections of veins. Such clotting is not uncommon in varicose veins, and in those irritated by intravenous infusion, and is termed thrombophlebitis. Heat, redness and pain are felt over the affected vein, and the temperature rises if the condition is extensive. Local warmth and support give comfort, and antibiotics can be given if there is infection.

A more dangerous condition is the clotting that may occur in normal veins, especially in the deep veins of the leg. Such clotting is encouraged by pressure on the veins (e.g. those of the calves). Patients who lie in bed with little movement and slack muscles are most liable. Low blood-pressure, slowing of the circulation and dehydration are contributory causes.

Deep vein thrombosis should be prevented if possible by regular movement,

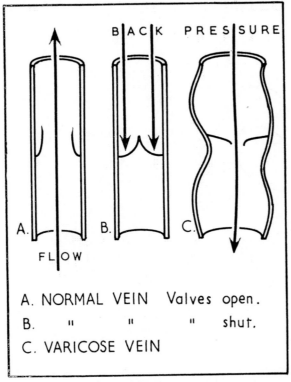

Fig. 30. In a dilated vein, the valves are unable to prevent backward flow of blood.

active or passive, of the legs by bed-fast patients. We have noticed that movement of the diaphragm helps the return of blood from the legs to the heart, so deep breathing exercises should be taught and regularly carried out.

The signs of venous thrombosis in the legs may be minimal—a little tenderness on pressure, swelling of the ankle, slight rises of temperature. If thrombosis is diagnosed, drugs to lower the clotting power of the blood (anticoagulants) are often prescribed. The method of giving them is along these lines.

1. **Heparin** by intravenous injection will lower the coagulation time immediately. Since it must be given at least 6 hourly, it is usual to introduce a needle of the butterfly type into the vein and strap it into place, to avoid frequent vein punctures. An initial dose of 15,000 units, followed by 10,000 units 6 hourly for

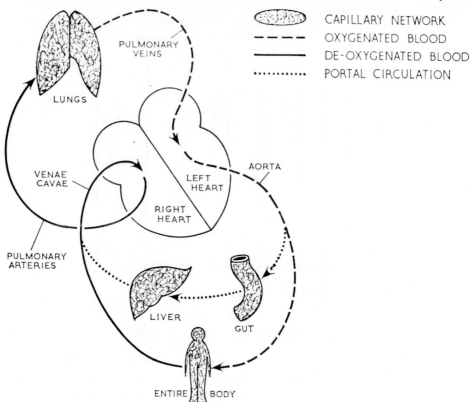

Fig. 31. A diagrammatic representation of the path taken by the blood.

24 to 36 hours is a common dose. If bleeding occurs, the action of heparin can be halted by protamine sulphate intravenously.

2. Oral anticoagulants act by antagonizing vitamin K the precursor of prothrombin. The dose is controlled by estimating the blood prothrombin time, which should be kept within two or two and a half times the control value. Daily estimation is necessary until the dose has been stabilized. Warfarin is the most used oral anticoagulant because it is the safest. It acts in thirty-six to forty-eight hours, when heparin is discontinued. If bleeding occurs a few doses

can be omitted, or if it is at all serious vitamin K_1 (Phytomenadine) can be given intravenously.

The great danger of deep venous thrombosis is that portions of the clot may detach and move upwards towards the heart. Moving fragments in the blood are known as emboli, and these emboli will, if they arise in the leg veins, pass up the inferior vena cava, through the right heart and into the pulmonary artery. This serious condition is pulmonary embolism.

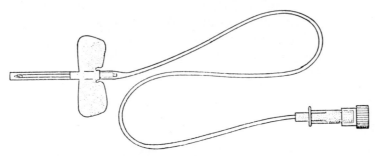

Fig. 32. Butterfly needle.

PULMONARY EMBOLISM

An embolus can reach the lungs from two places:
1. the veins, usually in the legs,
2. the right side of the heart, where clotting may occur, usually in the atrium of patients with heart disease.

The effects are the same. If the clot is a small one, it passes into one or other pulmonary artery, and is finally halted in a vessel too small to allow it to go farther. It cuts off the circulation to a portion of lung, this area being termed an *infarct*. Symptoms may include faintness and breathlessness, and later slight fever, tachycardia, rapid shallow breathing, pain in the chest and blood-stained sputum. The treatment is that described above for thrombosis, in the hope of preventing further emboli arising.

Massive embolism may cause death at once, or within a few minutes. In rather less severe cases, the patient feels intense pain in the abdomen and chest and may ask urgently for a bedpan, or may vomit. He becomes cyanosed, intensely breathless, and may lose consciousness. The nurse may suspect what has happened, though other events, such as coronary thrombosis, may produce similar symptoms. Her course of action will be the same whatever the cause.

The physician is summoned urgently, and the patient is told if conscious that help is coming and all will be well. He is kept at rest and oxygen is given if he is blue or breathless. If the pulse can be felt, a five-minute chart is kept, and sterile syringes and needles for intravenous injection are prepared. If the heart stops, external cardiac massage and artificial respiration would usually be begun.

Intravenous Leparin is usually given, and since respiratory depression allows acid to accumulate in the blood 1 dl of 7·5% sodium bicarbonate is administered. For a patient very gravely ill, the operation of pulmonary embolectomy may be considered, but unless bypass facilities are available in the theatre this operation carries a very high mortality. Drug therapy with streptokinase or urokinase is designed to dissolve the clot in the pulmonary arteries and may be used if the patient has no undue tendency to bleed. It is believed that 2000 to 3000 people die every year in this country from pulimonary embolism, so it can be seen that there is a great opportunity to save lives by prevention of the venous thrombosis that gives rise to embolism.

ARTERIES

Arteries are thicker-walled than veins, since they have to withstand a pressure during ventricular contraction of around 120 mm. of mercury. They are lined with the smooth layer of endothelium that is continuous throughout the circulatory system. The thickness of the wall is due to the middle coat, or tunica media. In the larger arteries this contains a good deal of elastic tissue, which

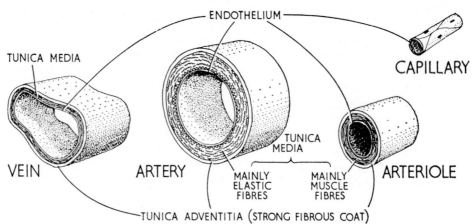

Fig. 33. *Veins* are comparatively thin walled and are easily compressed.
Large arteries contain much elastic tissue.
Arterioles have muscular middle coats, and help regulate the blood pressure.
Capillaries consist of a single layer of cells.

permits them to expand to receive the blood put out by each heart contraction. The smaller arteries, or *arterioles*, have a muscular middle coat. This enables them to expand to increase the blood supply to any structure that needs it, and by contraction to increase the blood-pressure.

Changes in arteries take place with increasing age, or because of disease processes. They may be summarized as follows.

1. HYPERTENSION (page 110)

Rise in the blood pressure is caused by increased resistance in the arteries, usually by spasm of the muscular middle coat.

2. ARTERIOSCLEROSIS

Hardening of the arteries is a common accompaniment of old age. Where arteries can be felt (e.g. the radial artery at the wrist), the vessel can be felt as a firm tube, and the pulse is "hard" or difficult to obliterate by pressure from the fingers. A moderate degree of arteriosclerosis need not shorten life, unless it is combined with another form of arterial disease. It is sometimes seen in a severe form in the arteries of the legs, when by restricting the blood-flow to the muscles and skin it may cause pain on walking (i.e. intermittent claudication), or threaten gangrene (page 115).

3. ATHEROMA

This is a condition affecting the intima or lining of the arteries. Plaques of fatty material, especially cholesterol, appear inside the arteries, narrowing them so that blood-flow is diminished, and roughen them so that clotting tends to occur.

The arteries most often affected are the aorta, and the coronary, cerebral and renal arteries, so that atheroma causes coronary thrombosis, strokes, and renal failure, all of which are important causes of invalidism and death.

Deaths from atheroma, especially from coronary disease, have increased alarmingly during this century. Before the First World War, coronary thrombosis was uncommon except in elderly men of the professional and middle class. Now it is seen in all classes at an increasingly early age, and numbers of women are affected.

Atheroma is uncommon in poorer countries, where the diet is low in fat and protein, but as material conditions improve, the incidence of atheroma increases. Much attention has been paid to the role of animal fats in causing atheroma, and in 1976 the Royal College of Physicians supported the view that a high intake of fats derived from meat and dairy produce should be avoided, and that polyunsaturated fats such as sunflower seed oil and corn oil should be used instead. This advice would be most valuable to those with a family history of arterial and coronary disease. In general, lack of exercise, over-eating and cigarette smoking appear to favour the onset of arterial disease.

4. INFLAMMATORY DISEASE
e.g. thromboangiitis obliterans, or Buerger's disease (page 117).

5. VASOMOTOR CONDITIONS
In which there is arterial spasm, especially in the fingers and toes.

HYPERTENSION
The blood-pressure depends on the amount of blood put out by the heart, and the resistance of the arterial walls. In a healthy young adult, the pressure during systole (heart contraction) is about 120 mm. of mercury, during diastole it falls to 80 mm. of mercury. The figure varies slightly from one person to another, and is influenced by emotion, exercise, and age as well as by disease. It is also possible to obtain a false reading by careless or imperfect technique.

If there are special instructions about the patient's position, these must be followed, the doctor may wish to know what the blood-pressure is before he gets up in the morning and again after he has risen. The patient must be sitting or lying, relaxed and at ease, and the arm is bared; if the sleeve is tight, the arm must be slipped out of it. The sphygmomanometer stands beside him on an even surface, about the level of the heart, and turned so that the patient does not see the scale. The cuff is applied with the rubber bag over the front of the arm where the brachial artery lies, and with the straight edge of the material uppermost. It is wound smoothly into place, and the end tucked in.

An approximate reading of the systolic pressure can be obtained by inflating the cuff while feeling the radial pulse and noting the point at which it disappears. The cuff must be completely deflated before taking the full reading. It is then inflated until the mercury rises about 30 mm. above the pressure found by palpation. A stethoscope is now applied above the elbow on the inner side of the biceps where the brachial artery lies, and the pressure gradually allowed to fall. The level at which the first sound of the pulse is heard is the systolic pressure. As the cuff deflates, the sounds become loud and knocking, then suddenly drop to a muffled tone; the level at this point is the diastolic pressure. The result should be recorded at once. A series of recordings is more informative than a single reading.

The point at which the blood-pressure is considered to be abnormally high is not easy to define. The best definition is perhaps a diastolic pressure persistently above 95 mm. Hg. in an adult at rest. In someone under forty, a pressure of 160/95 mm. Hg. would be thought abnormal. In a man of sixty, it would be thought within normal limits. As a rough guide, physicians would consider that hypertension was present if the systolic pressure exceeded 100 + the age + 20.

Hypertension is thought of as **primary** or **essential**, when there is no cause at present identifiable, and secondary when some other underlying disease is found to be present.

Secondary hypertension is uncommon compared with the primary forms. All patients presenting with symptoms should be most thoroughly examined to exclude associated conditions which may be causing the rise of blood pressure. Disorders which may cause hypertension include:

1. Congenital abnormalities of which coarctation of the aorta is the most important.

2. Kidney disease. e.g. acute or chronic nephritis, pyelitis, and chronic prostatic obstruction. Damage to renal vessels causes release of renin, which activates angiotensin. This substance raises the blood pressure by stimulating the sympathetic nervous system. Treatment of the cause must obviously be the main aim, but even if this can be removed the blood pressure may not return to normal, and continued medical treatment will be needed.

3. Toxaemia and hypertension of pregnancy. A gynaecological textbook should be consulted for details. These patients may be young, and treatment is energetically undertaken. The obstetrician has stricter criteria on hypertension than the physician, since there is a risk to the fetus. Results of treatment are good, but hypertension may recur in subsequent pregnancies.

4. Tumours of the adrenal gland and pituitary.

Hypertension, whether primary or secondary, may also be classed as benign or essential, in which the course of the disease is long; and malignant, in which the pressure rises rapidly, with early involvement of other organs. Neither term is especially appropriate, since essential hypertension reduces the life expectancy, so is not precisely benign. Malignant hypertension is not caused by cancer; the name refers to the rapid downhill course if the patient is not treated.

ESSENTIAL HYPERTENSION

This condition is common in the elderly, and may or may not be associated with atheroma. It is often found on routine examination in apparently healthy people, and many physicians would say that there are no symptoms until other organs begin to feel the strain of the high blood-pressure. Such complaints as memory failure, fatigue and headache, which are sometimes complained of, are found too, in those who do not have hypertension.

The effects of a raised blood-pressure are however usually felt in time by four organs. These are:

1. *The heart*, which has to eject blood with each beat against increased resistance. When the left ventricle is no longer able to keep up this increased effort, signs of left ventricular failure (page 124) begin to appear. Heart failure is by far the most common important result of hypertension.

2. *The brain*. Headache; vertigo; nausea and vomiting; and strokes due to cerebral haemorrhage or cerebral thrombosis (page 385) may occur.

3. *The kidneys*. Renal failure is called uraemia (page 228) and is the ultimate cause of death in a few instances.

4. *The eyes*. Haemorrhages from retinal vessels and spasm of these arteries may progressively interfere with sight.

Treatment. This will depend on the doctor's knowledge of his patient's age, history, his occupation, home circumstances, and temperament, and whether examination shows any of the complications mentioned above.

The life led should be quiet, but moderate activity is desirable, and restrictions which reduce the patient to anxious boredom are avoided. Unaccustomed violent exercise is bad, and os is worry and tension. A sedative such as diazepain 5 or 10 mg twice a day may relieve anxiety and allow relaxation

Overweight must be corrected, and if activity has been restricted, it should be pointed out that the intake must be reduced or the weight will rise. Alcohol need not be banned, provided it is used with moderation, but it is a source of calories and therefore liable to increase the weight.

Drug treatment. The blood pressure is a function of the cardiac output and of the peripheral resistance. Many other factors influence it, especially hormones. The sympathetic half of the autonomic system supplies the nerve fibres that constrict the arterioles, and so raises the blood pressure by increasing the peripheral resistance.

SYMPATHETIC NERVOUS SYSTEM

Constricts arterioles and so raises blood-pressure.

Quickens heart beat.

Dilates pupils.

PARASYMPATHETIC NERVOUS SYSTEM

Causes secretion from the digestive glands and promotes peristalsis.

Slows heart beat.

Constricts pupils.

A variety of drugs acting on the autonomic system have been synthesized to be used in the treatment of hypertension, and the newer ones have a selective action, so that they do not stimulate the parasympathetic system, and cause unwanted side effects.

In mild cases, a diuretic alone may be adequate, and one of the thiadiazine group (e.g. bendiothiazide given with potassium) is usually preferred, but if there is moderate hypertension, another drug will have to be used as well. Propanolol is a popualr one, and is safe unless the patient is asthmatic or liable to go into heart failure. It takes several weeks to attain its full effects. Bethanidine and guanethidine lower the blood pressure without stimulating the parasympathetic, and thus causing bowel upsets and dryness of the mouth. The fall in blood pressure is greater when standing than when lying, and patients may feel faint when rising from bed, unless warned to do this slowly by sitting on the edge of the bed for a time first. Diarrhoea is sometimes troublesome. Methyldopa is less likely to cause postural hypotension, but drowsiness and depression not uncommon, and some people do not respond to it.

Patients who are receiving these drugs should be seen regularly, the blood pressure estimated, and enquiries made about possible side effects. Drugs have to be taken over long periods, and encouragement will help patients to persevere.

MALIGNANT HYPERTENSION

Without treatment this condition may run a fatal course within months. The blood pressure is very high and rises progressively; if the eyes are examined with the ophthalmoscope there are haemorrhages in the fundi, the optic disc is swollen (papilloedema), and the arterioles are irregular and narrowed. There is albumin in the urine, and severe headache. Sight may be lost, and death occurs from renal failure and uraemia.

Such patients are medical emergencies requiring urgent treatment. Blood is taken for ures and electrolyte estimation, and treatment by intravenous hypo-

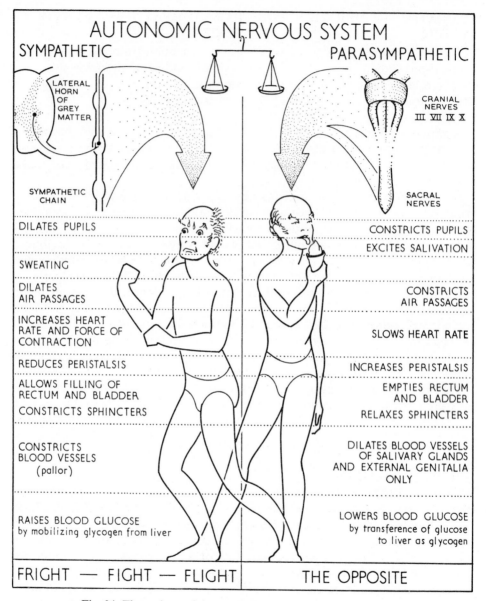

Fig. 34. The actions of the two halves of the autonomic system.

tensives is begun. If brain and kidney damage is not too far advanced, the outlook resembles that for milder forms of hypertension.

PERIPHERAL VASCULAR DISEASE

Disease of the peripheral arteries can be considered under three headings:

a) Arteriosclerotic disease.
b) Thrombo-angiitis obliterans (Buerger's Disease) (page 117).
c) Embolism.

A. ARTERIOSCLEROSIS

The patients are mainly elderly men, though women are also affected. Diabetics are especially prone to arteriosclerosis, and the leg arteries are the ones usually involved.

Signs and symptoms. At first the only signs may be that the limb is usually cold with a dull inelastic skin and brittle nails. As the condition progresses the patient feels pain, usually in the calf, on exercise. This is called intermittent claudication, and is a cramp felt when the blood supply is inadequate for the increased supply of oxygen needed by muscles at work. If the patient is walking he stops, and has to wait for the pain to pass away. If such a pain occurs at rest, it shows severe restriction of the blood supply. If it wakes him at night, the patient learns to seek relief by hanging the leg out of bed, so that gravity helps the blood flow.

Later, the patient feels pain especially in the foot and toes, even when the limb is at rest and blueness of the toes and discolored patches indicate that the circulation is grossly inadequate. These severe symptoms may come on gradually or occur quite suddenly as the result of arterial thrombosis or embolism.

Treatment. In mild cases, quite simple measures may be enough to prevent the limb deteriorating. The general health may need attention, and overweight must be treated. Such patients may be living alone, or with elderly frail wives, and the health visitor should be asked to call and see the domestic circumstances and offer detailed advice.

Cold should be avoided, and warm clothing should be worn. Woollen socks are better than nylons because they absorb moisture, and they should be well fitting and darns on the toes and heel must not be thick. Socks should be regularly washed, and if detergent is used it should be well rinsed out. Bed socks should be worn at night. Shoes must allow room for the toes.

Nails and corns should be trimmed by a chiropodist, since minor injuries may give rise to infection and precipitate gangrene. Feet should be regularly

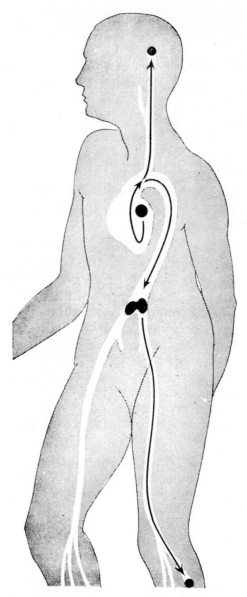

Fig. 35. Blood clot in the left atrium if it detaches gives rise to arterial embolism.

washed in warm water and thoroughly dried, especially between the toes. If tinea (athlete's foot) is present, it must be treated by regular dusting with a fungicidal powder.

Exercises to improve the circulation may be taught. The leg is raised above the horizontal for one minute, then hung over the side of the bed for a minute, while the ankle and toes are exercised. This is done four times, three or four times a day.

With more severe symptoms, admission to hospital will enable detailed examination to be made to determine the site and extent of the obstruction. The investigations may include arteriography if surgery is contemplated.

The aim of treatment is:

a) to reduce the need of the tissues for oxygen, and since this decreases as temperature falls, the affected limb is kept cool,
b) to encourage dilatation of the arteries, and avoid all stimuli that constrict them,
c) to avoid infection and any injury to tissues.

The patient is put to bed with the affected limb uncovered, and a fan may be used to keep it cool. The head of the bed may be raised, to allow gravity to assist the blood-flow. The rest of the body is kept warm, since vasodilation will affect the uncovered limb by reflex action. Smoking is forbidden, since nicotine is a vasoconstrictor, but because alcohol is a vasodilator a glass of beer may be ordered with lunch and supper.

The part most vulnerable to injury is the heel, and though only one limb is usually affected at first, the heel on the sound side must be carefully treated. Sorbo pads under the ankle may be used to keep the heels clear of the bed, or sheepskin heelguards may be effective. Frequent inspection for discoloration is essential, and gentle massage is used to promote circulation.

Lumbar sympathectomy is sometimes used in the hope of allowing the arteries to dilate by removing the constructing sympathetic action. It is of no avail if the artery walls are hardened.

In severe cases surgery will be required. The extent and site of the obstruction is identified, and the diseased part either replaced or bypassed. If gangrene appears, amputation becomes necessary.

B. THROMBO-ANGIITIS OBLITERANS

This condition is much less common a cause of peripheral arterial disease. It affects men almost exclusively, and usually begins earlier than arteriosclerotic disease. Cigarette smoking is thought to be important in precipitating it.

The symptoms are similar to those just described, but pain is often very severe, since not only the arteries but often the nerves are involved in inflammation. The cause is not known.

Treatment is on the lines already given, but sympathectomy is usually practised. The course is slow but usually progressive, and amputation is often required eventually, sometimes of both legs. Surgery to relieve the obstruction is not usually possible because the arteries affected are the smaller distal ones. Coronary and cerebral thromboses often occur in these patients.

C. ARTERIAL EMBOLISM

Blood clot in the left atrium may detach and pass into the aorta and lodge in a cerebral vessel, a leg artery, or even straddle the bifurcation of the aorta and obstruct the circulation to both legs. There is sudden acute pain, followed soon by loss of sensation and paralysis of the affected part.

Acute arterial obstruction is a surgical emergency because unless it is dealt with speedily, thrombosis spreads through the vessels beyond the obstruction and loss of the limb is inevitable. The surgeon will endeavour to remove the embolus. If embolectomy is successful, the condition of the heart must be assessed, and if possible treated. Anticoagulant therapy may help prevent further emboli from the left atrium.

VASOMOTOR CONDITIONS
RAYNAUD'S SYNDROME

In its mild forms, this condition is no more than an exaggerated response to cold. The arteries in the fingers and toes pass into spasm when the extremities are cold, so that they become white and "dead", and later blue. In severe cases ulceration and patches of neurosis indicate that there has been clotting of digital arteries. Results of treatment are poor; vasodilator drugs are ineffective, and sympathectomy is not now advised. Protection from the cold is the most effective measure to prevent attacks. People with warm living conditions are seldom affected.

Workers with pneumatic drills sometimes get a similar condition, but the introduction of machines with less vibration should make this less common.

CHILBLAINS

Chilblains are localized areas of vasodilatation on the fingers and toes, almost confined to areas with cold moist conditions. Shiny, irritable, bluish-red patches appear, especially in children and young people, and if severe the skin may break down. Protection from the cold will usually prevent them, and although no drugs are known to influence them, vitamin B is sometimes prescribed. Many kinds of treatment are described in folk-lore, but are valueless.

THE HEART

The heart is the pump which keeps the blood moving, and it is formed of three layers of tissue.

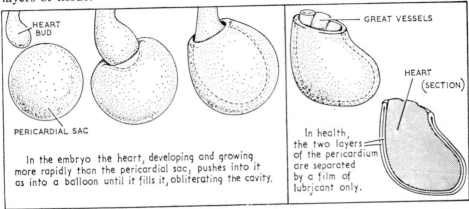

HEART BUD

GREAT VESSELS

HEART (SECTION)

PERICARDIAL SAC

In the embryo the heart, developing and growing more rapidly than the pericardial sac, pushes into it as into a balloon until it fills it, obliterating the cavity.

In health, the two layers of the pericardium are separated by a film of lubricant only.

Fig. 36. The relation of the pericardium to the heart.

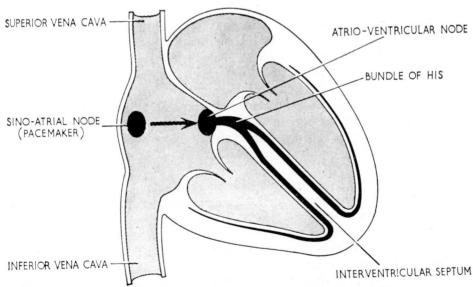

SUPERIOR VENA CAVA

ATRIO-VENTRICULAR NODE

BUNDLE OF HIS

SINO-ATRIAL NODE (PACEMAKER)

INFERIOR VENA CAVA

INTERVENTRICULAR SEPTUM

Fig. 37. The pathway of the conduction impulse in the heart.

1. The *pericardium*. The inner surfaces of this double serous membrane that covers the heart are smooth, so that friction is minimized. The firm outer layer prevents the heart expanding unduly during stress.

2. The *myocardium* or muscle layer is the driving force of the heart. The place from which heart contraction begins is between the entry of the venae cavae into the right atrium. This spot, the pacemaker, is called the sino-atrial (SA) node. From here, a wave of contraction crosses the atria, and reaches the atrioventricular (AV) node at the junction of the atria and ventricles. Thence the impulse passes down a specialized band of neuromuscular tissue, the *Bundle of His,* in the septum, and initiates contraction of the ventricles.

After contraction (systole), the myocardium rests (diastole), while the ventricles fill with blood from the atria. These two events form the cardiac cycle.

3. The *endocardium* is the smooth lining of the heart, which also forms the valves that direct the onward flow of the blood and prevent its return during diastole.

The heart muscle receives its blood supply from the right and left coronary arteries, which arise just outside the valves of the aorta, and run back over the surface of the heart. They are tortuous, to allow the heart to expand without straining them.

THE PULSE

The impulse of the heart beat is transmitted through the arteries, and can be felt by palpating an artery in a convenient site. The usual one is at the wrist, where the radial artery can be readily found. If this cannot be used because of injury or disease, the pulse can be taken from the facial or temporal artery.

The most accessible of the great arteries is the carotid, which can be felt between the larynx and the front border of the sternomastoid muscle. In cases of severe shock, when the pulse is too feeble to be felt in the wrist, it is found in the carotid arteries. When it is suspected that the heart has stopped the nurse feels for pulsation in the carotids and should be able to find these arteries quickly (Fig. 38).

The pulse is taken by counting the beats in a half minute, and multiplying by two to find the rate per minute. This time should not be shortened, since while holding the wrist one can notice the state of the skin, whether hot, cold or sweating, the tone of the underlying muscles; if the nail beds are normal in colour, or blue; if the patient is tensed or relaxed.

Of the pulse itself, the nurse notices not only the *rate,* but also the *rhythm, volume* and *tension.* The first three give information about the heart, the fourth about the artery.

Rate. The number of pulse beats per minute is the rate at which the heart is contracting. In a new-born baby it is around 130 per minute, and the rate falls throughout childhood, until in the adult it is 70 to 80 per minute. The rate is increased by exercise and by anxiety or excitement, as well as by disease

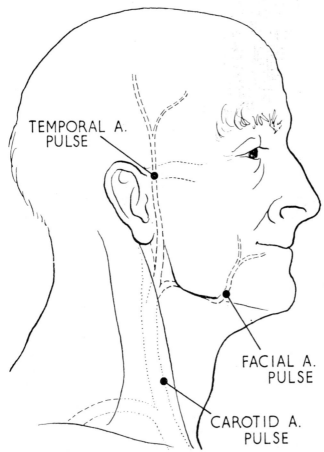

Fig. 38. Situation of the arterial pulses of the head and neck.

states (some kinds of shock; haemorrhage; infections; thyrotoxicosis; heart failure). Tachycardia means a fast heart rate. The opposite, bradycardia or slow heart rate, may be found in heart block, liver disease, or after administration of some drugs, especially morphine.

Rhythm. This should be regular, the beats following each other at equal intervals and with equal force.

The commonest cause of a change in rhythm is the *extra systole*, a beat interpolated by the heart after a normal one. There is then a slight pause followed by a forcible beat and normal rhythm is resumed. The patient is conscious of the strong beat, and this consciousness of the heart beat is called palpitation.

Occasional extra systoles occur in people with normal hearts, especially after a heavy meal, or following a debilitating illness. Sometimes, however, extra systoles are so frequent as to upset the normal rhythm completely, and are then of more serious import, especially if the heart is known to be diseased.

Coupling of the pulse means that beats occur in pairs with a pause following. It is caused by a relative overdosage with digitalis, and the nurse should be alert to notice this abnormality in patients having this drug.

Pulsus paradoxus. The pulse rate varies with the phases of respiration, becoming slower and weaker during inspiration, and fuller and faster during expiration. It is not uncommon in children with fevers, and if the respiration rate is fast the pulse may be difficult to count. It is not of serious import in these circumstances but is sometimes a symptom in serious heart conditions, such as constrictive pericarditis.

Pulsus alternans consists of alternate strong and weak beats. It may occur in left heart failure.

Atrial fibrillation is a fairly common cause of irregularity of the pulse, and is always serious. The atria lose their regular beat, and merely quiver. The AV node thus receives a shower of irregular stimuli, and the ventricles respond with contractions that are irregular in rhythm and force. Not all of these ventricular contractions are strong enough to be felt at the wrist, although they may be heard at the apex with a stethoscope. The pulse rate is therefore lower than the heart rate and the difference between the two is known as the *pulse deficit*.

To obtain a correct record of the apex and pulse rate, they must be taken simultaneously. One nurse locates the apex beat with a stethoscope, about $3\frac{1}{2}$ inches from the midline, just below the nipple. If the heart is enlarged, it may be further to the side. A second nurse feels the pulse, and holds a watch so that both can see it. When the first nurse can hear the heart beat well, she indicates the point at which both will start counting, and they continue for half a minute, multiplying by two to find the apex and radial rate per minute.

Heart block is a failure of conduction between the atria and the ventricles. The block occurs usually at regular intervals, so that the pulse, though abnormal, has a pattern of its own. A beat appears to be missing, since every second or third stimulus from the atria does not produce a ventricular contraction. In complete heart block, the atria and ventricles contract independently, and the pulse is regular, but with a very slow rate, usually 30 to 40. Heart block is caused by some form of heart disease, usually coronary thrombosis. It is not common, and the outlook depends on the underlying cause. An artificial pacemaker may be used to maintain a normal heart rate.

Volume. The volume of blood passing through the arteries is decided by the amount the heart puts out at each beat. It is increased by exercise, emotion, fever and increased intracranial pressure, and lowered by haemorrhage, shock and heart failure. It is only by experience that one can judge what is normal.

Tension. This quality refers to the compressibility of the pulse. An artery that has hardened and narrowed with age will give a pulse that is diminished in volume, but is difficult to obliterate by finger pressure. An infant's pulse is so soft that it can be compressed with a touch.

HEART FAILURE

The muscle of the normal heart is capable of maintaining its pumping action throughout a long lifetime, but there are many factors that may interfere with its action and lead to failure of its function. Some of these can be summarized thus:

1. **Obstruction of a coronary artery,** by atheroma or blood clot, which deprives part of the myocardium of its oxygen and nutriments.

2. **Toxic causes.** Many severe infections if not effectively treated may cause heart failure from the poisons that reach it in the blood stream. Acute rheumatism may be put in this group.

3. **Mechanical handicaps.** If there is *hypertension,* the heart must work harder to put blood out against the increased pressure. *Valvular disease* increases the work load of the heart; an incompetent valve allows backflow of blood, a stenosed or narrowed one impedes the onward flow. *Pericarditis* may embarrass the heart's action. Chronic lung disease (e.g. chronic bronchitis with emphysema, (page 187) increases the resistance to the flow of blood from the pulmonary artery, and can strain the right ventricle from which that artery arises. *Congenital defects* of the heart may lead to failure at a very early age.

4. **Rhythm disorders** such as atrial fibrillation or heart block reduce heart efficiency and may lead to failure.

The right and the left sides of the heart are separated from each other by the septum. Factors may affect one side more than the other; for instance, high blood-pressure imposes a strain on the left ventricle, while pulmonary emphysema is felt by the right ventricle. It is therefore possible for one side of the heart to fail.

If the right ventricle is incompetent, blood accumulates first in the right atrium, then in the great veins, which become distended. The liver enlarges, becoming tender and embarrassing the diaphragm. Pulsation can be seen in the jugular veins in the neck, and oedema collects in the lower parts of the body.

In left ventricular failure, congestion occurs in the left atrium, the pulmonary veins, and the lungs. In the early stages the patient becomes breathless on exertion, and later is awakened in the night with acute attacks of breathlessness, due to fluid accumulating in the lungs while the patient lies still in sleep. He may get out of bed in acute distress and restlessness. These attacks of nocturnal dyspnoea are sometimes called *cardiac asthma*. As the condition progresses, the increasing volume of blood in the lungs leaves less room for air, and the patient becomes increasingly breathless even at rest, and may be unable to breathe unless sitting up, i.e. *orthopnoea* appears.

Failure of the left ventricle soon affects the right ventricle via the lungs and pulmonary artery, and usually both sides are involved, the patient is said to have congestive failure.

CONGESTIVE HEART FAILURE

Since all organs rely for oxygen and nutrition on the heart, cardiac failure causes signs and symptoms in all systems, as shown below.

Cardio-vascular. The *pulse* is poor in volume, and irregularities of rhythm are common. *Palpitation* is usual. *Pain* in the centre of the chest is due to inadequacy of the coronary circulation. *Cyanosis* or blueness is best seen in the lips, ear lobes, nose and nail beds. *Oedema* of the dependent parts is due partly to circulatory failure, partly to the fact that the kidneys retain salt and water. Engorgement of the *veins* may be seen in the neck. *Clubbing* of the fingers accompanies long-standing disease of the chest, and therefore sometimes occurs with congestive heart failure.

Respiratory. *Dyspnoea* is always present, and the lungs may be so congested that the patient must sit up. (*Orthopnoea*). *Cough* with blood-stained sputum is especially seen in mitral stenosis, because the narrowed valve causes accumulation of blood in the lungs.

Gastrointestinal. *Anorexia* is caused by gastric congestion. *Constipation* is caused by the low intake, and by the breathlessness which makes evacuation difficult.

Renal. The *urine* is scanty, concentrated and may contain albumin. Salt and water excretion is low.

Because of the discomfort produced by all these symptoms, the patient finds rest and sleep difficult, complains of weariness and anxiety.

TREATMENT OF CONGESTIVE FAILURE

People with severe or acute congestive cardiac failure require hospital treatment. Their management may be considered under these headings.

Aims

1. to increase the heart's efficiency by rest and other suitable measures,
2. to relieve the patient of the oedema fluid in the lungs and legs,
3. to relieve his discomforts by all available nursing methods.

Bed. The patient will be nursed sitting up, and a back rest with a few well-placed pillows provides better support than a pile of soft pillows. A cardiac bedframe with the end dropped enables him to sit with the feet hanging down, encouraging movement of oedema away from the lungs and heart. Very breathless people often like to support the forearms on a bed table, since by fixing the shoulder girdle they may use muscles like pectoralis major to help them breathe.

A board at the end of the bed will keep the feet dorsiflexed, and a cradle should be supplied. If the hands and feet are cold, as they often are, socks can be given, and a flannelette blanket put next to the patient. A sputum carton should be within easy reach.

Observations. Temperature; pulse and apex rate; respiratory rate; presence of cyanosis, haemoptysis or pain; blood-pressure; appetite, sleep, and the mental state. Any change in the pulse, especially disorders of rhythm, should be reported.

An accurate fluid balance chart is kept, and the urine tested twice a week. It is not usually possible to weigh such a patient on admission, but if it is, a serial record of the weight will show if the oedema is regressing.

Hygiene. The nurse is completely responsible for the patient's toilet. Treatment of the skin overlying the ischial tuberosities must be regular and conscientious; two nurses are usually required for lifting a heavy oedematous patient, while a third attends to the pressure areas. The heels must not be neglected. When making the bed, the nurse should massage the calves in case clotting should take place in the veins.

Using a bedpan is difficult for a heavy breathless patient, and it may be found that a bedside commode is less fatiguing. Aperients are not commonly used; if constipation occurs, a suppository on alternate days is less disturbing.

Oxygen is usually given if cyanosis is present, and a disposable plastic mask is efficient.

Nursing. Absolute rest is required in the acute stage, and the patient must be fed until he is capable of doing it for himself. Drinks and sputum carton should be within easy reach, and nurses are alert to recognize the patient's needs and supply them.

Diet. A patient at absolute rest must have a low calorie diet (about 4200 kJ), or the weight will rise and increase the load on the heart. Sodium must be restricted, which means that intake of salt and sodium bicarbonate must be limited. This means that salt must not be added in the kitchen or at table; that foods like ham and kippers must not be allowed. Not more than half a pint of milk is given daily, salt-free butter is used, and if necessary salt-free bread (which can be obtained from many large bakers) must be eaten. This is a tasteless diet, and patients need encouragement to persevere with it.

Bulky foods which distend the stomach should not be given. Undue restriction of the fluid intake is not required if a low sodium diet is given.

Drugs. The remedies suitable for any underlying condition, such as hypertension or thyrotoxicosis, will be ordered.

Digitalis is a most valuable drug in many cases of heart failure, especially if atrial fibrillation is present. It is obtained from the foxglove, and the two commonest preparations are digitalis tablets, which are taken by mouth, and digoxin, which can be given by mouth or intravenously. Digitalis tablets contain 60 mg; the dose varies considerably, but 60 mg t.d.s. is an average dose. Digoxin is more powerful and more commonly used, and 0·25 mg t.d.s. might be ordered. The dose is adjusted by observing its effect.

The action of digitalis is to slow and strengthen the heart beat, and it depresses the bundle of His, so cutting off from the ventricle some of the smaller stimuli in atrial fibrillation. The heart beats more effectively and so venous congestion decreases. The urinary output rises, and so oedema lessens. Signs of intolerance are nausea, giddiness, a fall in the amount of urine, coupling of the pulse, and undue slowing of the heart. The nurse should take the pulse before giving each dose of digitalis, and if the heart rate falls below 60 should consult the physician before giving the dose, since he may wish to decrease or omit the digitalis.

Morphine is often ordered for cardiac pain, especially in coronary disease, and for the distressing breathlessness of left ventricular failure.

Diuretics are widely used, and a wide range of these are available, differing in their speed of action, their effects on potassium metabolism, and also in their cost.

Chlorothiazide (0·5 to 2 mg by mouth) is widely used. If continued for some time it may result in potassium deficiency, and potassium chloride is often administered with it.

Frusemide (Lasix) is another oral diuretic, with a rapid and intense action, which is usually complete in 4 to 6 hours. In some patients the total loss of water and salt is greater than with other oral diuretics, but as with chloro-thiazide, potassium is lost in the urine, and regular estimation of the serum electrolytes is necessary.

Ethacrynic acid (Edecrin) is another fast-acting diuretic. If it is given by intravenous injection, diuresis begins almost at once, so it is useful for patients with pulmonary oedema.

Spironolactone is an expensive diuretic which unlike the other diuretics described causes retention of potassium.

Aminophylline relaxes bronchial spasm, and is often used in left heart failure to help the breathing.

Other treatments. Withdrawing 500 ml of blood from a vein lowers the venous pressure, and may help the breathing considerably in acute left heart failure. The physician will not use venesection if the blood-pressure is low or there is anaemia.

Acupuncture is sometimes used to withdraw fluid from the legs. The patient should be prepared by keeping the legs hanging down for 24 hours beforehand to collect fluid. This can be drained either by insertion of Southey's tubes into the subcutaneous tissues, or by making multiple punctures into the skin with a no. 1 needle or a scalpel. In the latter case, maceration of the skin by the fluid running over it is prevented by applying a layer of Lassar's paste. When the procedure is stopped, the legs are elevated until the puncture holes are dry.

Convalescence. As the oedema lessens, and the heart improves, activity may be gradually resumed and light exercise is taken. In many cases, rest in hospital produces improvement which allows the patient to return home. The outlook depends on the cause of the failure, and how much damage the heart has sustained.

Life at home. The patient must be told that he can undertake activity that does not cause distress, but unusual physical or emotional strain should be avoided. If mounting the stairs causes breathlessness, he should sleep downstairs. Women who can walk on the level without effort may do the shopping, but should not carry heavy loads.

The health visitor will call, and offer advice and assess the need for a home help. Many patients are given weekly diuretic injections by the district nurse, and the general practitioner supervises the drug regime. From time to time, attacks of congestive failure may need treatment in hospital, but it is surprising how many people can live for long periods in comparative comfort after the first attack of congestive failure.

Heart surgery. A number of conditions that cause heart failure may be improved by surgery, which is now comparatively safe. Congenital defects can be repaired,

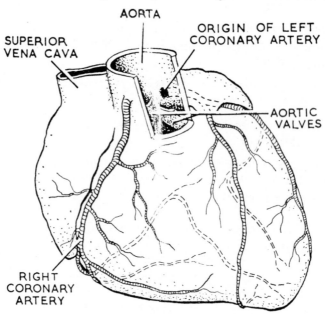

Fig. 39. The coronary arteries which supply the heart muscle arise just beyond the aortic valves.

mitral stenosis can be improved by valvotomy, incompetent valves can be replaced by artificial ones. Operation is not a desperate remedy only considered when the outlook is otherwise hopeless, but a method of treatment which is considered for any patient with a heart condition which may be relieved by surgery.

CORONARY ARTERY DISEASE

If atheroma (page 109) involves the coronary arteries, their lumen is narrowed, the blood-flow to the heart muscle is decreased, and when exercise increases the need of the muscle for oxygen, the diminished blood-flow cannot meet these extra demands. The muscle becomes *ischaemic* (short of blood) and severe cramp-like pain develops, called angina of effort.

ANGINA OF EFFORT (Angina pectoris)

Signs and symptoms. Pain is felt in the centre of the chest during exertion; early attacks may be slight, or the first one may be severe. Exposure to cold or a heavy meal may also trigger off an attack. The pain is intense and vice-like, sometimes radiating along the arms and up the neck, and accompanied by foreboding that death will occur. The patient stays motionless, pale and sweating, and as rest reduces heart activity, the pain passes away.

Treatment. Since coronary atheroma is associated with obesity, inactivity and smoking, sensible advice on the mode of life is given. Strenuous exercise must be avoided, though moderate regular activity is beneficial. The weight must be brought to an average level, and the patient is encouraged to give up smoking. Anxiety may be relieved by explanation that many years of useful life may follow. Glyceryl trinitrate tablets 0·5 mg. are given to relieve or prevent attacks. This drug is not effective if the tablets are swallowed whole; they should be put under the tongue, or crunched. Throbbing headache and flushing may occur, but the pain in the chest usually disappears in a minute or two with rest. Glyceryl trinitrate is very safe, and patients must be encouraged to make full use of it by taking it whenever extra exertion or stress is likely. Addiction does not occur.

Another useful group of drugs includes those that reduce activity of the sympathetic nervous system, especially its action in increasing the heart rate and raising the blood pressure. These drugs act selectively on those receptors (beta receptors) responsible for such actions, and are known colloquially as beta-blockers, and their action as beta-blockade. Oxprenolol (Trasicor) belongs to this class, and is often prescribed for angina.

While it is true that patients with angina may remain in reasonable health for years, there is the constant possibility that a clot will form within the diseased vessel, and that this coronary thrombosis will cut off the blood supply to part of the heart muscle.

CORONARY THROMBOSIS

Signs and symptoms. Severe pain resembling that of angina occurs in the middle of the chest, but unlike that of angina it often occurs when the patient is at rest, and does not soon pass off. There is pallor, sweating, a low blood-pressure, a rapid feeble pulse, dyspnoea and weakness. An electrocardiogram will show the extent of the damage to the heart. Between a half and three quarters of all deaths occur in the first hour and 60 per cent of deaths take place outside hospital. Nevertheless, many patients with mild symptoms are cared for at home by their general practitioner and community nurses, and do well.

Part of the myocardium has had its blood supply cut off and dies, and this area is called an infarct. What happens to the patient depends on the size of the area affected. If it is very large, sudden death occurs. If the patient survives the original thrombosis, during the next week or so, repair processes take place, and the muscle is slowly converted to scar tissue. The temperature is slightly raised, and there appears in the blood large quantities of an enzyme liberated when tissue is destroyed. This is glutamic oxaloacetic transaminase (SGOT). If the resulting scar is small, the patient may make a good recovery and resume a normal life; if it is large, the effects on the heart may be crippling.

Prevalence. Coronary heart disease is the most common type of heart disease in the United Kingdom, and the number of cases has risen steadily ever since the condition was first recognized. Below the age of forty five, men are affected about six times as often as women, but this difference steadily narrows as the age of patients rises. Quite often there is a family history of coronary disease.

Complications.

1. *Cardiogenic shock* is a condition with a high mortality. The patient is pale, the skin is cold, the blood pressure is very low, the urine output falls, and there is acute heart failure. Death is due to the inability of the heart to maintain circulation through the vital organs.

2. *Congestive heart failure* is common. Coronary disease affects the left ventricle, so the function of the left side of the heart is always impaired to some degree. If the infarct is a large one, and the ventricle cannot expel its contents efficiently, blood will accumulate first in the left atrium and then in the lungs. This overloading will soon affect the right side of the heart, and the signs of congestive failure appear. The treatment is described on page 124.

3. *Disturbances of rhythm* are the most frequent complications. Some are slight, but cardiac arrest and ventricular fibrillation may arise suddenly, and the patient will die unless these emergencies are detected at once and resuscitation (page 133) supplied.

4. *Embolism.* Blood clots may form on the inner surface of the infarct, and if these detach they may pass into the aorta, and reach any part of the body. Venous thrombosis occurs as the result of immobility in bed, and can give rise to pulmonary embolus.

5. *Rupture* of the heart is due to stretching of a thin infarct until it breaks. This is fatal.

Treatment in a Coronary Care Unit. If the patient can be admitted to a Coronary Care Unit, his chances of survival are better than if he goes to a general hospital ward. This is because the facilities for observation in a special unit help the staff to foresee the onset of serious complications, and to prevent them or treat them early.

The patient is put to bed in a comfortable semi-recumbent postion in which he can breath easily and pain is relieved by morphine or a similar drug. An ECG monitor is set up, and routine observations are begun. The heart rate is recorded half-hourly, and the arterial blood pressure hourly. If either is unsatisfactory these frequent observations are continued, but if they are stable the interval can be lengthened after six hours. Oxygen is given, and an intravenous drip infusion of 5 per cent dextrose is started, running very slowly in order not ot overload the right ventricle. This enables the staff to give drugs by the intravenous route; this is necessary because circulation through the tissues is so slow that drugs given by hypodermic injection remain at the site. It is also possible to combine intravenous infusion with monitoring of the central venous pressure, by passing a catheter along a vein into the superior vena cana. A three-way stopcock is inserted into the giving set, and a manometer scale graduated in cm of water is used to read the pressure when required. Comparison of the arterial blood pressure and central venous pressure is helpful in distinguishing the signs of heart failure from those of a fall in the circulatory volume. In some units the pressure in the left atrium is also recorded from a second intravenous catheter.

The ECG Monitor. The basic purpose is to give a visual display of the patient's heart activity. The simplest form is the oscilloscope, in which a bead of light moves across the screen, tracing the pattern or complex of electrical activity associated with each heart beat. It can also be set to give an audible bleep at each heart beat. Most units have a central screen at the nurses' station, on which tracings from all patients' monitors can be observed.

More sophisticated models show the whole complex at once. It appears on one side of the screen, and travels across it to disappear on the other. This movement can be stopped at will so that the picture can be examined. Some machines produce write-outs, either on demand or in response to abnormalities of the heart action. Various other facilities may be incorporated, such as alarm systems. Senior nurses in Coronary Care Units are trained to interpret ECGs, and instructed in what action they should take in the event of changes. Such action may be to observe for a further period, to send immediately for help, or to take action themselves in an acute emergency. Machines are not able to save lives, only to make available the information that enables the medical and nursing staff to do so.

A rise in the pulse rate may be a symptom of pain or fear, or herald the onset of left heart failure. Premature or ectopic beats occur occasionally in normal people, but if these show up frequently on the ECG, they should alert the staff to the possibility that ventricular tachycardia will follow and precipitate ventricular fibrillation, which will be fatal unless promptly treated.

It is not the function of a general textbook to teach the details of ECG reading, this ability comes from planned training in a unit. This account is of some of the means that are used in the treatment of arrhythmias that may occur with myocardial infarction. These are:-

1. **Drugs.** A selection of those frequently used would include *lignocaine*, which depresses excitability in the heart muscle, and is used if the ectopic beats mentioned above are frequent. *Beta-blockers*, such as oxprenolol, are often needed, especially if anxiety is present. If this is the case, tranquillizers such as *diazepam* are helpful. *Digitalis* may be prescribed to slow and strengthen the the heart beat. *Atropine* will increase the heart rate if this is too slow.

2. Defibrillation. Ventricular fibrillation is a dangerous condition which is treated by passing a synchronous direct current (DC) shock through the heart. This makes all the heart muscle temporarily refractory to further stimuli, after which it is hoped normal contraction will return. For best results the shock should be delivered within 30 seconds of the onset of fibrillation, so in all units there should be a nurse in charge who is trained to use the defibrillator if a doctor is not at hand. The defibrillator is a powerful and potentially dangerous instrument, and careless use might result in harm to staff or burns to the patient's chest. All staff involved should know the techniques and policies of the unit, and follow them implicitly. Perhaps the most important point is that no one should touch either the patient or his bed while the shock is being delivered.

3. Artifical pacing may be used to control ectopic beats, or heart block, or abnormal rates. In a coronary unit the pacemaker is usually a temporary expedient, and the most frequently used type is an intravenous electrode, which can be introduced through the subclavian vein under local anaesthesia, and the tip manoeuvred into the right atrium or right ventricle.

If progress is uneventful, the patient will not spend more than two or three days in the coronary care unit. ECG monitoring is only a part of his general care. Anxiety is lightened by calm efficiency as well as by drugs, and by giving him as much simple information as he is able to assimilate. He is kept quiet, clean and comfortable, the mouth is moistened and refreshed, and leg movements are undertaken to prevent thrombosis. Thrombosis occurs readily in people with myocardial infarction, and some units may use anticoagulant drugs. Relatives must have suitable access to the patient, and full knowledge of his progress.

On transfer to the ward, nursing observations will continue, and gradual mobilization is started at once by allowing the patient to feed himself and use a commode. The length of stay in hospital depends on the amount of damage to the heart muscle, but in most cases will not exceed a fortnight. The advice he is given on rehabilitation will greatly influence the quality of life after myocardial infarction.

Convalescence. Graduated exercise is part of the return to normal life. Sometimes anxiety inhibits the patient so much that he finds it difficult to resume any activity, but he must have an explanation of the value of activity. Life must not be strenuous, but there is no need to counsel retirement unless the heart shows signs of failure. The importance of over-indulgence in food, drink or smoking must be understood. Though many people live for years without incident after a myocardial infarct, a second thrombosis is quite common.

CARDIAC ARREST

Ventricular standstill or fibrillation can be promptly and adequately treated in an intensive care unit but sudden apparent "death" can occur in a variety of situations. All hospitals have a plan of procedure in this emergency, and even the most junior nurse should know whom to call, where the equipment is, and how to proceed until medical help arrives. The heart may not be irreparably damaged; it may stop in the same way as an engine stalls, and can be started again with prompt action.

If the heart stops, respiration ceases, consciousness is lost, and there is no carotid pulse (see diagram 38). Either the ventricles are in fibrillation or they

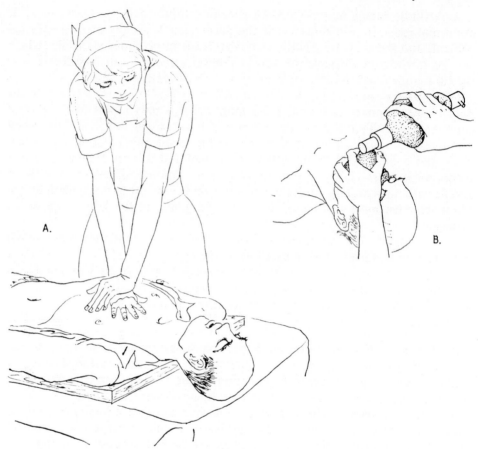

Fig. 40. Resuscitation.

A. External cardiac compression.

B. Artificial respiration. Notice how the nurse's left hand is holding the mask and keeping the patient's head extended simultaneously.

are at a standstill. These can only be distinguished by an electrocardiograph, but if oxygenation of the brain can be maintained until skilled help and equipment arrives, the diagnosis can be made and the correct treatment applied, which may result in recovery. Once the nurse has decided that cardiac arrest has occurred, the staff should proceed as follows:

    1. Call the doctor designated to deal with this emergency.

2. Lay the patient flat. A firm surface is necessary to perform cardiac massage effectively, and wards should have a board for slipping beneath the thorax. It may be time-consuming and dangerous to try to get the patient on to the floor.

3. The heart must be stimulated by external compression, and expired-air artificial respiration begun. If the nurse is alone, she must do both, inflating the lungs first, and then applying heart stimulation as described.

a) Artificial respiration. A Brook airway or a resuscitator bag should always be available. The lower part of the Brook airway is passed over the tongue into the pharynx, and the upper part is used by the resusatator to inflate the lungs. If the bag is used, an artificial airway must be inserted as a preliminary.The mask is applied over the face, making sure it fits well, the head is extended to keep an open airway, the bag is squeezed, and the chest seen to expand. Pressure on the bag is released to allow it to fill. This is repeated at a rate of 12 to 20 to the minute. The bag must be allowed time to refill, or the procedure is not effective.

If such a bag is not at once available, mouth to nose expired-air resuscitation is begun. Inflate the lungs, part the lips widely over the nose, blow steadily, and his chest should expand. Remove the mouth, and allow his chest to deflate. Repeat 12 to 20 times a minute. Deliberate and purposeful movements are the most effective.

b) External cardiac compression. Place the palm of one hand over the lower third of the sternum, put the other hand over it, and with firm pressure push the sternum 3 or 4 cm towards the backbone. Repeat rhythmically at a rate of 40 or 50 a minute. If performing artificial respiration yourself as well, allow one breath to 5 or 8 compressions. Continue until a pulse is felt in the neck, or the doctor arrives to take over resuscitation.

4. Prepare equipment for oxygen administration; intravenous injection and infusion; passing an endotracheal cuffed tube. Such emergency equipment should be kept in one place, together with the necessary drugs.

When the doctor arrives, he will with an electrocardiograph decide if the heart has stopped, or if it is in ventricular fibrillation. If it has stopped, he may give 10 ml. of 1 per cent calcium chloride intravenously, or apply stimulation from an artificial pacemaker. If the ventricles are in fibrillation, an electric defibrillator is used to send a shock through the heart that may make it revert to a normal rhythm.

During the time when there is no breathing, acid accumulates in the body, and sodium bicarbonate is given intravenously to correct this acidosis. After such an episode, continuous watch must be kept. The urinary output is recorded, since sometimes even if consciousness is regained, the kidneys do not resume their function, and uraemia follows.

136

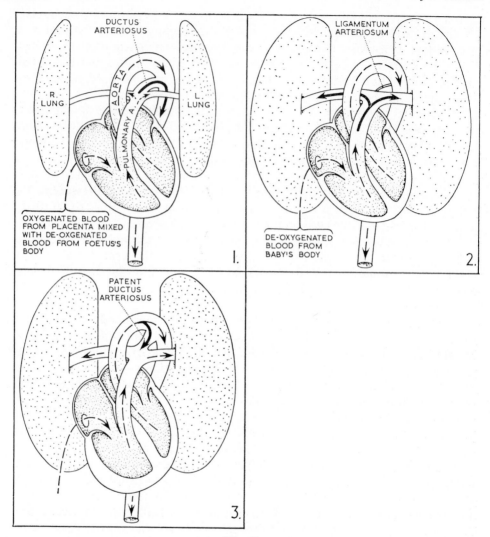

Fig. 41.

1. Before birth the unexpanded lungs need little blood so it is shunted from the pulmonary artery to the aorta via the ductus arteriosus.
2. At birth, the lungs expand and take over oxygenation of the blood. The ductus arteriosus constricts, and within a week should be completely closed.
3. If the ductus fails to close blood flows from the aorta into the pulmonary artery. The right ventricle must then work against increased pressure and may eventually fail.

CONGENITAL HEART DISEASE

The baby before it is born needs very little blood in its lungs, compared with the amount required when the lungs take on their work of oxygenating the blood. A passage between the aorta and pulmonary artery, the *ductus arteriosus*, and an opening between the right and left atria, the *foramen ovale*, provide for the temporary diversion of blood from the lungs. Both openings should close at or soon after birth; if they fail to do so they may give rise to trouble later. Other developmental faults may occur in the heart, as a result of German

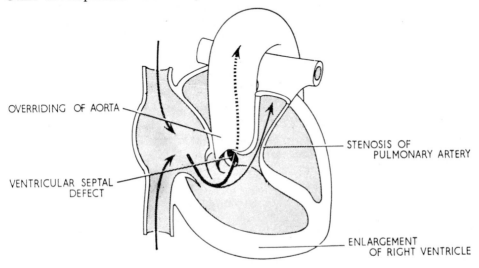

Fig. 42. Fallot's tetralogy.

measles in the mother in the first three months of pregnancy, or for unknown reasons. The result is congenital heart disease, of which the following are some of the more common varieties.

1. A persistent ductus arteriosus allows blood to pass from the aorta into the pulmonary artery, so that the left ventricle has to increase its output. Although there may be symptoms in early life, infection often occurs in the ductus (bacterial endocarditis) and there is a risk of heart failure. Closure by operation is simple and safe.

2. Coarctation of the aorta is a narrowing of the aorta usually just below the left subclavian artery. If the narrowed portion is short, the surgeon usually resects it and joins up the two ends.

3. Atrial septal defect allows blood to pass from the left atrium, through the hole into the right atrium, and thence into the lungs again. Symptoms are slight in early life, but heart failure usually supervenes later, and the defect should be repaired surgically.

4. Ventricular septal defect. Modern surgical techniques also allow this abnormality to be repaired if it is not too large.

5. Fallot's tetralogy. There is stenosis of the pulmonary artery, ventricular septal defect, the aorta overrides both ventricles, and the right ventricle is enlarged. Blood which should go into the lungs for oxygenation passes into the aorta, so that there is cyanosis. The patient is often described as a blue baby, and many fail to survive to childhood. Operation offers the only chance of survival to adult life.

SUBACUTE BACTERIAL ENDOCARDITIS

Subacute bacterial endocarditis is an infection of the heart lining and valves, usually by a streptococcus, which often inhabits the mouth and tonsils. It often arises after removal of an infected tooth, which allows streptococci to enter the circulation. These do not usually cause trouble unless the heart valves are diseased (e.g. after rheumatic fever) or there is a congenital deformity. In that case the interior of the heart and its valves may become covered with masses of infected fibrin. These masses are called vegetations, and from time to time fragments break off and enter the circulation.

Signs and symptoms. The first group is due to the septicaemia. There is fever, sweating, tachycardia, loss of weight, anaemia and a brownish discoloration of the skin. The organism can often be cultured from the blood. In addition, there is a second group due to the emboli that break off from the valves, and reach the skin, kidneys, lungs, brain and other organs. Small haemorrhages (petechiae) appear in the skin, there may be blood in the urine, and other signs depending on the organs involved. Damage to the valves may lead to heart failure.

Treatment. A full course of antibiotics is begun as soon as the diagnosis is made. If the organism can be grown from blood culture, its sensitivity is determined but otherwise penicillin is used. Treatment is continued until the temperature, blood culture and sedimentation rate are normal, and since the streptococcus is protected by layers of fibrin, this may take some weeks.

The patient should be given all the nursing care to enable him to remain at complete rest. The temperature rises and falls with bouts of shivering and sweating, and warm bed baths with frequent changes of linen are required. The urine is tested daily, and watch kept for signs of emboli. The patient is encouraged to drink freely, and a light high protein, high calorie diet is given. Eggs, milk, malted milk, sweetened fruit juices, complan or casilan, fish and minced chicken are suitable items.

The prognosis depends on what the condition of the heart is once the infection is brought under control, as it usually can be. Sometimes, however, the heart has been so severely damaged that congestive failure eventually supervenes.

PERICARDITIS

Inflammation of the pericardium can be produced by a variety of causes, including rheumatic fever, tuberculosis, myocardial infarction, and infection by pus-producing organisms, such as cause pneumonia. There is also a kind known as benign pericarditis, in which no obvious cause is found, although there is often a story of an upper respiratory infection.

In the early stages, pericarditis is "dry", with pain in the centre of the chest as a leading sign. In many cases, fluid appears between the two layers of pericardium, and when such an effusion develops it interferes with the return of blood to the heart. The patient looks and feels gravely ill—dyspnoeic and restless.

The treatment of pericarditis is in general that of its cause. Effusions are aspirated only if they are large enough to embarrass the heart. Some tuberculous pericardial infections result in the formation of dense fibrous tissue with calcified plaques, which encloses the heart in a stiff case, impeding the return of blood and causing oedema of the lower part of the body. This constrictive pericarditis is treated by the surgeon, who frees the heart as far as possible.

INVESTIGATIONS OF THE HEART

Some or all of the following methods may be used to find the cause, extent and best treatment for heart disease.

a) Records of the pulse, sleeping and waking. Apex/radial rates if there is irregularity.
b) Examination of the heart by stethoscope (auscultation).
c) X-ray examination will show the size and shape of the heart. Angiocardiography involves injection of radio-opaque dyes to outline the heart chambers and great vessels.
d) Electrocardiography. Each part of the heart cycle is accompanied by changes in the electrical activity of the heart. These changes can be detected by electrodes applied to the outside of the body; these changes cause movement in a galvanometer, and these are recorded on graph paper.

Electrocardiography is especially valuable in the diagnosis of coronary disease and in distinguishing between various disturbances of rhythm.

e) Cardiac catheterization. A flexible radio-opaque plastic catheter is introduced into a vein in the bend of the elbow and pushed onwards until it enters the superior vena cava and then the right atrium. Its passage can be watched on a screen, as it passes through the right ventricle into the pulmonary artery. Blood samples can be withdrawn at various points, and pressures read. Anatomical abnormalities can be detected, and the output of the heart found. Such an examination is usually made if heart surgery is being considered. Catheterization of the left heart can be effected by puncturing the femoral artery in the groin. It is potentially more dangerous than examination of the right side of the heart, and watch should be kept on the monitor for cardial irregularities.

Chapter 7

Diseases of the Blood

All the processes of the body depend on fluids for their performance. Oxygen and foodstuffs are carried to the cells by fluid; the digestive juices are fluids, the excretion of protein wastes is by means of the fluid secretion of the kidneys. The basic fluid from which these processes derive is the blood, of which an adult has up to 7 litres in the blood vessels.

Every minute the heart ejects into the great arteries 5 litres of blood, which passes through the arteries to reach the body tissues via the capillaries, and then returns to the heart for dispatch to the lungs.

COMPOSITION

The blood has the following ingredients:

1. **Water.**
2. **Blood cells.** These will be considered in detail below. By far the most numerous are the red blood cells which give the blood its colour but the white cells are also of great importance.
3. **Foodstuffs.** Amino-acids, glucose and fatty acids are transported by the blood.
4. **Waste products.** The results of all metabolism, principally urea and carbon dioxide, are carried away by the blood for disposal in the urine, by the lungs or the skin.
5. **Proteins.** The blood proteins—albumin, globulin, and fibrinogen—are soluble. Their function is by the osmotic pressure of their large molecules to keep up the volume of the blood. If their level falls, fluid from the blood leaves the vessels and accumulates in the tissues.
6. **Hormones.** Chemical secretions from the endocrine glands (ch. 11) reach their destinations via the blood.
7. **Salts.** The most abundant salt is sodium chloride, of which there is 0·9 g in every 100 ml (1dl) of blood. Calcium and phosphates are of great importance too. The salt content of the blood constantly tends to change as salts are used in digestion and the sweat, and absorbed in varying amounts from the alimentary tract. The salt level is continually and accurately adjusted by the kidney, since the cells of the blood are sensitive to the salts around them. Were this too high,

water would be drawn out of the cells, which would shrink and perish. If it were too weak, the cells would absorb water until finally they burst. A solution of the same salt concentration as the blood is called *isotonic*. A solution of 0·9 g of sodium chloride in 100 ml. of water is isotonic with the blood, and is called *normal saline*. A full discussion of the other salts in the blood, and their functions, will be found in chapter 3.

BLOOD GROUPS

Transfusion of blood from one person to another has been attempted from early times, but in some cases resulted in the death of the recipient. The reason is that there are different blood groups, and blood from an individual of one group may be incompatible with that of another. The substances chiefly responsible for this reaction are two factors referred to as A and B. These are found in the red cells, and are called **agglutinogens.** Everyone carries in the blood cells **one** of these factors, or **both** of them, or neither. On this basis, people belong to one of four blood groups.

Group AB carries both factors in the red blood cell.
Group A   carries only A.
Group B   carries only B.
Group O   has neither.

Linked with the presence or otherwise of these substances in the red cells are two plasma factors called **agglutinins.** If agglutinin anti-A is present in the plasma of a patient, and he receives a transfusion of blood from a Group A donor, the incoming red cells carrying the A agglutinogen will be clumped together as they enter the circulation, with grave consequences described below. The

Group	Agglutinogen in the red cells	Agglutinins in the plasma
A	A	Anti-B
B	B	Anti-A
AB	AB	None
O	None	Anti-A and Anti-B

description of the factors found in the blood of people of different groups may therefore be expanded, as follows.

Group O people constitute 46 per cent of the population. They have in their plasma agglutinins capable of clumping red cells which carry either factor A or B or both. They are therefore unable to receive a transfusion from a donor from any other group than their own without harmful effects. On the other hand, since Group O red cells carry no agglutinogen at all, blood from donors of this group is not clumped by the plasma of recipients from groups AB, A or B. In other words, Group O people cannot receive transfusions from any but Group O donors, but they can give blood to people of all other groups, within certain limits.

These limits depend on the size of the transfusion. In the ordinary way, only a bottle or so of blood is given, and the volume of the donor blood is small compared with that of the recipient, and the only clumping effect of practical importance is the action of the recipients plasma on the incoming cells. In cases of massive haemorrhage (for instance, bleeding from oesophageal varicose veins), where very large volumes of blood may be given, the effect of the agglutinin in the donor's plasma on the recipient's cells becomes important. For instance, the plasma of a Group O donor contains agglutinins Anti A and Anti B, and if large quantities are given to a patient of group A or B, or AB, the recipient's cells will be damaged by the incoming plasma. Although Group O blood can be given in an emergency to anyone, the blood group of the patient must be ascertained, and subsequently he should receive blood from a donor of his own group.

If transfusion of incompatible blood is given, pain is felt in the back, the patient begins to shiver, and a rigor with high fever occurs. The pain is due to blocking of the kidney capillaries by the clumped cells. Haemoglobin is released from them, so that the urine becomes dark red, and eventually, if more than a little blood has been given, anuria results because of necrosis of the kidney tubules.

Such reactions should not occur, since all transfusion centres and hospitals take stringent precautions as follows:

a) All donor blood is grouped and labelled.
b) All those requiring transfusion have the blood group ascertained.
c) When the blood group is known, the patient's blood is cross-matched with (i.e. tested directly against) the bottles of blood intended for him. These bottles are then labelled by the pathologist with the full name of the patient, and such other particulars (ward, registry number) as are appropriate in the local circumstances.

d) When blood is given, the particulars of the patient and the details on the bottle must be checked against each other. Special precautions must be taken in accident departments, where the names of victims may not be known. The same routine is observed when bottles are changed.

If the nurse suspects that her patient is receiving incompatible blood, she should check her patient's particulars against the label on the bottle, and if these differ should stop the transfusion and call the doctor. If the bottle appears to be the correct one she should summon the doctor, and slow the transfusion rate till he arrives.

BLOOD GROUPING

Clumping is visible to the naked eye if a small quantity of blood is mixed with an antagonistic serum, and this enables blood to be assigned to its correct group. Only two tubes are required, containing anti-serum A and B. A drop of each is placed on a white tile, and to each is added a drop of blood. If clumping occurs, small red dots like cayenne pepper become visible to the naked eye. Clumping may be seen in one specimen, in both, or in neither, and on this basis the blood may be assigned to its correct group. In the diagram below, the plus sign indicates agglutination.

	Anti-serum A	Anti-serum B
Blood may be Group O	−	−
A	+	−
B	−	+
AB	+	+

The other important substance pertaining to blood groups is the Rhesus factor. Most people in Britain possess this, and are said to be Rhesus positive; the minority who do not are Rhesus negative. While no immediate harm follows transfusion of Rhesus positive blood to a Rhesus negative recipient, the eventual result may be disastrous, as is described on page 16.

RED BLOOD CELLS

The red cells, and three-quarters of the white ones, are made within the bones of the skeleton. Bone is hard and dense on the outside, and in the shafts of

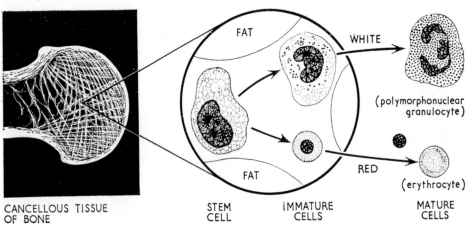

Fig. 43. In bone marrow are made the red cells, and some white cells, the polymorphs. Developing cells in bone marrow are different from the mature cells in the circulation.

long bones, but in the ends of long bones, and in the centre of flat and irregular bones is a more open, lighter-textured bone, the cancellous tissue. Its spaces are filled with the most actively proliferating tissue in the body, *bone marrow*, which makes most of the blood cells. Children who have to increase their store of blood cells as they grow, make cells throughout all the marrow in the skeleton; in adults, blood cell formation or *haemopoiesis* takes place almost entirely in the bones of the trunk, though in an emergency or in disease, the marrow of the long bones may begin to function once more.

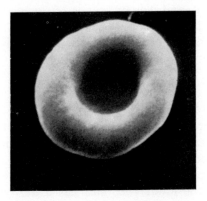

Fig. 44. Scanning electron micrograph of a red blood cell. Magnification 5,500.
(By kind permission of Dr. A. J. Salsbury)

Red cells pass through several stages in the marrow, and finally the nucleus breaks up and disappears before they enter the circulation. These mature red cells, or *erythrocytes* are golden when seen singly under the microscope, but are present in such numbers that they colour the blood scarlet. There are about five million such cells in every cubic millimetre of blood, which is quite a small bead. To give some reality to such a figure, it would take three months to count five million, counting two a second for 16 hours a day.

Erythrocytes are flattened discs, circular when seen from above, and thinner in the centre than at the edges. They are all about the same size (7·2 μ 1/1000 mm), and consist of a cell-membrane enclosing **haemoglobin.** This substance consists of a protein (globin) and haem, a coloured substance or

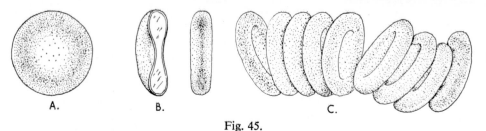

A.   B.   C.

Fig. 45.

Erythrocytes are A. circular
                 B. flattened
                 C. tend to adhere to each other in rouleaux when blood is shed.

pigment containing four atoms of iron. It unites readily with oxygen in the lungs to form oxyhaemoglobin, and it is by means of oxyhaemoglobin thus formed that the tissues receive their oxygen. When the oxygen has been given off, the reduced haemoglobin that is formed becomes perceptibly bluer in colour, and if it is present in appreciable amounts, the blueness of the tissues that results is called *cyanosis*.

ERYTHROCYTE SEDIMENTATION RATE

If citrated blood is allowed to stand, the red blood cells sink down and a clear portion of plasma appears at the top. The fall in the first hour, measured in millimetres, is the erythrocyte sedimentation rate.

The sedimentation tube is graduated in millimetres and centimetres from 0 at the top to 19 at the lower end, and has a narrow bore. It is filled to the 0 mark by suction with citrated blood, and then fastened upright in its stand. An hour later the level of the top of the red cells is read. Normally the fall is less than 10 mm. but it is increased in pregnancy, during infections, in anaemia, and in malignant disease.

The estimation of the sedimentation rate is most useful in chronic inflammatory states like rheumatoid arthritis, to indicate whether activity is declining or not.

The causes of a rise in the sedimentation rate are partly in the plasma and partly in the red cells. The amount of fibrinogen in the plasma increases in the

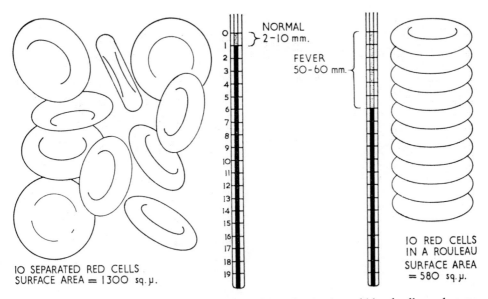

Fig. 46. Changes in the plasma increase rouleau formation in the red blood cells, and cause a rise in the sedimentation rate.

conditions mentioned above, and this rise causes an increased tendency to rouleau formation in the red cells. In rouleaux their surface area decreases, they take up less space, and so sink further down the tube. The rise in the sedimentation rate in anaemia is because the proportion of cells to plasma is decreased.

In order that red cells may be formed in adequate numbers, the following are necessary:

1. *Healthy bone marrow.*
2. *Protein in the diet.*
3. *Iron.* The total amount of iron in an average adult is 3–4 g, and of this

65 per cent is found in the haemoglobin. Most of the rest is stored in the liver, spleen and bone marrow, and some is found in the plasma bound to a protein, transferrin. A constant amount (0·5–1·0 mg) is lost daily in the urine and faeces, and in the normal shedding of the upper layers of the skin, and this loss must be made good or iron deficiency will result. Adult men resuire no more than 1 mg of iron daily to replace this, unless they are losing blood, by some route. Women

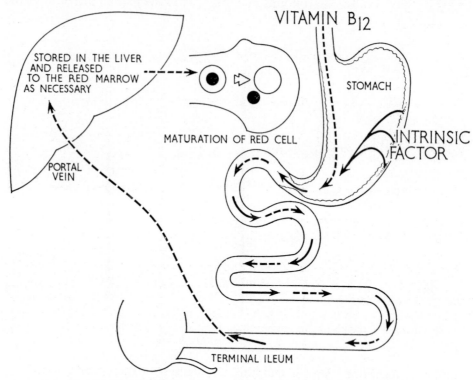

Fig. 47. The absorption and use of cyanocobalamin (vitamin B_{12}).

however, must make good the loss sustained in menstruation and through pregnancy and growing children must also have extra iron.

The foods that contain most iron are red meat, especially liver; eggs; oatmeal; and legumes like peas, beans and lentils. There are also foods that have no iron in themselves, but acquire it from the "tin" used in canning them, or in preparing them; raisins, sardines and black treacle are examples. Many factors are known to affect the absorption of iron. Absorption increases when the iron stores of the body are low, when ascorbic acid (vitamin C) is present and when, alcohol is taken. If iron is given in high dosage, the percentage taken up falls.

4. *Vitamin B$_{12}$* (cyanocobalamin). This vitamin is necessary for the maturing of red cells, and is always present in adequate amounts in the diet in temperate climates. It is only absorbed however, if there is present in the stomach a secretion called the intrinsic factor. The vitamin and the intrinsic factor are absorbed from the last part of the small intestine, the terminal ileum. Anaemia will result if vitamin B$_{12}$ is not available, either because it is missing from the diet, or because there is no intrinsic factor to facilitate its absorption. Folic acid is another member of the vitamin B group with a part to play in blood formation.

5. *Vitamin C.*
6. *Thyroxine.* This is the hormone of the thyroid gland.
7. Traces of substances like copper and manganese appear necessary.

The survival time of erythrocytes in the circulation is known quite accurately because they can be labelled with radioactive isotopes, and it is 120 days. After this they are aged and break up. The cells lining the spleen, the lymph glands and the bone marrow, which together form the **reticulo-endothelial system,** break down the haemoglobin released from the red cells. The globin is returned to the protein pool; the haem is split into iron and bilirubin. The iron is retained for re-use. The *bilirubin* is changed by the liver into a water-soluble form, and excreted in the bile. In the colon this is changed by bacterial action into *stercobilinogen,* and gives the stools their characteristic colour. Some of this stercobilinogen is reabsorbed into the blood and excreted in the urine, when it is called *urobilinogen.*

As long as red cell formation and red cell breakdown, or *haemolysis,* proceed at the same rate, the number of cells in the blood remains constant. This number can be reduced by either of these causes.

A. Loss of blood, acute or chronic.
B. Diminished production of red cells, due to a lack of one of the substances named above.
C. Increased breakup, or haemolysis, of red cells.

In each case, the result is **anaemia,** which means a reduction in the number of the red cells, or their haemoglobin content, or of both of these.

ANAEMIA

The haemoglobin is 100 per cent when there is 14·8 g of this substance in every 100 ml of blood. The haemoglobin values accepted as normal for the two sexes are:

Men   95–115 per cent or 14–17 g per 100 ml (1dl).
Women   82–105 per cent or 12–15·5 g per 100 ml (1dl).

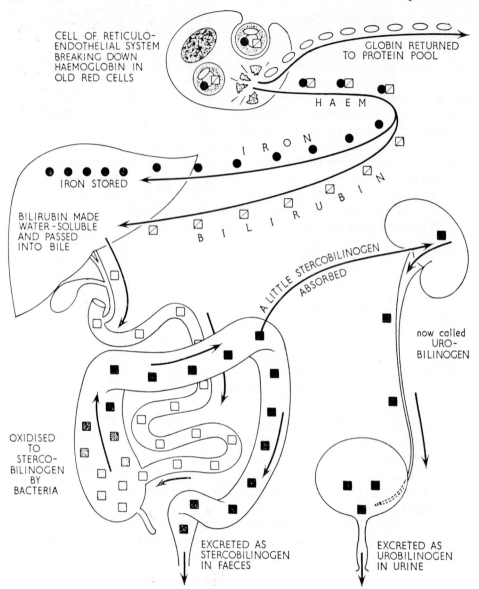

CELL OF RETICULO-
ENDOTHELIAL SYSTEM
BREAKING DOWN
HAEMOGLOBIN IN
OLD RED CELLS

GLOBIN RETURNED
TO PROTEIN POOL

H A E M

I R O N

IRON STORED

B I L I R U B I N

BILIRUBIN MADE
WATER-SOLUBLE
AND PASSED
INTO BILE

A LITTLE STERCOBILINOGEN
ABSORBED

now called
URO-
BILINOGEN

OXIDISED
TO
STERCO-
BILINOGEN
BY
BACTERIA

EXCRETED AS
STERCOBILINOGEN
IN FAECES

EXCRETED AS
UROBILINOGEN
IN URINE

Fig. 48. The metabolism of haemoglobin.

Minor variations are perfectly normal, but if the level falls by more than 15 per cent, anaemia is present. The organs which need most oxygen are the brain, heart and muscles, and a diminution of the haemoglobin affects all three, and causes the signs common to all types of anaemia.

Signs and symptoms

Brain; headache, fainting attacks.

Heart; palpitation, pain in the middle of the chest known as angina; breathlessness on exertion, swelling of the ankles.

Muscles; fatigue (the patient is easily tired by exercise); lethargy (a disinclination to undertake exertion); pain in the calves, causing limping, or intermittent claudication.

Since the haemoglobin in the tissues is reduced, there is *pallor* not only in the skin, but in the mucous membranes of the mouth and conjunctiva, and the nail beds. In addition, each different type of anaemia has its characteristic signs.

INVESTIGATIONS

If the history and appearance suggest that a patient is anaemic, the physician begins a series of investigations to decide, is this patient indeed anaemic? If so, what is the type of anaemia? And finally, how did it arise in this particular patient? The diagnosis and the cause may often be found quickly, but in some cases many of the investigations below may be required.The student who needs details of these should consult a medical textbook.

1. *BLOOD*

a) *Haemoglobin.* Unless there is a fall of more than 1·5 g per dl from the normal for the sex, the patient is not considered anaemic.

b) *Red cell count.* Sometimes this is greatly reduced, but the cells may be smaller than normal (*microcytic*) or larger (*macrocytic*), so that their number may not by itself give a true picture of the degree of anaemia.

c) *Packed cell volume* or *haematocrit*. This figure gives the total volume of the red cells. From these three figures (the haemoglobin, red cell count and haematocrit) can be calculated the next figure:

d) *Mean corpuscular haemoglobin concentration.* This tells us the amount of haemoglobin in each cell.

e) *Mean corpuscular volume*, or how big the red cells are.

There is no need for the nurse to memorize such terms as the last three,

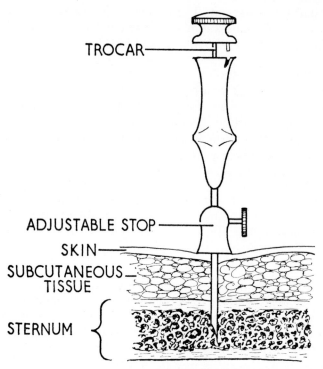

TROCAR

ADJUSTABLE STOP

SKIN

SUBCUTANEOUS
TISSUE

STERNUM

Fig. 49. Sternal puncture. The trocar is removed, and bone marrow aspirated through the
cannula with a syringe.

but since she will often see them on report forms, she may well ask what
they mean.

f) *Reticulocyte count.* The last stage of red cell formation in the bone marrow
is the reticulocyte, in which the nucleus is in process of breaking up.
Such cells do not normally appear in the circulation in any numbers, and
if the reticulocyte count rises it shows that immature forms are entering
the circulation. This is normal after a haemorrhage, or in the course of
treatment of anaemia.

g) *White blood cell count.* Sometimes the state of the bone marrow causes a
fall not only in the number of the red cells, but in that of the other cells
made there, the white cells and the platelets.

2. *GASTRIC JUICE*

Test meal. Normal gastric juice contains hydrochloric acid, usually after food has been taken, and always after an injection of *histamine.* If a Ryle's tube is passed into the stomach, a sample of the fasting juice can be obtained, and the response of the stomach to food and to histamine injection can be ascertained. Histamine increases the output of hydrochloric acid from the normal gastric mucous membrane, but in some kinds of anaemia (e.g. Pernicious anaemia, page 158) acid may be lacking, and may not be secreted even after histamine injection, i.e. the patient has a *histamine-fast achlorhydria.* A form of test meal which does not involve the use of tube may give the information wanted. The "meal" consists of an ion-exchange resin, Diagnex blue. When this is immersed in acid, as in the normal stomach, the blue part of the resin is released, absorbed into the blood stream, and excreted into the urine by the kidneys. Blue dye in the urine indicates that there is acid in the stomach. If there is no gastric acid, as occurs in some kinds of anaemia, there will be no blue dye in the urine.

3. *SCHILLING TEST*

In order to form red blood cells vitamin B_{12} (cyanocobalamine) or extrinsic factor is needed. This occurs in meat and animal products, but can only be absorbed if the stomach produces the intrinsic factor. In pernicious anaemia intrinsic factor is absent, and this can be demonstrated by the Schilling test. This consists of "labelling" vitamin B_{12} with radioactive cobalt, which the patient is asked to drink. At the same time a large dose of unlabelled vitamin is injected intramuscularly to raise the level in the blood, so that it will be excreted by the kidney. The urine is collected and its radioactivity measured. This tells us how much of the oral dose has been absorbed. The test can be done with and without giving also intrinsic factor by mouth. If there is virtually no absorption when the vitamin is given alone, but normal absorption if intrinsic factor is given as well, we know that the defect is lack of intrinsic factor, i.e. the patient has pernicious anaemia (page 158).

4. *THE BONE MARROW*

If it is thought that the anaemia is due to failure of manufacture in the bone marrow, a little marrow can be withdrawn from the sternum, or the iliac crest, or occasionally the spinous process of a lumbar vertebra. The trocar and cannula used has an adjustable stop to prevent too deep penetration. It is introduced into the cancellous tissue where the marrow is found, the trocar is

taken out, and a syringe used to withdraw a few drops for examination. A
certain amount of force is necessary to introduce the needle, and careful
explanation, and even a sedative, may be required. A small dressing is applied
to the puncture-hole, and the patient is asked not to get it wet for a few days
while washing.

5. URINE

More than the normal amount of urobilinogen in the urine indicates that more
than the normal amount of bilirubin is being produced, and that therefore
haemolysis is proceeding faster than usual.

6. STOOLS

If the stools are normal in colour, bilirubin is being excreted normally in the
bile. *Melaena* or altered blood in the stools may indicate a cause for the anaemia,
as may fresh blood from haemorrhoids. The nurse may be asked to collect stools
to test for the presence of hidden or *occult blood*. Examination of the stools is
of great importance; loss of blood from the gastro-intestinal tract may escape
notice, whereas bleeding of any other kind (e.g. in excessive menstrual loss) is
obvious.

7. CENTRAL NERVOUS SYSTEM

The nurse may be asked to assist in a neurological examination, since both
sensory and motor upset is seen in one important kind of anaemia, pernicious
anæmia (page 158).

VARIETIES OF ANAEMIA

Anaemia may occur as a result of some other condition. If secondary deposits
of malignant growth replace bone marrow they interfere with its blood-forming
function; conditions like leukaemia (p 167) and lymphadenoma (p 170) are
causes of anaemia. In nephritis, the affected kidneys may not produce the
erythropoietin that stimulates the bone marrow to produce red cells. Patients
with artificial heart valves will be anaemic unless given iron, because the life of
the red cells is shortened by trauma from the plastic valve. Anaemia is always
a great problem in the management of patients on renal dialysis, because of the
physical effects of the kidney machine on the cells. Apart from such conditions,
anaemias can be grouped under these headings:-

  1. Iron deficiency anaemias, due to inadequate supply a excessive bleeding.

2. Anaemias associated with vitamin B_{12} and folic acid deficiency.
3. Haemolytic anaemias
4. Aplastic anaemia due to bone marrow failure.

IRON DEFICIENCY ANAEMIA

This is the most frequent kind, very common where the standard of nutrition is poor, less so in developed countries. One or all of three factors may produce it; insufficient iron is taken in the food, iron is imperfectly absorbed, or there is chronic blood loss which drains the iron stores.

Chronic bleeding, as from piles, peptic ulcer, or excessive menstrual loss takes place quite slowly, and the body adapts to the declining haemoglobin level. The patient may remain at work in spite of severe anaemia, with all the signs described below. Sometimes the patient may be unaware that bleeding is taking place, as with the chronic ooze from the gastro-intestinal tract that may accompany long-continued taking of aspirin. People with ulcerative colitis are always at risk from anaemia because of blood loss in the frequent stools. In each case the cause of the bleeding must be sought and corrected if possible.

Acute bleeding may be external, i.e. blood may be lost from a cut vessel, or by haematemesis (vomiting blood); haemoptysis (coughing up blood); loss of blood in the stools. It can also occur internally into the peritoneal or other body cavity, or into a fracture haematoma. The signs and symptoms associated with acute bleeding are a *low temperature and blood pressure;* a *pulse* rising in rate and diminishing in volume; *pallor, sweating, fainting* and *anxiety; respiration* interrupted by sighs, gasps, and (especially in gastric haemorrhage) yawning.

The source of the bleeding must be identified and arrested. Before and after this, the nurse will record the temperature, pulse, respiraton every 15 minutes, and the blood pressure hourly until stable. Measurements of fluid lost by any route are important. Blood transfusion will usually be necessary as an emergency measure.

People with many different kinds of gastro-intestinal disease may find extra difficulty in absorbing iron. The following are some of these conditions.

1. Partial gastrectomy, or short-circuit operations on the small intestine.
2. Resection of small gut, which of course shortens the length of the absorbing part of the intestine.

3. Coeliac disease (page 261) in children, or steatorrhoea (page 260) in adults.
4. Chronic inflammation of the small intestine, e.g. Crohn's disease (page 259).

A deficiency of iron in the diet may be due to economic causes; to apathy or indifference in the old; and to strict dietetic rules (e.g. some vegetarians omit dairy produce as well as meat from their intake). Over the whole world un-

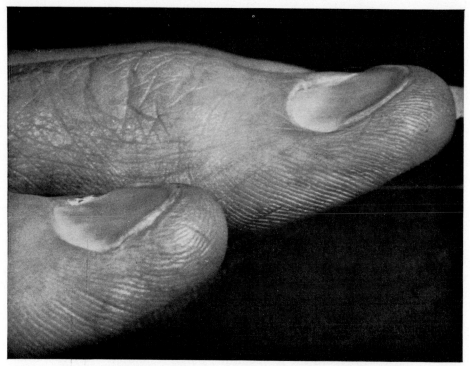

Fig. 50. Spoon-shaped fingernails in chronic iron-deficiency anaemia.

doubtedly the prime cause is poverty that limits the kind and amount of food taken.

People presenting with anaemia may need simple advice on food, or a session with the dietitian. The health visitor will be able to counsel vulnerable people at home, and meals-on-wheels may be needed for the old. All those with iron deficiency anaemia will have iron prescribed.

Iron is not an easy substance to absorb; many people complain of abdominal

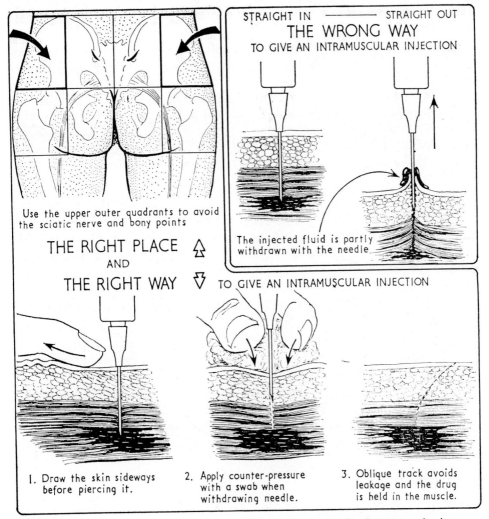

Fig. 51. Precautions to prevent staining of the skin when giving intramuscular iron.

pain, diarrhoea or constipation while taking it. Ferrous sulphate is the least expensive, and can usually be tolerated if taken after meals. One or two tablets of 0·2 g each t.d.s. is a common dose. If this kind of iron cannot be tolerated, ferrous gluconate, ferrous fumarate or ferrous succinate may be prescribed, though they are more expensive, and not more effective. Patients should be warned that iron tablets are poisonous to children, and that such drugs should be kept locked up.

If oral iron cannot be tolerated, or is ineffective, iron may be given by intravenous or intramuscular injection. The nurse who is asked to give intramuscular iron must remember that it will cause long-lasting staining of the skin unless given with great care. The gluteal muscles are the best site, since any other will be visible in beach attire; the skin should be drawn to one side before inserting the needle, which must penetrate deeply into muscle. The drug is given slowly to prevent fluid welling up into the superficial tissues along the needle track, and for the same reason counter-pressure with a swab should be made while withdrawing the needle.

DISORDERS OF VITAMIN B_{12} AND FOLIC ACID METABOLISM

Normal blood formation depends not only on the supply or iron, but on provision of vitamin B_{12} (cyanocobalamin) and folic acid. If these are not forthcoming, anaemia results. The red cells are much reduced in number, and variable in shape and size, but mostly larger than usual.

Anaemia due to lack of vitamin B_{12} or folic acid arises in several ways, two of which are of outstanding importance.

1. The diet may be deficient in either B_{12} or folic acid or both. This nutritional anaemia is the most common in the tropics and is often accompanied by other signs of inadequate diet.

2. Even if the intake of vitamin B_{12} is normal, this vitamin cannot be absorbed unless the stomach mucosa secretes the *intrinsic factor*. If this factor is missing. Addisonian or **pernicious anaemia** results. This is the most important anaemia of this group in temperate climates.

PERNICIOUS ANAEMIA

This name is a memento of the days when the cause and treatment of this disease were unknown, and the outlook hopeless. Today, long-term treatment can enable the patient to lead a normal life. Men with pernicious anaemia are rather more liable to develop stomach cancer than the average.

Aetiology. This disease affects almost exclusively adults, usually over 45, women somewhat outnumbering the men. There appears to be an inherited tendency.

Signs and symptoms. The patient usually appears well-nourished, and the skin may be lemon-yellow, due to pallor combined with slight jaundice caused by excessive break-up of the abnormal red cells. In addition to the general signs of anaemia, there may be a sore, red tongue and mental irritability. A histamine test meal will show absolute achlorhydria. Nervous signs such as tingling or weakness of hands and feet are caused by degeneration of both sensory and motor fibres in the spinal cord. This condition, *subacute combined degeneration of the cord*, is often associated with pernicious anaemia, and in untreated people may be severe enough to cause paralysis.

Treatment. If the haemoglobin level is very low, the patient should be kept in bed. His diet should be easily digestible, with adequate protein and iron-containing foods. Mouth toilet should be undertaken. Blood transfusion is reserved for severe cases; it is liable to overload the right heart and induce heart failure unless given slowly. Packed cells are used rather than whole blood.

The missing vitamin must be supplied, and is usually now given as hydroxo-cobolamin, which is better retained than cyanocobalamin. 250 mg every two months is given by intramuscular injection.

TROPICAL MACROCYTIC ANAEMIA

This kind of anaemia is caused by taking a diet poor in protein and fruits over a long period, and can be cured by folic acid 5–10 mg daily, and a good mixed diet. Since chronic undernourishment is widespread in many tropical countries this may be advice very difficult to follow, and industrial and agricultural progress leading to a higher general standard of living must be the main lines of attack on this disease.

Adequate supply of Vitamin C. People who are grossly short of this vitamin have scurvy (page 35) and anaemia is always present. Elderly people may, through apathy or lack of money for an adequate diet, be so deprived of vitamin C that they become anaemic. Vitamin C is said to assist the absorption of iron, and people with iron-deficiency anaemia may benefit from taking vitamin C as ascorbic acid, though not all physicians find the evidence for this convincing.

Anaemia due to increased haemolysis. If the pace at which red cells are broken down is greater than the ability of the bone marrow to make good the loss, anaemia results. Since there is an abnormally high amount of bilirubin in the tissues, the liver cannot wholly excrete the excess, and the patient is jaundiced as well as anaemic.

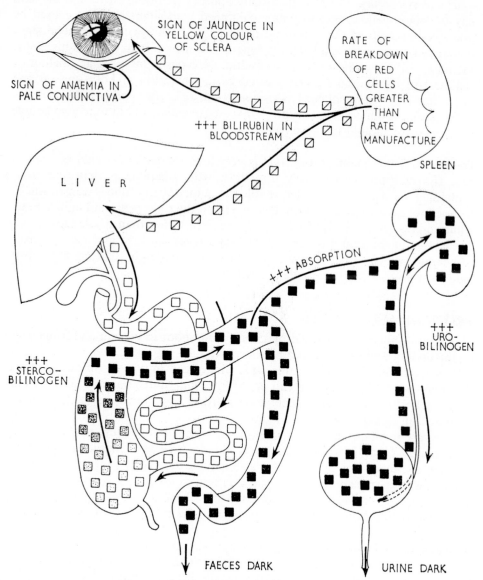

Fig. 52. The metabolism of bilirubin in haemolytic anaemia.

a) *CONGENITAL HAEMOLYTIC ANAEMIA* (*acholuric jaundice*)

This is an inherited disease, in which the red cells are spheres in section and are unduly fragile, and so break up in shorter time than normal cells. The first signs appear in early childhood, and are often only moderately severe. Anaemia and jaundice are usually mild, but at intervals both may become suddenly worse. During such crises transfusion may be required.

If symptoms are severe splenectomy (removal of the spleen) will usually cure them, but if they are only mild no treatment may be required.

b) *HEREDITARY ABNORMALITIES OF HAEMOGLOBIN*

The protein part of haemoglobin is, like all proteins, made of amino-acids. If these are linked in an unusual order, unusual forms of haemoglobin are formed. Haemoglobin S is a form found only in negroes, and it forms crystals which make the red cells sickle-shaped and fragile. People with only a small proportion of their cells affected may show no symptoms but those with many affected suffer from *sickle-cell anaemia*. People from Mediterranean countries may suffer from an anaemia caused by another haemoglobin abnormality; this is Cooley's anaemia, or thalassaemia. Neither kind of anaemia can be cured, and repeated transfusion may be necessary in severe cases.

c) *HAEMOLYTIC ANAEMIA OF THE NEWBORN* (*Icterus gravis neonatorum*)

During her first pregnancy, small amounts of Rhesus + cells may cross the placenta into the maternal circulation, but although Rhesus + cells are antigens to a Rhesus—person, the amounts involved are not large enough to provoke antibody formation. During labour, however, the uterine contractions will force significant amounts of the foetal blood into the mother's circulation, and ten days or so after delivery she begins to make Rhesus antibodies. The first baby will thus escape harm, but if a second Rhesus + child is conceived, the small amounts of its cells leaking into its mother's bloodstream initiate a rapid rise in the antibody already in her blood. IgG molecules are small enough to cross the placenta into the baby's circulation, and will break down its blood cells. If untreated, the child may die in utero, or suffer severe brain damage, or develop haemolytic anaemia with jaundice soon after birth.

This state of affairs can be prevented by giving the mother an injection of anti-Rhesus antibody from another woman immediately after delivery. This suppresses her own antibody synthesis, and if she receives passive immunization like this after each delivery, her babies will be unaffected. If she does not receive

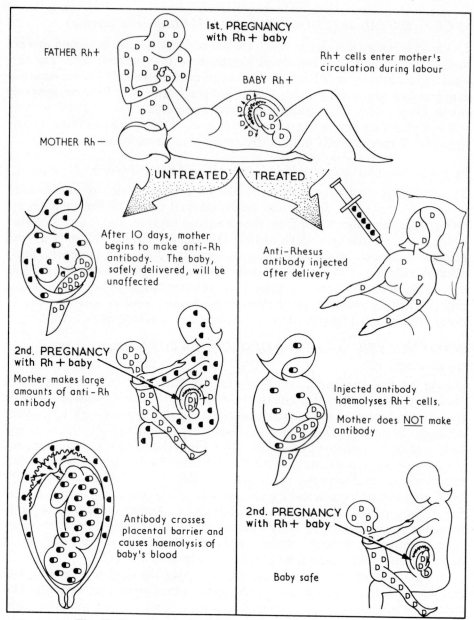

FATHER Rh+

MOTHER Rh−

1st. PREGNANCY
with Rh + baby

Rh+ cells enter mother's
circulation during labour

BABY Rh+

UNTREATED   TREATED

After 10 days, mother
begins to make anti-Rh
antibody. The baby,
safely delivered, will be
unaffected

Anti-Rhesus
antibody injected
after delivery

2nd. PREGNANCY
with Rh + baby

Mother makes large
amounts of anti-Rh
antibody

Injected antibody
haemolyses Rh+ cells.

Mother does NOT make
antibody

Antibody crosses
placental barrier and
causes haemolysis of
baby's blood

2nd. PREGNANCY
with Rh+ baby

Baby safe

Fig. 53. Pregnancy in the Rh-ve woman with a Rh+ husband.

treatment after her first Rhesus + pregnancy, special precautions must be taken over all subsequent deliveries.

The presence of antibody in the mother's blood can be detected by Coombs' test, and this test is performed on all Rhesus negative women during pregnancy. If Coombs' test is positive, the patient must be delivered in hospital, and the baby treated by exchange transfusion if affected. A syringe with a two-way tap is used to withdraw a syringeful of the baby's blood from the umbilical vein, and a syringeful of compatible Rhesus negative blood given instead. This is repeated until about 80 ml. of blood per pound body weight has been exchanged. The transfusion may be repeated later. The effect of the antibody tends to disappear after the first few weeks of life, and if the baby can be kept healthy in the neonatal period, it should do well.

d) INCOMPATIBLE TRANSFUSION

If blood of an incompatible group or sub-group is given to a patient, the incoming cells undergo haemolysis in the blood vessels. Symptoms arise very quickly; there is shivering (sometimes a rigor), nausea and vomiting, the skin is livid and cold, and pain is felt in the back. The temperature and pulse rate rise. The cells may be haemolysed so quickly that haemoglobin cannot be completely broken down, and it appears in the urine, colouring it red. Anuria may occur, and jaundice soon develops.

This catastrophe can be avoided by an efficient checking system. Blood for transfusion should be directly cross-matched with the recipient's blood, and labelled by the pathologist with the full name and registry number of the patient. Each new bottle must be carefully checked by the nurse to ensure that it carries the patient's name, and is labelled with the same blood group as the patient's. People undergoing operations should have their name attached to the wrist, so that accidents cannot occur in the theatre. Most troubles occur from failure to observe the safety precautions.

No patient should be left alone during a transfusion, and observation during the first half-hour is especially important. The temperature and pulse should be taken hourly, and the urine inspected. The physician should be informed of any unusual symptoms.

e) HAEMOLYTIC ANAEMIA DUE TO INFECTION OR TOXINS

The most important anaemia of this kind is caused by malaria. The organism responsible invades the red blood cells, and at intervals of two, three or four days, depending on the type, the cells rupture and release into the blood stream the next stage of the parasite. The prevention of malaria is an important function of public health services in many parts of the world, especially in the tropics.

Many drugs depress the bone marrow and cause anaemia, and sometimes this is haemolytic in type.

f) *AUTO-IMMUNE HAEMOLYTIC ANAEMIA*

On rare occasions the patient may make antibodies directed against his own red cells, which leads to their premature destruction, just as antibodies formed against Rhesus positive red cells in haemolytic disease of the newborn leads to a haemolytic anaemia. This may arise in the course of other diseases, particularly auto-immune diseases such as systemic lupus erythematosus (page 52), malignant diseases of lymphocytes (chronic lymphocytic leukaemia), and certain infections such as glandular fever (infectious mononucleosis), myco- plasma pneumonia, and syphilis. It may also occur without the presence of any other disease, and the treatment consists of giving corticosteroids, such as prednisone, sometimes splenectomy, and more recently by using immuno- suppressive drugs (page 176).

APLASTIC ANAEMIA

Aplasia means failure of formation; occasionally people are seen with anaemia due to cessation of cell formation by the bone marrow for no apparent reason. Sternal puncture shows no activity at all in the bone marrow. Though recovery can occur, the outlook is poor.

Aplasia due to drugs (such as chloramphenicol or cytotoxic drugs (page 176)), or to radiotherapy, may improve when the drug or treatment is stopped.

POLYCYTHAEMIA VERA

The number of red cells normally increases when the oxygen supply is reduced, in order to make up for this deficiency, so that people who live on mountain tops have a higher red cell count than those who live at sea level. There is also an uncommon blood disease in which the red cell count rises from the normal 5 million to levels as high as 13 million. Patients are usually middle-aged and over, with dusky-red faces, they complain of headache, dizziness and noises in the head. If the condition is not treated successfully, hypertension, heart failure and cerebro-vascular accidents may occur.

Treatment. Removal by venesection of up to 1 litre of blood is helpful in an emergency, but more lasting effects will follow the administration of an intra- venous injection of radioactive phosphorus.

WHITE BLOOD CELLS

The blood of an adult contains in every cubic millimetre 4 to 11,000 cells (4 to 11 $\times$ 10^9/l.) which are colourless in life, and so are called the white cells, or **leucocytes.** Of these, three-quaters are made in the bone marrow. These are the polymorphonuclear leucocytes, or **polymorphs.** Their name refers to the many shapes the nucleus can sssume, and they are also known as **granulocytes** because of the granules in their cell-substance.

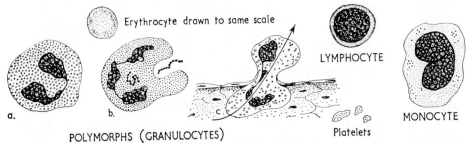

Fig. 54. White blood cells. a, b and c are all polymorphonuclear granulocytes; their granules vary in size and staining properties. b is engulfing streptococci (phagocytosis). c is migrating through a capillary to a site of infection.

These cells show some variation in the way they take up stains, but all have the function of taking in small particles (e.g. bacteria, cell débris) and disposing of them. For this reason they are called phagocytes (eating cells). They accumulate in areas where infection is present, and their number rises quickly when septic infection occurs. This rise is called leucocytosis, and is a normal and desirable physical response to infection, so that a count of the polymorphs in the blood may help in diagnosis, and in forecasting how the patient is coping with his illness. Pus is a mixture of bacteria, tissue débris and dead polymorphs.

The **lymphocytes** are made not in the bone marrow but by the lymphatic glands all over the body. There are 1 to 3000 per cubic millimetre (1 to 3 $\times$ 10^9/l), and they are concerned in antibody production, and so form part of the body's reaction to bacterial invasion.

The **monocytes** are not numerous, and only form 3–10 per cent of all white cells. The **platelets** (150 to 400,000 per cubic millimetre or 150 to 400 10^9/l.) are concerned with clotting (page 171). Clotting is highly desirable when the tissues are injured, in order to stop bleeding, but when it occurs inside the arteries or veins, it can cause serious harm.

A white blood count is often requested by the physician; a differential white

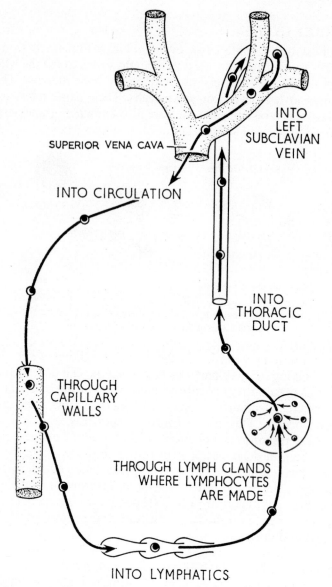

SUPERIOR VENA CAVA

INTO LEFT SUBCLAVIAN VEIN

INTO CIRCULATION

INTO THORACIC DUCT

THROUGH CAPILLARY WALLS

THROUGH LYMPH GLANDS WHERE LYMPHOCYTES ARE MADE

INTO LYMPHATICS

Fig. 55. The circulation of the lymphocytes. These are made in the lymphatic glands, reach the blood by the thoracic and right lymphatic ducts, and may leave the capillaries and pass through the tissue spaces to rejoin the lymphatic system.

count is one which gives the numbers of each kind of white cell, and is a help in the diagnosis of many conditions. Some of the more common conditions that affect the white cells are given below.

AGRANULOCYTOSIS

Polymorphs or granulocytes only live for 1 to 2 weeks, so the effect of injury to the bone marrow is seen first by the white cells, not by the longer-lived red ones. Factors that may cause such injury to the marrow are radiotherapy; many drugs, such as the sulphonamides, carbimazole, phenylbutazone, chlorpromazine, gold; while in some cases (as in aplastic anaemia) no cause may be known.

Signs and symptoms. The onset is often sudden, with fever, sore throat, and ulceration of the mouth and fauces. This is due to the invasion of the tissues by the normal bacterial inhabitants of the mouth, permitted by the diminishing number of phagocytes. The white cell count shows a small number of polymorphs (leucopenia) or even a complete absence (**agranulocytosis**).

Prevention. Close surveillance and regular blood check is necessary for patients during radiotherapy or drug treatment. Such people should be told to consult the physician at once if they get any infection, particularly a sore throat.

Treatment. If the cause of the condition is a drug or radiotherapy, this must be stopped. To protect the patient from infection, an antibiotic such as oral penicillin (e.g. phenoxymethylpenicillin or penicillin V) is given. The patient must be protected from further infections, such as colds, and nursed at complete rest to conserve his strength. His food should be soft, with plenty of protein, and casilan is a useful supplement. Aspirin mucilage before meals may make swallowing less painful.

The most difficult nursing problem is the care of the ulcerated mouth, which must be treated as often as possible. If cleaning in the usual way causes pain or bleeding, irrigation with a Dakin's squirt filled with glycothymoline may be tried. An emulsion of nystatin with honey, which the patient uses to rinse the mouth, and then swallows, may be useful in reducing infection due to thrush and promoting comfort.

LEUKAEMIA

This term (meaning "white blood") is applied to a group of diseases in which there is an abnormal increase in the circulating white cells of the blood, and an overgrowth of the tissues that produce them. The cause is unknown, and treatment can at the moment do no more than prolong life or make it more comfortable. These diseases are often described as "cancers" of the blood, and the new cells are invasive. It is known that exposure to radiation increases the likelihood of leukaemia, and many workers believe that a virus may prove to be at least partly responsible.

Leukaemia can affect either of the three kinds of white cells previously described—granulocytes, monocytes and lymphocytes. It may also appear as an acute or a chronic disease.

ACUTE LEUKAEMIA

This disease may be divided into two main groups. First, acute lymphoblastic leukaemia, due to a malignant change in primitive lymphocytes, which is most commonly encountered in children. This used to run a rapidly fatal course, but now with intensive modern treatment, half the patients will survive five years, and a few may even be cured. Secondly, acute myeloid leukaemia, a malignancy of primitive bone marrow cells, which is commoner in adults, and still has a bad prognosis, although with modern treatment this is improving.

Signs and symptoms. The onset is often sudden, and resembles that of an acute infectious disease. The signs can be considered under four headings.

a) There are no normal polymorphs, so infections occur as in agranulocytosis, and fever and sore throat are usual.
b) There is a reduction in the number of platelets, so that bleeding from the nose and gums and into the skin is frequent, increasing the anaemia, and raising many nursing problems.
c) Reduction in the number of red cells causes anaemia, with all the signs previously described.
d) Enlargement of the lymph nodes and spleen occurs.

Pain in the limbs and joints may be distressing. The diagnosis is usually made on the blood count, but marrow puncture may be necessary.

The aim of treatment has changed recently. One used to try to alleviate symptoms by combating infections with antibiotics, giving blood transfusions for anaemia, and a variety of cytotoxic drugs and prednisone in order to produce a remission for a variable period of time. Death was thought to be inevitable, and the parents and relatives had to be supported throughout the rest of the patient's life. Now the aim, even if it is only rarely achieved, is to cure the disease. For this reason treatment should be intensive, and is best carried out in special centres where much experience has been gained in the use of cytotoxic drugs. Nevertheless relatives still need great support, and not surprisingly, they often press for more or different treatment, seeking help in unorthodox quarters, and refusing to believe that the outcome may be fatal. This attitude is natural, and is not necessarily a criticism of the medical and nursing staff.

CHRONIC LEUKAEMIA
MYELOID OR GRANULOCYTIC

This is seen in those of 30 or over, and affects men and women equally. The onset is gradual, as leukaemic tissue spreads throughout the cancellous bones of the body, the liver, and the spleen. Anaemia gradually increases, and causes marked weariness and lethargy. Enlargement of the spleen, and in the later stages bleeding from the mucous membranes may be troublesome. Irregular fever is common.

Treatment. A course of X-ray treatment to the spleen or of the cytotoxic drugs will reduce the white cell count and make the patient more comfortable, and both methods will probably be used during the few years in which the disease runs its course. Blood transfusion makes the patient feel better, and Myleran improves the symptoms.

The nurse caring for such a patient must never be depressed by the hopeless outlook, but seek to relieve her patient's discomforts as they arise. A patient who is in pain, or cannot sleep, is depressed and despairing; if the mouth is sore or dirty, the appetite disappears and nutrition suffers. The patient should be allowed to do as much as he feels he can manage, since whether he gets up or stays in bed will not affect the outcome.

LYMPHATIC LEUKAEMIA

The general picture is similar, but enlargement of lymph glands is more prominent, and it is the lymphocytes which are increased in number. The course of the disease tends to be longer than in the myeloid type, and some elderly patients may survive for many years. The most effective drug is Leukeran.

THE RETICULOSES

The diseases discussed above are notable for the changes in the circulating blood; there is another group of malignant diseases in which the changes are in the cells of the reticulo-endothelial system that line the lymph glands, bone marrow, liver and spleen. They include reticulo-sarcoma, which is eventually fatal, and lymphadenoma, or Hodgkin's disease.

LYMPHADENOMA (Hodgkin's Disease)

The cause is not yet known. If only one or two glands are affected, radiotherapy will cure the majority of patients. Widespread disease used to be fatal, but most patients respond to modern chemotherapy, and some may even be cured.

Signs and symptoms. The first sign is usually swelling of a group of lymphatic glands, often in the neck or axilla, or groin. These are painless, and there are none of the signs of acute inflammation. Enlargement of glands in the abdomen or chest may cause jaundice, breathlessness, difficulty in swallowing, and other symptoms depending on the position of the glands.

Progressive anaemia causes increasing weakness and languor in the terminal stages, as with any malignant disease. Not unnaturally, resentment and despair may also be encountered.

Diagnosis. A gland biopsy will confirm the diagnosis.

Treatment. The size of the glands, and the effects due to their pressure, can be reduced either by radiotherapy, which is always used in early cases, or by the use of cytotoxic drugs (see page 176). The courses of these have to be repeated at increasing intervals, and their effect become less. The drugs most effective are those of the nitrogen mustard group, and cyclophosphamide may be useful. The method of administration is described on page 176. Blood transfusion will help the weakness and relieve the effects of the anaemia.

The task of the nurse is to help relieve the symptoms, both of the disease, and those that complicate the treatment. A diet containing enough protein, appetizing but not bulky, will do much to maintain well-being. In some patients there are intermittent attacks of high fever, when such measures as tepid sponging and the use of electric fans may be necessary.

Nurses often feel much distressed by the fate of these patients, who are often of their own age, and to whom they naturally become attached during the long course of this illness. They must try to take an objective view, using their technical skill and imagination to help alleviate their patient's discomforts.

GLANDULAR FEVER OR INFECTIOUS MONONUCLEOSIS

This is a mildly infectious disease and appears to be caused by a virus. The incubation period is about a week, and since it is a disease of young adults, student nurses are not uncommonly affected, so it is more common in hospitals than in the general community.

Signs and symptoms. Fever, headache, sore throat, fatigue, and sometimes a rash occur early in the disease. This is soon followed by enlargement of lymph glands, and the appearance of an increased number of monocytes in the blood. The Paul Bunnell test is a blood test which often helps to establish the diagnosis. The disease usually runs a short course, but the patient may feel ill and show persistent changes in the blood for weeks or even months.

Treatment. There is no specific treatment, and the patient will recover completely. Simple analgesics for the sore throat and headache are indicated, and rest in bed will be needed until the fever subsides. Mild depression is often experienced long after the acute stage is over, and convalescents find it difficult to raise energy or enthusiasm. They should be assured that this is only a temporary phase, and will right itself.

CLOTTING AND BLEEDING

The power of the blood to clot is a vital protection against loss of blood from injuries. It is important that injuries to vessels, whether large or small, should be sealed against blood loss, just as it is important that clotting should not take place under inappropriate conditions, for instance inside the circulatory system.

In order to understand diseases that are characterized by bleeding, it is necessary to know the outlines of the process by which clotting is believed to

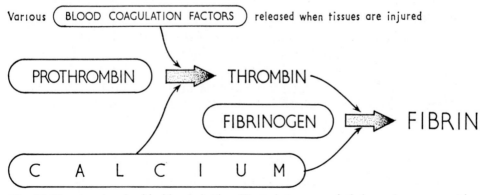

Fig. 56. The steps involved in blood clotting. The substances encircled are always present in the blood and the process is triggered off by injury.

occur. It is started by the production in the blood of **thrombokinase** (also called thromboplastin) which should appear when blood flows over rough or unusual surface. **Calcium,** a normal blood constituent, is necessary for the next step, which is the change of **prothrombin,** which is always present in the blood, to **thrombin.** This substance converts the soluble protein **fibrinogen** into threads of insoluble **fibrin,** which entangle the blood cells and produce the clot.

The production of thrombokinase is due to the blood platelets, which must be present in adequate numbers if clotting is to occur normally. In addition, there are other factors in the blood, whose absence may lead to bleeding.

CONDITIONS CAUSING BLEEDING
These may be classified as under.

1. Those due to absence of a clotting factor, e.g. haemophilia (page 174).
2. Those due to low prothrombin levels, e.g.
   a) in patients receiving drugs such as heparin and phenindione to prevent clotting in the blood vessels.
   b) in patients deficient in vitamin K, from which prothrombin is formed,
   c) in patients with low platelet counts, as in leukaemia.

3. Those due to capillary defects, allowing the escape of red cells into the tissues, e.g.
   a) in patients with scurvy (page 35).
   b) in patients with allergic and other unknown causes.

Areas of bleeding into skin or mucous membrane are known as **purpura.**

PURPURA
Purpura is caused by bleeding into the skin. The lesions produced may be of any size, the very small ones being termed **petechiae**. If red areas in the skin are pressed with a watch glass or glass spatula, those due merely to dilatation of capillaries will become white, but purpuric rashes are unchanged because blood has actually been released into the skin. Bleeding may occur not only into the skin, but from mucous membranes, into joints and internal organs in some of the more severe varieties.

The purpuras may be divided into two groups:
A. Those due to changes in the capillaries, allowing the escape of blood.
B. Those due to diminution in the number of platelets in the blood. This group can again be subdivided into purpuras of unknown cause, and

those which are due to diseases affecting the bone marrow in which the platelets are made.

A. **Purpura due to capillary changes.** *Senile Purpura* affects the forearms and the backs of the hands of elderly men and women, and is due to weakening of vessels with age. No treatment is required, but enquiry should be made to find if the diet is good, since some old people living alone may take insufficient vitamin C, and in **scurvy** (page 35) which is caused by lack of this vitamin, bleeding is a prominent feature. Infections such as bacterial endocarditis, septicaemia, typhoid and measles may cause purpura. **Drug rashes** may sometimes come into this category, but are more often erythematous eruptions like measles. The purpura seen in those taking **corticosteroids** is due to a diminution in the amount of connective tissue supporting the capillaries. The treatment is that of the condition which caused the purpura.

B. **Purpura due to decreased number of platelets.** The number of platelets in the blood varies quite widely in health (250,000 to 450,000 per c. mm). They normally survive about 8–10 days, but this period may be greatly shortened in blood diseases. If the number drops below 40,000 per c. mm. signs of purpura will occur. The **bleeding** time is always prolonged; this is estimated by pricking the finger, and drying the blood produced by applying the edge of a filter paper without pressure every 30 seconds. Normally the blood ceases to appear in 2 to 5 minutes, but in patients with a reduced number of platelets **(thrombocytopenia)** the bleeding time may be prolonged for an hour or more. If the sphygmomanometer cuff is applied to the upper arm and the pressure kept slightly above the diastolic level for five minutes to occlude venous return, but allow blood flow through the artery, purpuric spots appear on the forearm.

Thrombocytopenia commonly occurs in patients whose bone marrow is diseased, or has been irradiated, e.g. those with leukaemia, or extensive secondary deposits of malignant disease in bone, and the bleeding caused, especially from the mouth, causes many nursing problems. In addition, there are conditions in which the cause of the thrombocytopenia is unknown.

Idiopathic thrombocytopenic purpura is most common in children, but also affects adults. The first attack is sometimes the only one, but the condition may become chronic, or may recur at intervals. There is no fever, but purpuric patches occur in the skin and there is bleeding from the mouth, nose, stomach or urinary tract. The tourniquet test is positive, and the platelets are much reduced in number.

Careful investigation is made to ensure that the purpura is not secondary to some other condition, such as leukaemia. Full examination of the blood and usually marrow puncture is required.

Treatment. Treatment during an attack is by transfusion of blood, or platelet suspensions. If the condition does not resolve speedily, corticosteroids are given, though the reason for their effectiveness is not known. It is often possible to reduce the dose eventually to a low level, or to give up the drug altogether.

If the condition is chronic or severe, splenectomy may be performed, and is often effective, though here again, the reason is not known.

Henoch's purpura (anaphylactoid purpura) differs from the above condition in its mode of onset, and in the fact that the platelet level is normal. The capillaries are inflamed, and masses of polymorphs collect around them.

The patients are mostly children under the age of seven, and Henoch's purpura is rare above the age of thirty. The child feels ill for a few days with vague symptoms and fever. Small purpuric spots appear, especially on the extensor surfaces of the limbs. Bleeding also occurs under the periosteum of limb bones, into joints, and into the intestine. The last may cause colic, vomiting, and blood in the stools. These children may be admitted to surgical wards with a diagnosis of intussusception, or telescoping of part of the bowel into the section next to it. The nurse who puts the child to bed may notice purpuric spots and must of course report these. It is of course possible that intussusception may occur in a child with purpura, and records of the changes in the temperature and pulse, and of anything passed per rectum must be accurately kept.

The most serious complication, apart from the acute abdominal one described above, is nephritis. This is treated on the lines described in chapter 8. There is no specific treatment for Henoch's purpura, and attention is given to relieving the symptoms as they arise.

HAEMOPHILIA

This hereditary blood disease is rare, but widely known because of its transmission in the line of monarchs in Europe, especially in Spain and Russia. It is presumed to be due to the congenital absence of a clotting factor, and the gene responsible is a sex-linked one, transmitted by women but only becoming manifest in their sons.

Signs and symptoms. Early in childhood, abnormal bleeding from trivial injuries is apparent, and haemorrhage from cuts or following dental extraction may be long-lasting and even fatal if appropriate treatment is not available. Bleeding into joints is common and may cause crippling, while bleeding from the nose is frequent.

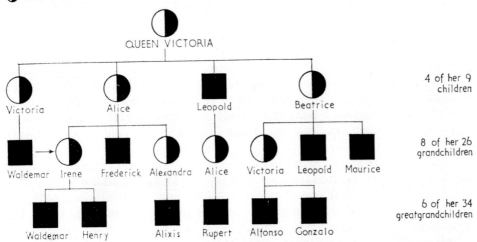

Fig. 57. Queen Victoria was a carrier of haemophilia and this chart indicates the effect on her descendents.

Though not a common disease, it is often well known to nurses because of the frequent and lengthy visits to hospital by haemophiliacs with bleeding episodes.

Treatment. Recently it has become possible to concentrate the anti-haemophilic globulin (AHb) by precipitation in the cold, so that a large amount of AHb is available in a small volume of cryo-precipitate. This means that bleeding can be stopped without massive transfusions that might cause heart failure, and is particularly useful in treating the joints. In order to prevent joint destruction and deformity, patients should report immediately if haemorrhage occurs in the joints, or even if they suspect it. AHb is given intravenously. Joints should be kept at rest on a splint, and iced compresses applied. If bleeding is occurring from a wound, application of styptics like Russell Viper venom, adrenaline, or plastic foam dressings can be tried.

There is no cure for haemophilia; patients must try to avoid injuries that may cause bleeding, and should carry a card giving details of their disease. Sufferers and female carriers of the gene would be well advised not to have children. Haemophiliacs do not pass the disease to their sons, but their daughters will carry the gene and transmit it to their sons.

CYTOTOXIC DRUGS

The use of cytotoxic drugs has been mentioned several times in the treatment of diseases involving the white blood cells. Although the use of these drugs is by no means confined to such diseases as lymphadenoma and leukaemia, it is here that some of the greatest successes of these drugs is to be seen, so that it is convenient to discuss them here.

Once it had been proved possible to destroy the bacteria in the body without harming the tissues, the possibility of finding drugs that would kill cancer cells without irreparably damaging the normal cells was explored. Such an action depends on the fact that body cells divide and reproduce at different speeds. Nerve cells, for instance, last us all our lives, whereas white blood cells are replaced every three weeks.

The fastest cells in this respect are bone marrow cells and cancer cells, while the skin is another one that replaces itself rapidly. Drugs which are cell-poisons, or which interfere with the power of cells to divide may be useful when malignant cells are more sensitive to them than are the cells of the bone marrow. The dose must be the highest that will not cause serious damage to these blood-forming cells, or disappearance of the leucocytes from the blood will occur. This condition is **agranulocytosis,** described on page 167.

It must be emphasized that cure cannot yet be commonly expected from the use of cytotoxic drugs. Nevertheless, there is some evidence to suggest that in some diseases e.g. acute lymphoblastic, Hodgkin's disease and choriocarcinoma, some patients may well be cured. Their action is less than that of a course of radiotherapy, but they may make a great difference to the comfort of the patient, and to the length of life. Some of the substances currently used are described below.

Cell poisons damage the nuclear acids on which cells depend for existence. They include:

a) Nitrogen mustard preparations. All these are related to mustard gas. They include Mustine and phenylalanine mustard (Melphalan). Mustine is a blistering agent and so is given intravenously. Severe nausea and vomiting will result unless the patient is well prepared. A sedative like amylobarbitone is given beforehand, and an anti-emetic like chlorpromazine (Largactil) or perphenazine. The stomach should be empty. An intravenous infusion is set up, and the drug given well diluted. Melphalan may be given by mouth.

Cyclophosphamide (Endoxan) is often used with some success for lymphadenoma and the other reticuloses. Loss of hair may follow prolonged treatment showing that the skin is vulnerable to such drugs.

Chlorambucil (Leukeran). This drug is given by mouth. Leucopenia occurs more often with this drug than with others.

b) Thiotepa. This is said to have a larger margin of safety than others.

c) Busulphan (Myeleran) is used for chronic myeloid leukaemia and may bring relief for some time.

Antimetabolites are substances that interfere with the chemical life of cells. They include:

a) 6-mercuptopurine, which is used for acute leukaemia.

b) Methotrexate.

Other drugs which have an action that is not fully understood include colchicine, vinblastine and vincristine. The corticosteroids (page 322) are effective in reducing the lymphatic swelling in lymphatic leukaemia. Until recently these drugs were used as single agents, but if this is done the disease inevitably becomes resistant to the drug. The trend now is to use the agents known to be effective in any particular malignant disease in combination, in courses lasting a few days or weeks, with periods without treatment to allow time for the normal tissues to recover.

Cancer of the breast, and the prostate gland, and chorion-cancer of the uterus may be improved by drug treatment, and for accounts of these a surgical textbook should be consulted.

LOCAL CHEMOTHERAPY

The safest way to expose a single growth to a high concentration of a cytotoxic drug is to inject it into the artery that supplies the growth. Perfusion implies that the drug is introduced into the artery to the part, while the venous blood is discharged into a pump for recirculation. Growths of the limbs are suitable for treatment in this way, since the blood supply to these parts can be most effectively isolated. Growths of the head and neck can be treated by infusion.

The bottle must hang at a height of about 3 metres in order to overcome the pressure in the artery, and junctions must be wired together to prevent tubing and connections being forced apart. Some damage to the skin is commonly experienced.

Although cytotoxic drugs are not able at the moment to effect a cure in malignant disease, there are grounds for hope that big improvements in this field of treatment are to be expected.

Chapter 8

Diseases of the Respiratory System

The diseases of the respiratory system which bring people under the care of the physician are mostly infections, or the late results of infections. Such diseases are caused by a large assortment of viruses and bacteria, and are particularly prevalent in cool moist areas with high atmospheric pollution from industrial processes. Infections of the upper air passages are generally less important than those of the lungs and bronchioles, but since the mucous membrane of the respiratory tract is continuous throughout the system, spread from one part to another is possible. In order to understand how this spread may occur, and the meaning of some respiratory symptoms, a few facts of anatomy and physiology must be recalled.

ANATOMY AND PHYSIOLOGY

The purpose of breathing is to expose the blood in the capillary network of the lungs to the air in the alveoli, so that it can be replenished with oxygen and discharge carbon dioxide.

If this process is interfered with, the amount of reduced haemoglobin in the tissues rises, and causes blueness or **cyanosis.** This may be central in cause (extensive pneumonia, congenital communications between the right and left sides of the heart), or peripheral, as in heart failure and shock, when the blood stagnates in the extremities and loses its oxygen. Peripheral cyanosis is best seen in the lips, nail beds, and lobes of the ears.

Air is drawn into the chest because the intercostal muscles that connect the ribs and diaphragm (which divides the chest from the abdomen) increase the capacity of the chest by their action during inspiration. Pressure falls within the chest as a result of this increase in size, and air flows into it down the air passages. The inner wall of the chest and the diaphragm are covered with a smooth layer of membrane, the **pleura.** This is reflected from the root of each lung over the lung surface, and these two layers normally lie in contact with each other and move in unison, so that the lung surface is kept in contact with the chest wall. The elastic lungs are thus stretched when the thorax enlarges in inspiration, and compressed as the ribs descend in expiration.

Breathing is a reflex act, and the stimulus to breathing is the amount of

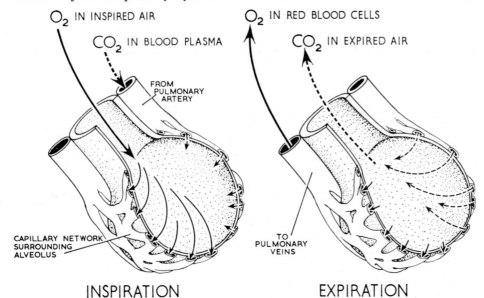

Fig. 58. Exchange of gases between blood and the alveoli.

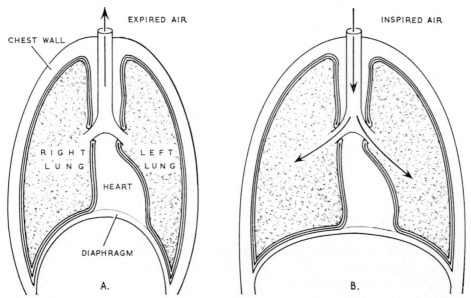

Fig. 59. The movements of the chest wall and diaphragm during expiration and inspiration.

carbon dioxide in the blood passing through the respiratory centre in the medulla. In the normal person, accumulation of carbon dioxide or other acids in the blood will stimulate the respiratory centre to increased activity in order to wash this excess acid out of the blood stream.

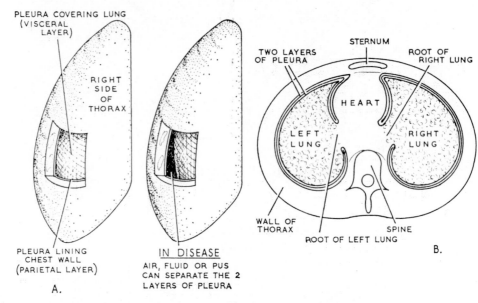

Fig. 60.

A. As long as the pleural space is airtight, the lung is held stretched and in contact with the chest wall.

B. Each lung is separately enclosed in an airtight pleural sac.

If air separates the two layers, the lung collapses. Blood, fluid or pus may also collect in the pleural cavity and compress the lung.

The passages through which the air passes on its way to and from the lungs are:

1. **The nose.** Much of the interior of the nose is occupied by the three turbinate processes on each side. Air is drawn along the spaces between these processes and is brought into close contact with the mucous membrane, deriving warmth from its thick capillary network and moisture from its mucous glands. If the nose is obstructed or more air is required, the mouth will be used to draw in more air.

2. **The pharynx,** into which both nose and mouth open.

3. **The larynx.** This has a double function, for the passage of air, and for speech.

4. **The trachea** runs down the front of the neck, and is kept open by rings of

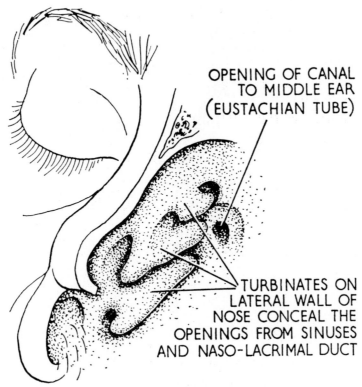

OPENING OF CANAL
TO MIDDLE EAR
(EUSTACHIAN TUBE)

TURBINATES ON
LATERAL WALL OF
NOSE CONCEAL THE
OPENINGS FROM SINUSES
AND NASO-LACRIMAL DUCT

Fig. 61. The side wall of the nose.

cartilage to allow the free passage of air. These rings do not meet at the back, behind which lies the oesophagus.

5. **The bronchi.** The trachea divides into a right and left bronchus, one going to each lung. The whole of the upper respiratory tract is lined with ciliated mucous membrane. Cilia are minute processes on the surface of the cells, and these beat upwards to carry the secretions of the tract up to the pharynx, whence they are normally removed by swallowing.

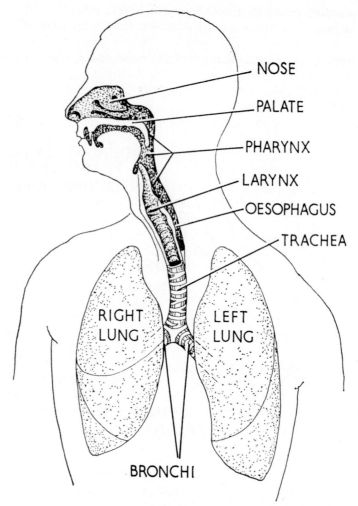

Fig. 62. The organs of the respiratory system.

RESPIRATORY SYMPTOMS
TYPES OF RESPIRATION

Men use the diaphragm predominantly in breathing, women their intercostal muscles. The rate, rhythm and depth of respiration are affected by many disease processes in the lungs, heart, abdomen and brain. A rise in the respiratory rate always occurs when the temperature is high, in order to meet the increased needs of the body for oxygen.

In acute abdominal conditions, the breathing becomes **shallow** in order not to disturb the painful abdomen. Pleurisy also causes shallow respiration, because movement of the inflamed pleural membranes over each other is painful. **Deep** breathing is produced if the respiratory centre in the medulla is stimulated by excess acid, as in diabetic coma (page 317).

Unusual sounds are produced during breathing if there is obstruction in the airway by secretion or new growth. Patients who have had a stroke often show **stertorous** breathing because the paralysed cheek and throat muscles vibrate with respiration.

Prolonged **wheezy** *expiration* is produced when the muscles of the bronchi are in spasm, as in asthma and some cases of chronic bronchitis and emphysema. Effort is required to force the air past the obstruction.

Irregular breathing always originates in the medullary respiratory centre, which may be influenced by increased intracranial pressure, or by changes in the blood reaching the medulla. It is an important sign, and its onset should be reported immediately. The best known form of irregular breathing is **Cheyne-Stokes** respiration, which occurs when the medulla is only responsive to a high level of carbon dioxide. The breathing becomes quicker and deeper till it reaches a maximum then diminishes until there is a period when breathing ceases. Carbon dioxide then accumulates in the blood until it reaches a level high enough to stimulate respiration again. This kind of breathing is usually only heard when the patient is asleep, and the night nurse will notice that the patient stirs and almost wakes as the breathing reaches its maximum. Cheyne-Stokes respiration is seen in heart failure, uraemia and some cerebral conditions, such as raised intracranial pressure.

COUGH

Coughing is stimulated by irritation of the nerve endings in the respiratory tract or the pleura. The vocal cords are closed, so that pressure builds up in the trachea, the cords fly open and the air is violently expelled. A dry cough occurs at the beginning of many infections, whether trivial as in bronchitis or serious, as in **tuberculosis.** The character of the cough is often an aid to diagnosis, a child with measles, for instance, has a hard brassy cough which may suggest what the illness is before the rash appears.

Sputum produced in the early stages of inflammation is mucoid, but as the infection progresses it becomes muco-purulent. If an abscess forms in the lung, its contents are eventually discharged into a bronchus and the sputum coughed

up will be purulent and may be very offensive indeed. Acute left heart failure
will cause oedema of the lung, and very large quantities of watery sputum are
produced.

Coughing up blood is called **haemoptysis.** Streaks of blood are not often seen
in the sputum of patients with infections of the respiratory tract, but are
common in mitral stenosis, or carcinoma of the bronchus. In the early stages
of pulmonary tuberculosis, small quantities of bright blood are often coughed
up, while in the later destructive stages of the disease haemoptysis may be
severe.

THE COMMON COLD

Cause. This is a virus infection.

Aetiology. Colds are commonest in temperate climates with cool wet winters,
where they are most frequent in autumn and winter, but may occur throughout
the year. Most people in Britain have one or two colds a year.

Course. Sneezing, sore throat and nasal congestion are the earliest signs. The
nasal mucous membrane is congested and soon begins to discharge mucus.
The sense of smell is lost, food seems tasteless, sleep is disturbed by the necessity
for mouth-breathing and there is often headache, and partial deafness due to
blocking of the Eustachian tube by inflammation. The temperature is usually
normal, but may show a slight rise. The nasal discharge becomes opaque and
often purulent in a day or so, but soon diminishes and the cold gradually
disappears.

Infection may spread along the mucosa to the nasal sinuses, the larynx,
trachea and bronchi, and the treatment of these conditions will be considered
later.

Treatment. There is no specific cure for a cold and since several viruses are
involved, active immunization is not yet practicable. Symptoms, however, can
be treated, and comfort given during the day or two that the condition lasts.
A day off work in a warm room is helpful in preventing complications, and the
spread of infection to others, but is perhaps a counsel of perfection. Ephedrine
nasal drops may improve the airway, steam inhalers are comforting, soluble
aspirin 300 mg. four-hourly relieves headache, and antiseptic or soothing
lozenges, e.g. Strepsils, are liked. A hot bath before retiring to a warm bed with
a glass of hot milk (with or without a little whisky or brandy) will promote
sleep. A little petroleum jelly applied to the nostrils at night will prevent

soreness due to the discharge. There is as yet no firm evidence that vitamin C is effective in preventing or aborting colds, but many put faith in it.

Sinusitis, usually due to a secondary infection, is indicated by fever, headache, pain over the maxillary antrum and purulent nasal discharge. The patient should be kept in a warm room, ephedrine nasal drops and steam inhalations are given four-hourly, and an antibiotic such as ampicillin prescribed. Watch must be kept lest the infection spreads; middle ear disease, for instance, may be caused via the Eustachian tube, and post-nasal discharge may cause laryngitis and bronchitis.

If sinusitis does not clear within a few days, an X-ray of the sinuses is taken, and may show a fluid level in one or both maxillary antra. If medical treatment cannot resolve this, puncture and washout of the antrum may have to be undertaken by an ear, nose and throat surgeon.

LARYNGITIS

Inflammation of the larynx may be due to any of these causes:

a) Infection. Laryngitis is often part of an upper respiratory inflammation, and also may occur in chronic infections such as pulmonary tuberculosis (page 203) if there are organisms in the sputum. Laryngitis may also be a feature of early tuberculosis.

b) Trauma, e.g. over-use of the voice, as by politicians during a general election.

c) Chemical irritation or scalds. Children are liable to injury from trying to drink from teapots or kettles.

d) Allergy. Sensitivity reactions may cause swelling in any area, and is especially important around the larynx.

Acute inflammation is by far the commonest cause, and produces hoarseness or actual loss of voice, soreness and often a dry painful cough. It usually responds quickly to a period of silence, rest in a warm room with a steam kettle, antiseptic lozenges and a linctus to subdue the cough. Smoking is forbidden.

In such simple cases, the only function of the larynx that is affected is speech, but it will be recalled that the larynx is also part of the airway, and that severe swelling may cause obstruction. This is especially a risk with scalds of the throat in children. The nurse must be vigilant to notice dyspnoea and report it, since tracheostomy may be required at short notice.

Tracheitis is often associated with inflammation of the larynx or the bronchi and causes pain behind the sternum, with a painful cough dry at first but later yielding a little stiff sputum. The treatment is as for acute bronchitis.

BRONCHITIS

ACUTE BRONCHITIS

Cause. Many organisms may infect the bronchi, e.g. viruses, streptococci, staphylococci.

Aetiology. Bronchitis is most common in highly industrialized areas of cold foggy climates in autumn and winter. It occurs as a complication of infectious diseases in which there is inflammation of the nasopharynx—scarlet fever, measles, whooping cough. It affects people of all ages, and is usually only dangerous to the old and the very young, and those weakened by some other disease.

Course. The patient feels generally ill, with back and joint pains and headache. There is a raw feeling in the centre of the chest, and the temperature rises a degree or two. The dry painful cough becomes increasingly productive as mucus is poured out by the inflamed bronchi, and the breathing becomes bubbly. Soon the sputum becomes infected and may become copious, but the cough is now less painful. Normally the inflammation now begins to subside, and in a week or ten days the bronchitis has resolved.

Treatment. A fit person having a mild attack requires only comfort and nursing care. Bed rest is advisable in the early days, and until the temperature has settled the patient should remain in a warm bedroom. A steam kettle to moisten the air will soothe the cough in the dry stage and encourage expectoration later. If a kettle is not available, four-hourly inhalations are given. At first a linctus is used to soothe the useless cough, and when sputum is produced a spoonful of a mixture of equal parts lemon juice and honey is appreciated. Food need not be pressed if the appetite is poor, but fluids must be taken in abundance. A sedative may be required to ensure sleep at night.

   If the patient is frail, or the attack is a severe one, a broad-spectrum antibiotic like tetracycline will probably be prescribed to limit the infection.

Complications. An extensive infection may develop into bronchopneumonia (page 194). The event most to be feared, however, is that bronchitis will return each winter, and that eventually the condition will become chronic.

CHRONIC BRONCHITIS

Chronic bronchitis is a common and important disease in Britain, causing loss of working hours and invalidism, and leading in many cases to death from heart failure. It is a disease of industrial areas and is most prevalent in the lower income groups.

The usual history is of winter colds which go to the chest and cause a productive cough. After a few years, this respiratory infection lasts throughout the winter, and finally the summer interval shortens until there is cough with sputum throughout the year. The patient becomes increasingly short of breath, and cyanosis occurs during coughing bouts. Often the chest feels tight and breathing is wheezy because of spasm of the bronchi.

Breathing in is a muscular effort involving raising the ribs and lowering the diaphragm; breathing out is performed by allowing the ribs to fall and compress the elastic lungs. If the bronchi are obstructed by spasm and retained sputum, expiration becomes progressively more difficult, and the lungs become increasingly distended with air. The chest becomes barrel-shaped, and the accessory muscles of respiration, such as the sternomastoids, are prominent. The walls of the alveoli or air sacs are ruptured by the increased pressure, which means that the area over which oxygenation of the blood takes place gets smaller (Fig. 58). This condition is called emphysema, and marks an advanced stage of respiratory disease. The distended rigid lungs cause a rise of pressure in the pulmonary artery which is trying to force blood into the lungs, and this rise of pressure in turn causes strain on the right ventricle, and leads to right heart failure, which is a common cause of death in chronic bronchitis.

Prevention. Advice that may be given to those with winter coughs on how to avoid chronic bronchitis is as follows:
1. Give up smoking.
2. Sleep in a warm bedroom, and on cold or foggy nights keep the windows closed.
3. Avoid ill-ventilated crowded places where respiratory infection may be contracted.
4. Do not work in dusty occupations.
5. Stay indoors during foggy weather, or if a cold has been caught.
6. Live in a non-industrial area.
7. Spend the winter in a warm climate.

Unfortunately, it will be obvious that to the wage-earners who form the bulk of those prone to chronic bronchitis, only the first three or four items are of much practical application.

Treatment. Although treatment will not cure chronic bronchitis, it will delay its advance and relieve some of the discomforts it causes. The main points are:

1. Reduction of infection. Tetracycline 250 mg four times a day if there is a cold, or the symptoms become more acute. Sometimes the physician may order a prolonged course of antibiotics during the winter, and in this case watch must be kept for side effects such as diarrhoea, and soreness of the mouth.

If chronic sinusitis is present, it must be treated, or it will keep reinfecting the chest.

2. Relief of bronchial spasm. Tightness of the chest and wheezing show that the plain muscle of the bronchi is constricted, narrowing the tubes and making expiration still more difficult. Ephedrine 60 mg twice a day, or an inhaler of isoprenaline or salbutamol may give relief.

3. Breathing exercises. These are especially helpful if there is emphysema by ensuring full use of the remaining lung tissue.

4. Cough mixtures. The drugs often prescribed as expectorants are not highly esteemed today, but many bronchitics find benefit in Mist. Sodium Chloride (N.F.) which is a mixture containing salt and sodium bicarbonate. It is taken on rising, with a glass of hot water, and may assist in the expulsion of sputum that has accumulated during the night. This mixture is not of course allowed to those having a low sodium diet, e.g. those with congestive heart failure. If cough is troublesome in the night, a linctus (such as Linctus Codeine (N.F.) 4–8 ml.) can be taken. A linctus should not be diluted but sipped a drop or two at a time. It should not be taken by bronchitics during the day, except on special social occasions, or it will cause retention of sputum and increase of infection.

5. General measures. The advice given above on avoiding exposure to fog and giving up smoking is important. In addition, any dental sepsis should be dealt with, and an adequate diet with plenty of fluids taken.

Chronic bronchitics seen in hospital are mostly those with acute exacerbation of their infection, incapacitating emphysema with cyanosis, or right heart failure. If they require oxygen, it should be given with a mask such as the Venturi pattern, which gives oxygen at a concentration of not more than 30 per cent. The reason for this is that the respiratory centre in such patients has become insensitive to carbon dioxide, which is the normal respiratory stimulus, and relies instead on oxygen lack. If this lack (or **anoxia**) is abolished by giving a high concentration of oxygen, carbon dioxide narcosis may follow.

The patient has a good colour, but begins to sweat, muscular twitching occurs, and eventually coma supervenes. Alert observation of all bronchitics having oxygen is necessary.

An anaesthetic is a risk to bronchitics, and if such a patient has to have an operation, he must give up smoking altogether. Antibiotic cover is given, and breathing exercises are practised before and after operation.

INFLUENZA

Cause. Influenza is caused by several viruses; an attack by one of these gives no protection against the others. Occasionally influenza occurs in pandemic form, and spreads around the world. There was such a pandemic in 1918, which caused many deaths, and another in 1957.

Course. The onset is sudden, and the main symptoms are general ones—shivering, headache, back and joint pains. A cough is usually present, but respiratory symptoms are relatively slight. The fever continues for several days, and convalescence is often slow. Depression is often a marked feature of the convalescent stage, and it may be weeks before energy and good spirits are regained.

Treatment. There is no effective treatment for the infection, but the symptoms can be relieved. Soluble aspirin 0·6 g. four-hourly is probably the most useful drug, since it relieves the pain in the back and head.

Prevention. Vaccines are available, and in an epidemic in which the type of virus is known may provide protection.

Complications. Virus and secondary bacterial pneumonia is the most feared complication, and it is more prevalent in some epidemics than in others. The treatment is given in the next section.

PNEUMONIA

Pneumonia means inflammation of lung tissue. There are many organisms that may be responsible for pneumonia, and the amount of lung involved varies from case to case. It may produce many widespread patches, involve one segment of a lobe, or affect one or more lobes in one or both lungs. The classification used here is one that should make the methods of treatment easier to understand. The pneumonias may be thought of as falling into two main groups.

    A. Those due to a specific infecting organism.
    B. Those due to retention of secretions, or inhalation of infected secretion.

PNEUMONIA DUE TO SPECIFIC ORGANISMS

Such organisms may be:

1. Pneumococci. Pneumococcal pneumonia is quite common, and runs a typical course. Its treatment is described in detail below.
2. Staphylococci. Pneumonia of this type occurs in staphylococcal septicaemia, or as a complication of influenza. Lung abscess is a quite common complication of this infection.
3. Friedländer's bacillus is not a common cause of pneumonia, but usually gives rise to a serious illness.
4. Streptococci.
5. Viruses. Pneumonia may follow influenza, more often in some epidemics than in others. There was a very high mortality in 1918 from pneumonia in the influenzal epidemic, but it was mostly due to secondary bacterial invasion, and since these bacterial infections can now be cured with antibiotics, such a high death-rate is not likely to occur again.

   Psittacosis is a virus disease contracted from parrots and budgerigars, causing general illness, patches of pneumonia and enlargement of the spleen.

   The viruses of measles and smallpox may cause pneumonia, but in such cases there is usually secondary bacterial infection.
6. Tubercle bacilli. The treatment of tuberculous pneumonia is along the lines subsequently described for pulmonary tuberculosis.

Pneumonia localized in one or more lobes is called **lobar pneumonia;** if patches of infection are scattered throughout the lung it is called **bronchopneumonia**.

The treatment of pneumonia in this group consists of

a) identifying the organism responsible, and giving the appropriate antibiotic if one is available,

b) giving the supportive treatment required by an ill person,

c) relieving the discomforts by appropriate nursing measures.

PNEUMOCOCCAL PNEUMONIA

The pneumococcus usually causes lobar pneumonia.

Aetiology. It affects all age groups, including children, but is most common in adults between 20 and 40. Lobar pneumonia occurs all over the world but in temperate climates is most common during the winter.

Course. The symptoms appear suddenly, with shivering or even a rigor that sends the temperature up rapidly, while the respiration rate rises even more markedly. Breathing is shallow because pleurisy develops over the inflamed lobe, and chest movement is painful. There is a dry cough, often cut short with a little groan because of the pain. The face is flushed, herpes (or cold sores) may appear on the lips, and the general picture is of acute distress. Before antibiotic therapy was available, lobar pneumonia ran a severe course for a week or ten days with continuous fever which often ended in a sudden fall with drenching sweat. If the disease was extensive or the patient frail the outcome was not infrequently fatal. Effective treatment has greatly changed the prognosis and the course of the disease.

Treatment. The patient is put to bed comfortably supported with pillows to make breathing easier, and these investigations made to determine the severity of the disease and the appropriate treatment.

1. Chest X-ray, which will show the consolidated lobe.
2. Blood culture, which may reveal the pneumococcus.
3. White cell count. The normal leucocyte count is 5–8000 per 10^9l., and the response to a septic infection should be a rise of up to 20,000, and such a rise indicates that the patient's physical resistance is satisfactory.
4. Sputum culture and the sensitivity of any organism to antibiotics.
5. The temperature, pulse and respiration rate are taken four-hourly, and the fluid intake and output recorded.

Pain and distress are best relieved at the outset by morphine 15 mg Linctus codeine is given to suppress the cough, which at first produces only a little mucus tinged orange by red blood cells. An antibiotic such as penicillin, tetracycline or ampicillin is given at once.

The appetite will be lost and food need not be pressed, but every endeavour must be made to keep the fluid intake adequate. Drinking stimulates the cough and increases the dyspnoea, and the patient is exhausted after a few sips. Fluids should be offered in small amounts, and the patient's likes are more important than the energy value. Sympathetic persistence by the nurse is indicated. Sleep will be disturbed, and a sedative is usually needed. Warm sponging and attention to the dry mouth will promote comfort.

Cyanosis is often seen in lobar pneumonia, and oxygen may be required. Response to antibiotics is, however, rapid and within twenty-four hours the temperature usually begins to fall, and is normal or subnormal. The affected lobe is still solid, and it will be two or three weeks before natural repair processes have cleared it, so it must not be thought that recovery is complete because there is no pyrexia. The patient may get up when the temperature has been normal for four or five days, but must remain under care until an X-ray shows that the chest is clear. Convalescence is necessary before a return to work.

Complications

1. *Delayed resolution.* Sometimes instead of clearing in the usual time, the affected lobe remains congested and opaque to X-rays. Provided the health is

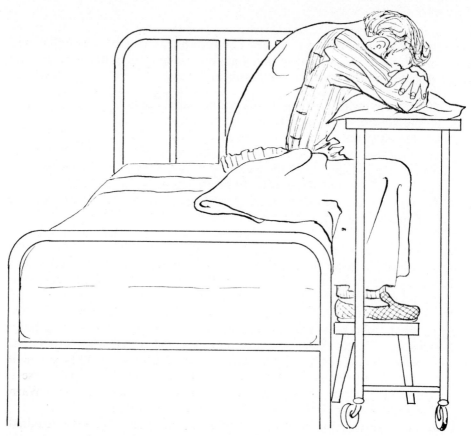

Fig. 63. The best position for chest aspiration. It is comfortable for the patient and convenient for the physician.

good and there are no adverse symptoms, anxiety need not be felt, and serial X-rays will show a gradual clearing. If resolution does not progress, there may be some other condition keeping the pneumonia active, and in an elderly patient this may be carcinoma of the bronchus. Bronchoscopy or bronchography may be undertaken to help in diagnosis.

2. *Pleural effusion.* In the second week, the temperature may rise, breathing becomes embarrassed, and an X-ray shows a fluid level on the affected side. Chest aspiration is performed daily, a culture made, and benzyl penicillin injected into the pleural cavity. In most cases the amount of fluid gradually decreases, and eventually the condition resolves. Occasionally the fluid becomes grossly infected and the next stage is reached.

3. *Empyema.* This is a collection of pus in the pleural cavity, and if the pleural effusion has been well treated, it will be well localized. Aspiration should be continued until the fluid becomes thick, and then surgical drainage and insertion of a tube is necessary. The aim is to obliterate the abscess cavity; to encourage the lung to expand to fill this space, and to achieve good function in the lung. The patient must be encouraged by the physiotherapist and the nurse to attain expansion by chest exercises and deep breathing.

4. *Lung abscess.* The temperature rises again after a period of normality, and may fluctuate markedly, with sweating and shivering. The patient feels ill, and the breath may be offensive. If an X-ray is taken at this stage an opaque patch will be seen.

The abscess will rupture into a bronchus, and very offensive pus is coughed up, sometimes mixed with blood. An X-ray now will show a cavity with a fluid level. The temperature now falls and the patient feels better. Treatment must however be energetic and continued until healing is complete, or the abscess may become chronic. If this occurs, offensive pus is coughed up in large quantities, extensive destruction of lung tissue may occur, and pus may gain entry to a blood vessel and pass via the pulmonary vein and left heart to the brain, causing cerebral abscess.

Treatment is by antibiotics and postural drainage. The attitude that the patient must assume in order to empty the abscess by gravity is determined, and this position must be adopted for periods during the day while the physiotherapist percusses the chest over the cavity. If possible the patient should sleep in this position.

Lung abscess may be caused by inhalation of septic material or vomit following operation, and the treatment is the same. It may also occur in connection with carcinoma of bronchus.

PNEUMONIA DUE TO RETENTION OF SECRETIONS

In all varieties of pneumonia in this group there is infected secretion in the lungs, and its evacuation forms an important part of treatment. Some of the commoner varieties are:

1. **Hypostatic pneumonia.** This is a common complication of all conditions in which people lie flat for long periods in medical and surgical illnesses unless measures are taken to avert it. Secretions accumulate in the bases of the lungs, and if they are not expectorated will become infected. It is an especial

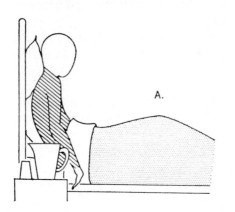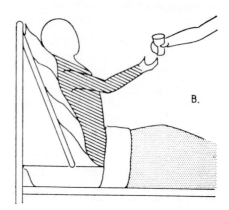

Fig. 64.

A. A poor position for the patient with chest infection; chest expansion is hindered. An ill patient is too listless to pour himself a drink.

B. Correct position. Constant encouragement by the nurse ensures a good fluid intake.

danger to the old, and to those with poor respiratory movement. It is a very frequent complication of any illness or accident (such as fracture of the neck of the femur) which confines old people to bed. Those who have had strokes, or severe haematemesis with shock, are vulnerable people in medical wards.

People at risk should be encouraged to do deep breathing exercises if they are able. Those who are unconscious should be turned from side to side hourly or two hourly and percussion applied to the chest. If it is possible to sit the patient up, this should be done. Patients must not be allowed to sink into the pillows with the spine flexed, but should sit with the back well supported so that chest expansion is not restricted.

2. **Post-operative pneumonia.** Pain after abdominal operations may make breathing shallow and predispose to bronchopneumonia. Large doses of

morphine by depressing respiration may have the same effect. Men are more liable to this complication than women because they use the diaphragm relatively more, and because heavy smokers are more likely to be men.

To prevent post-operative pneumonia, breathing and coughing exercises should be taught before operation, and smoking discouraged. Enough post-operative analgesic is given to permit deep breathing, and coughing if the incision is supported. The patient should sit up as soon as his condition permits.

3. **Pneumonia secondary to carcinoma of bronchus.** A new growth of a bronchus may cause retention of secretion behind the obstruction and so give rise to pneumonia, sometimes before the growth is suspected. Cancer of bronchus is discussed on page 209.

4. **Aspiration pneumonia,** which is described in the following section. The methods by which one may hope to avert pneumonia due to retained secretion have been described under the appropriate heading. Should pneumonia arise, it will be treated on these lines.

The aims of treatment in all pneumonias in this section are:

1. to give the antibiotic appropriate to the infecting organism,
2. to encourage the expectoration of the infected secretions,
3. to maintain the general condition and promote comfort.

ASPIRATION PNEUMONIA

Unless precautions are taken, patients during unconsciousness may inhale stomach contents, pus from a peritonsillar abscess, or blood from an operation on the mouth or tonsils. Large quantities may cause death by obstructing the airway, smaller amounts will cause severe pneumonia.

The usual kind of aspiration pneumonia is however a less dramatic affair, and is due to the entry of bacteria from the sinuses or other part of the upper respiratory tract. Following a cold or similar episode, the temperature rises and the patient begins to cough and feel generally ill. An X-ray shows a patch of consolidation.

This kind of pneumonia is common in winter. The patient is put to bed, and sputum specimen sent for culture. Steam inhalations will help to loosen sputum, and an antibiotic like tetracycline or ampicillin is given until the results of sputum sensitivity are known. A dry cough may be checked by a linctus, especially at night, and a hypnotic may be necessary to allow sleep. Plenty of fluid should be taken.

The most important part of the treatment, apart from the antibiotic, is physiotherapy. Postural drainage of the chest implies putting the patient in a position in which the affected part of the lung can drain by gravity. After a quarter of an hour in this position, deep breathing and coughing exercises and percussion of the chest are given, to encourage the coughing up of sputum and re-expansion of the lung.

The temperature usually falls to normal or subnormal in a day or two, but the test of recovery is re-expansion of the lung as seen on an X-ray. This should occur in two or three weeks, but may take longer. If resolution is unduly delayed, it is possible that some lung condition is maintaining the pneumonia. Carcinoma of bronchus and bronchiectasis have to be considered.

COLLAPSE OF THE LUNG

It will be recalled that the lung surface is normally kept in contact with the chest walls and diaphragm by the adherence of the two layers of the pleura. The elastic lung is kept slightly on the stretch and even during expiration there is air in the bronchioles and alveoli. Collapse of all or part of a lung means that it becomes airless and solid.

Collapse may be brought about in two ways.

A. Absorption collapse. Blockage of a bronchus by mucus or by pressure from a growth means that air cannot enter the part supplied by this bronchus; the air already in it is absorbed, and the tissue collapses.

B. Relaxation collapse. Air enters the pleural cavity, either through a wound in the chest wall, or from the lung itself. Air in the pleural cavity is called **pneumothorax.** If it is the result of a disease process, it is called a **spontaneous pneumothorax.** It was formerly a custom to introduce air into the pleural cavity in order to collapse and thus rest a tuberculous lung. This procedure, now fallen into disuse, was called induction of an **artificial** pneumothorax.

ABSORPTION COLLAPSE

A typical and not uncommon example of this kind of collapse occurs after operations on the chest or abdomen. These make coughing painful, so that there is difficulty in clearing the bronchial secretions, while the atropine or hyoscine used pre-operatively to dry the airway makes the mucus thicker. The temperature, pulse and respiration rate all rise suddenly and markedly, the patient is flushed, uneasy and anxious. A chest X-ray will reveal the collapsed portion of lung.

Prevention is important. Breathing and coughing exercises should be taught before operation, and if there is any infection postural drainage and percussion of the chest will be required, and an antibiotic may be ordered. As soon as

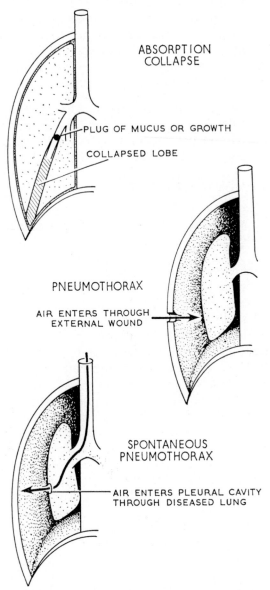

ABSORPTION
COLLAPSE

PLUG OF MUCUS OR GROWTH

COLLAPSED LOBE

PNEUMOTHORAX

AIR ENTERS THROUGH
EXTERNAL WOUND

SPONTANEOUS
PNEUMOTHORAX

AIR ENTERS PLEURAL CAVITY
THROUGH DISEASED LUNG

Fig. 65. Some causes of collapse of the lung.

consciousness is regained after the anaesthetic, the wound should be supported and the patient encouraged to cough and breathe deeply. Enough analgesic should be given to allow free coughing, but not so much as to depress the respiratory centre. The patient should be sat up with the chest well expanded and not allowed to sink with curved spine into his pillows. The fluid intake should be kept high so that the sputum is loosened.

Treatment of pulmonary collapse is urgent. The patient should be given morphine 10 mg, laid flat on the sound side and the foot of the bed is raised. The chest is percussed and the patient encouraged to cough. If the plug of mucus is not coughed up, it must be aspirated with a bronchoscope.

SPONTANEOUS PNEUMOTHORAX

In young people, this is usually due to the rupture of a small cyst or vesicle on the lung surface, allowing air to escape from the lung and separate the two layers of the pleura. In older patients it is usually associated with emphysema (page 187).

When it occurs, there is often a sharp pain in the chest and the patient may faint. Difficulty in breathing is usual. The patient is admitted to hospital if symptoms are marked, given a sedative, and nursed at rest comfortably supported in bed. Usually the lung heals, and the air in the pleural cavity is gradually absorbed. If the pneumothorax is large, a needle attached to Stott's apparatus is inserted, the pressure in the pleural cavity read from the manometer, and some of the air withdrawn. Another method of treatment is to insert a catheter through the chest wall by means of a trocar and cannula, and connect it to a bottle with a water seal, through which air is expelled when the patient coughs. Several types of valve are made, which can be attached to the catheter, and allow air to escape from the chest but not return to it. This method of treatment allows the patient mobility and obviates the risk of fluid being syphoned into the chest from a carelessly handled water seal jar. However, the air cannot be seen escaping, the intrapleural pressure cannot be measured, and it is even possible to insert the valve the wrong way round, and thus cause a tension pneumothorax.

Occasionally the opening between the lung and the pleural cavity has a valve action, so that more air is forced into the pleural cavity at each breath, and a **tension pneumothorax** develops. The patient becomes increasingly dyspnoeic and cyanosed as the mediastinum is displaced by the rising pressure. Relief of the tension by the insertion of a needle or trocar and cannula as described above must be undertaken at once, or the patient will die.

BRONCHIECTASIS

The pathological change in bronchiectasis is dilatation of the bronchioles. It usually follows absorption collapse of a portion of lung due to blockage of a bronchus by sputum during measles or whooping cough. Foreign bodies in the bronchus are another cause of collapse leading to bronchiectasis. If this collapsed tissue is not re-expanded by effective treatment, neighbouring parts of the lung are stretched to take up the space formerly occupied by the airless portion. Sputum accumulates in the dilated bronchioles, and becomes infected. This infection harms the cilia of the mucous membrane which becomes less capable of moving the sputum upwards. Bronchiectasis is usually comparatively localized but may affect both lungs.

Bronchiectasis is now less common than it used to be, especially in its severer forms, because pneumonia can be more effectively treated. Whooping cough can now be prevented by immunization, and it is hoped that measles will soon be in the same category.

Course. The patient is usually a child or young person when first seen. The chief complaint is of a productive cough, the sputum being often abundant, foul smelling, and containing streaks of blood. When the patient wakes and moves in the morning, sputum which has accumulated in the night in the dilated bronchioles spills over into normal ones, coughing is stimulated and large amounts of sputum are produced. Irregular fever is common and there are acute episodes in which the temperature rises sharply. Anaemia is often found. A child is usually under the size normal for the age, and is handicapped both socially and scholastically by frequent absences from school. If a major portion of lung is affected, there may be breathlessness and cyanosis on exertion.

Treatment. The general condition is assessed from records of the temperature and pulse, the weight, and the haemoglobin level. The amount of the sputum is recorded, and the organisms present and their sensitivity to antibiotics established. The extent of the local condition is discovered by bronchography. Radio-opaque oil is introduced into the bronchus, and by positioning of the patient is allowed to run into each lobe.

The infected sputum must be drained as completely as possible by **postural drainage.** The patient is put into a position in which gravity helps in the expulsion of the sputum. This position is assumed for periods ordered by the physician; for instance ten minutes several times a day, and during this time percussion of the chest by the physiotherapist or the nurse is performed. Antibiotics are ordered if appropriate. If sinus infection is present, it must be treated.

General measures to improve the health include a diet with plenty of protein and perhaps vitamin supplements; a good fluid intake; iron if anaemia is present; general and breathing exercises to aid lung expansion. These measures may be sufficient to keep the patient in good health, provided he undertakes postural drainage regularly.

If the disease is strictly localized, surgical excision of the affected lobe (**lobectomy**) offers good prospects of a complete cure. The patient is prepared for operation by a course of the medical treatment outlined above.

BRONCHIAL ASTHMA

Bronchial asthma is characterized by recurrent attacks of dyspnoea, chiefly expiratory. The underlying cause is spasm of the plain muscle of the bronchioles. Air is drawn into the lungs with some difficulty, but expiration is prolonged, laborious and wheezing, since breathing out is normally due not to muscular effort but to the elastic recoil of the lung as the rib cage descends.

Aetiology. Asthma may first show itself at any age, even in infants, and in most patients the first attack occurs before the age of 25. Not uncommonly, however, it first manifests itself in middle age. Men are more often affected than women. Several factors may appear to be implicated in causing this disease.

1. *Allergy.* Asthmatic attacks may be due to sensitivity to substances inhaled, such as dust or debris from the coats of horses, dogs, cats and other animals and birds, and pollen from grasses; to articles of food, such as shellfish, eggs or soft fruits; to drugs, especially aspirin; and to sera, such as antitetanus serum. It was at one time thought that allergy was the predominant feature in asthma, but this view is now changing, and it is believed that other causes may be just as important. In some, allergy is undoubtedly the basic cause, as in Besnier's syndrome in which the patient has eczema, hay fever and asthma in sequence or together.

2. *Heredity.* A tendency to allergic conditions is undoubtedly hereditary, and among the family of a young asthmatic will often be found others with asthma, hay fever or eczema.

3. *Infections.* Those who suffer their first asthma attack as adults usually have it following bronchitis, or pneumonia. In any asthmatic, a head cold or sinusitis will usually trigger off an attack.

4. *Nervous factors.* It is well known to asthmatics that fatigue, anxiety, frustration or anger will start an attack, and since the cause of the bronchospasm must be overaction of the vagus nerve, it is not surprising that impulses from the brain or autonomic system should have such an influence.

Symptoms. Between attacks, the asthmatic patient may be free of symptoms, although if the condition is of long standing, there is usually some "tightness" of the chest in the intervals. An asthmatic attack may occur at any time, but is most common in the small hours of the morning. Those who have had few or no attacks are intensely frightened and restless, feeling that they are about to suffocate. People who have had them before know what to expect, and endure them stoically until time or treatment brings the attack to an end.

The patient is often wakened by oppression and tightness of the chest, and since his chief difficulty is in expiration he adopts a position in which by fixing his shoulder girdle he can bring his accessory muscles of respiration to bear on the chest. He sits up in bed and puts his elbows on his knees, or sits on the edge of the bed and rests his hands on the mattress, or sits astride a chair with his forearms on the chair-back. Breathing is laboured, with a short inspiration, and a prolonged slow wheezy expiration. He is pale, tense, sweating, cannot speak, and concentrates all his energies on breathing. The chest is distended, and the violent efforts at breathing seem to make little difference to its size. At this stage however he begins to cough, and may expectorate small firm pellets which are coils of the thick mucus which have accumulated in the spastic bronchioles. After this the attack soon subsides, and he may soon fall asleep.

Sometimes the attack does not subside, or may quickly be followed by another. This dangerous and exhausting condition is called status asthmaticus, and usually requires treatment in hospital.

Treatment. This may be considered under two headings:
  a) the management that will reduce the number and severity of the attacks,
  b) the treatment during the paroxysm.

Management. A thorough investigation of all the circumstances that cause attacks is made. In highly strung children the nervous factor is often predominant; children who are well at home may get a severe attack on return to boarding school or vice versa. Anxious and over-protective parents must be reassured, and they and the child encouraged to believe that this is a disability that can be dealt with, and must not be allowed to dominate their lives. Many children finally become free of asthma as they grow up.

The patient's occupation and hobbies should be considered as being the environment that causes attacks. Dust is always irritating and should be avoided. Feather-filled pillows and eiderdowns may cause nocturnal asthma, and the patient should use latex pillows and a terylene-filled quilt. Family pets such as dogs and cats may have to be found another home. Heavy meals late at night are bad, and the diet should not include any foods to which the patient is sensitive.

Asthmatics usually react severely to sera, such as antitetanus serum, and should not be given it except in an emergency. Aspirin should not generally be prescribed, and morphine is highly dangerous, especially during an attack, when by inhibiting the respiratory centre it may cause death.

Holidays in the mountains are often attended with no attacks at all, perhaps because of the dust free air, but on return home attacks may be resumed.

In older patients in whom the asthma is secondary to other chest conditions, such as bronchitis, the appropriate treatment for such infections is given, and examination of the heart and circulatory system is made lest the nocturnal attacks of breathlessness are due to left heart failure, and not to bronchial asthma. An antispasmodic such as ephedrine or isoprenaline may be ordered at night in order to ward off attacks.

Drugs used in asthma. The actions of these may be classified under three headings:

1. Drugs that initate the action of the sympathetic system. Adrenaline up to 1·0 ml can be given by subcutaneous injection. It is less used now that other drugs are available, because of the tachycardia and palpitation it may cause. Ephedrine by mouth is effective in preventing attacks. Isoprenaline can be given as a sublingual tablet, or by nebulizer or aerosol spray. Orciprenaline and salbutamol are slower to act than isoprenaline, but last longer. Salbutamol (Ventolin) is probably the safest of the three.
2. Corticosteroids are important in the management of status asthmaticus, and used too for chronic asthmatics.
3. Sodium cromoglycate prevents the release of the substances that cause the bronchial constriction and mucosal swelling. It is given as a powder from a special inhaler, which even children can learn to manage.

Nebulizers and aerosols are very widely used to ward off attacks, and since they are not without dangers patients must be clearly instructed in their use. Though the dose is usually metered, patients who do not receive quick relief may repeat it at short intervals. Sudden death has occurred in asthmatics using them, and it is thought that this is due to overuse of aerosols containing isoprenaline.

Treatment during an attack. One of the drugs in paragraph 1 or 2 is given, preferably by inhaler for rapid effect. Oxygen is of little value, except in status asthmaticus.

The patient should be supported in a comfortable position during an attack, and calm confidence should be shown that the attack will soon pass. When it is over the patient may be soaked in sweat; he is rubbed down with a towel, given a dry pair of pyjamas, the pillows are turned, and he is encouraged to sleep.

Status asthmaticus can usually be relieved by adrenaline, aminophylline, or steroids such as prednisone. A 1 ml syringe of adrenaline 1 in 1000 can be used; the needle is inserted subcutaneously, and 0·1 ml injected every minute or two. Intravenous aminophylline or even hydrocortisone hemisuccinate may be required for severe dyspnoea. In less acute cases prednisone 5 mg four times a day may be effective. Most physicians would prefer not to prescribe prednisone for asthmatics except in emergencies, because of the well-known side effects of long periods of administration of drugs with a steroid effect.

HAY FEVER

Hay fever is the result of an allergic reaction of the mucous membrane of the upper respiratory tract to pollen, especially that of grasses. In this country timothy grass is a very common cause. Hay fever usually begins in adolescence, and may persist throughout life. From May to July the sufferer gets swelling of the nasal mucosa, with watery discharge and sneezing. Because the conjunctival sac is connected with the nose by the naso-lacrimal duct the eyes are also affected and photophobia (dislike of light) is common.

IgE is made in response to the allergen and becomes attached to the mast cells in the respiratory tract. Subsequent exposure to the pollen causes these mast cells to release histamine, which releases fluid from the capillaries into the tissues—this causes the symptoms.

Mitigation of attacks can sometimes be obtained by hyposensitization with increasing doses of pollen extract before the season begins. This course will have to be repeated every year.

Treatment consists of preventing histamine release by giving sodium cromoglycate, a drug apparently without side effects. This seems likely to supersede treatment by antihistamines, which may cause drowsiness and dryness of the mucous membranes.

TUBERCULOSIS

There are strains of tubercle bacilli that infect men, cattle, birds and reptiles, but the only ones that produce disease in man are the first two. The human type is usually inhaled, and causes disease of the lung, whence it may spread to many other organs. The bovine strain is swallowed in infected milk, and causes abdominal infection, with spread to bones and joints. Bovine tuberculosis has become rare in western countries, due to pasteurization of milk, which destroys the bacillus, and eradication of tuberculosis in cattle. Pulmonary tuberculosis has declined steadily in incidence from the beginning of the century in the west because of rising social, economic and hygienic standards, and mass radio-graphy which permitted early diagnosis. The introduction of drugs active against the tubercle bacilli caused a very steep fall in the numbers affected, but hopes that it might be reduced to an insignificant level have not been realized. 10,000 new cases are notified annually in the United Kingdom, and over a thousand people die, while throughout the world it is estimated that three million people die every year. Although there is now a range of drugs active

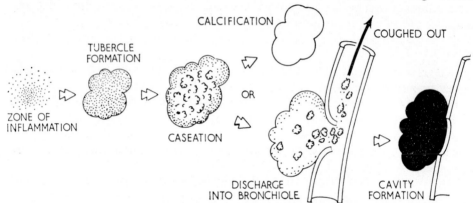

Fig. 66. The progress of tuberculous infection.

against tuberculosis, many countries do not have the medical resources to trace cases, nor the ability to budget for the drugs required to treat them. Tubercu-losis is one of the most important infectious diseases in the world.

When the bacilli gain entry to the tissues they set up a surrounding zone of inflammation. If the body is unable to overcome this infection, this focus may spread and amalgamate with neighbouring lesions until it forms a tubercle that is visible to the naked eye. The centre of the tubercle breaks down to form a cheesy material, a process known as **caseation.** If the disease is checked at this stage, the lesion will calcify and remain inactive. If it extends, the tubercle may ulcerate into a neighbouring vessel or passage, such as a bronchus, when the caseous material will be discharged, and a **cavity** will remain. In this way extensive destruction of tissue may occur, and infectious material may be dis-charged which may spread the disease to others. Infection may spread along the lymphatics to cause tuberculosis of the regional glands.

PULMONARY TUBERCULOSIS

A first infection is known as **primary tuberculosis.** A small lesion occurs in a lung, and the mediastinal lymph glands enlarge. Unless the patient has been exposed to a very heavy infection, the illness is slight and may pass quite unnoticed, since there may be no general symptoms, and usually healing occurs. The tissues have however been sensitized to the tubercle bacilli. If a preparation (tuberculin) is prepared from killed bacilli and injected into the skin, a red swelling will appear. This is the basis of the Mantoux test. Someone who has had a primary infection will continue to show a positive Mantoux reaction. At one time most people living in towns became Mantoux positive in childhood, but now this is uncommon unless immunization has been performed.

If primary tuberculosis occurs in an infant, or if a child is exposed to very heavy infection, extensive disease may result. Bacilli may gain entry to the blood stream, and cause **miliary tuberculosis.** "Milia" means millet seed, and refers to the vast number of small tubercles scattered throughout the body, especially in the lungs and over the meninges. Tuberculous meningitis is described in Chapter 14.

The treatment of miliary tuberculosis is on the same lines as other forms, and if diagnosis is made early and treatment is energetic, the prognosis is good even in this severe disease.

TUBERCULOUS CERVICAL LYMPHADENITIS

If the tubercle bacillus lodges on the tonsils, the cervical lymph glands become infected, and caseation takes place. Pus may track through the fascia and form a cold abscess under the skin. This condition used to be not uncommon when unpasteurized milk was drunk by children, but is now rare. Treatment will usually resolve it, and surgical excision of the glands, once a standard procedure, is now not needed.

POST PRIMARY TUBERCULOSIS

Any infection occurring after the primary episode, which as we have seen is usually not severe, is called post primary tuberculosis. It is what the lay public knows as "T.B.", and usually attacks the lungs, especially the upper lobes. The way in which the disease process advances has been described, and may eventually result in cavities in the lung, from which infected sputum is coughed up. This infected material may cause tracheitis and laryngitis, and if the sputum is swallowed, gastritis occurs and tuberculous ulcers may occur in the small intestine. Fistula-in-ano is not uncommon.

Progress of the disease is normally quite slow, except where the patient has unusually low resistance, and it may become arrested at any stage. Sometimes healing is accompanied by the formation of so much fibrous tissue that lung function is grossly restricted, and may end in heart failure.

Symptoms. In the early stages, there may be no symptoms, and the first complaints are vague. The patient feels tired, loses weight, sweats at night, and may have a slight rise of temperature in the evenings. Cough is at first dry and racking, but later mucoid sputum is produced. Haemoptysis often occurs quite early, and is rarely more than slight, but it is always alarming, and usually induces the patient to visit the doctor at once. Sometimes pleurisy is an early symptom, and acute pleurisy in a young adult (other than one recovering from pneumonia) is usually tuberculous.

If the disease is advanced, loss of weight and fever are noticeable, and haemoptysis occurring at this stage is often profuse, and may cause death.

Investigations. X-rays of the chest will often reveal the disease before the patient has any symptoms. If a lesion is found, it is usually desirable to admit the patient to hospital for a complete assessment of his condition. He is weighed on admission, and thereafter weekly. His temperature is charted four hourly, in order to detect a small occasional rise. The blood sedimentation rate is estimated; this is usually raised above the normal 2 to 8 mm. in the first hour, and a series of estimations may be valuable in assessing improvement or otherwise. The sputum is examined for tubercle bacilli, repeatedly if the first tests are negative. Sputum may not be forthcoming if it is small in amount and the patient swallows it. In this case, the physician may ask the nurse to pass a Ryle's tube into the stomach before breakfast, inject a few millilitres of normal saline, and withdraw the resting juice. Examination of this may reveal the tubercle bacillus, which is not destroyed by the stomach acid like most bacteria. In doubtful cases, the Mantoux reaction may be ascertained, since if this is negative, the patient is unlikely to have tuberculosis.

Treatment. This may be considered under three headings:
   a) General care.
   b) Anti-tuberculous drugs.
   c) Local treatment of the lung.

General care. In very early cases, where living conditions are suitable, the patient may be nursed at home, but usually his treatment is best undertaken in hospital. Rest in bed is important, since exercise increases respiratory movement and may interfere with healing. Mental relaxation is important, but may be difficult to ensure. The diagnosis is usually a great shock, even though tuberculosis no longer takes years to heal as once it did. The patient must be given a full explanation of the likely course of his disease, and his anxieties about the health and financial affairs of his family will be relieved by the measures described under social aspects. A sedative such as diazepam 5 mg b.d. may enable him to relax. As the condition improves, he may be allowed up for toilet purposes, and gradually begin to undertake light activity.

Free ventilation is essential, and it may be possible to nurse the patient on a verandah. The bedclothes must be just sufficient to keep him warm under these conditions, since overheating and a stuffy atmosphere causes night sweats. Fresh air will also lessen the likelihood of spread to others if tubercle bacilli are being coughed up. Direct sunlight for long periods is not advisable during the active stage of the disease.

The diet must be generous, especially in protein, and in the early stages when the appetite is poor it may need tempting. Overweight however is not desirable, and the patient is weighed weekly. Vitamin supplements may be prescribed if the nutritional state is poor. A dry useless cough is checked by means of a linctus.

Patients are taught to use a sputum carton, and given a box of tissues and a bag for their disposal. Sputum cartons can be weighed in order to estimate the amount of sputum, and the cartons are incinerated. If tubercle bacilli are being coughed up, precautions to prevent spread of infection are taken. Gowns and masks are worn by the staff when making the bed or performing similar services involving close attendance, and crockery is sterilized after use. Staff who are still Mantoux negative should not be allowed to nurse patients with open tuberculosis, and regular chest X-rays should be taken of those engaged in nursing them.

Drug treatment. The three classical anti-tuberculous drugs are streptomycin, isoniazid (INAH) and para-amino salicylic acid (PAS). At least two, and sometimes all three are combined in a course, since drug-resistant forms of the tubercle bacillus appear readily, and this means that not only is the patient more difficult to cure, but if he infects someone else, this person's disease will be resistant to therapy from the start.

If sputum is available, a culture is made for ascertaining sensitivity of the organism to drugs, but the results will not be available for two or three months, and treatment must be begun at once. Streptomycin is given by intramuscular injection; the daily dose does not exceed 1 g. and the total dose is usually in the region of 70 g. Deafness and giddiness due to damage to the auditory nerve may follow a relative overdose, and complaints of either symptom must be reported at once. Nurses readily become sensitized to streptomycin if they get it on their hands or faces, so gloves should be worn while preparing and giving the injection, and the amount in the syringe must be adjusted with the needle tip still in the phial.

PAS is given by mouth, often in cachets because of its disagreeable taste. A common dose is 12 g. daily. It often produces nausea and diarrhoea, and patients often feel great aversion to taking it, especially as it may be given for a year or two. They may need supervision and encouragement. INAH is comparatively non-toxic except in high doses, when pyridoxine is given to avoid nerve symptoms. If PAS and INAH are both being given, they may be combined in sachets or granules. This means taking four sachets three times a day, and it can be seen, what a burden this is, especially as after the early stages of treatment the patient feels well.

Once the course of streptomycin has been completed, the other two drugs are given together, and are usually continued for two years after the disease has become inactive, with a two years minimum. When the results of sensitivity tests are known, or if the usual drugs are badly tolerated, it may be necessary to change to one of the newer drugs. Though these are usually known as "second-line" drugs in the attack on tuberculosis, they may be used from the beginning in situations where drug-resistant strains are prevalent.

Rifampicin is the most important; it is a bactericidal drug which can be given by mouth. It is well tolerated, except for a tendency to lower the platelet count. Ethambutol is often given with it, and patients receiving this drug must be warned to report to their doctor if they notice any impairment of sight or of colour vision. Other drugs which may be used are thiacetazone, cycloserine, prothionamide and pyrazinamide. For the toxic effects of these and other anti-tuberculous drugs a pharmacological book should be consulted.

Local treatment of the lung. Before the introduction of effective drugs, it was the custom to rest the lung by collapsing it, either by introducing air into the pleural cavity (artificial pneumothorax) or by resection of ribs which allowed collapse of the chest wall (thoracoplasty). It is not likely that either procedure will be used today. Resection of a lobe or a segment is used occasionally for patients with localized destructive disease which does not respond to general and drug treatment.

Patients with acute pleurisy are often ill and in great discomfort on admission. They should be nursed at complete rest comfortably supported in bed. If effusion is present, fluid is usually withdrawn for examination, and perhaps for injection into a guinea-pig to establish the diagnosis. Unless there is a large amount of fluid which embarrasses breathing, it is not usual to aspirate it, and general treatment with a course of drugs should be effective.

Prevention of tuberculosis. The factors other than effective treatment which have produced the decline in tuberculosis in this country are as follows:

1. Better social conditions have led to less overcrowding, and higher wages have enabled the worst-paid sections of the community to take a better diet and open-air holidays.
2. Pasteurization of milk and eradication of tuberculosis from dairy herds has eliminated bovine forms of the disease.
3. Mass radiography has enabled the detection of early cases.
4. Public health workers and tuberculosis dispensaries have traced contacts and educated patients in hygiene.
5. More effective treatment has encouraged people to seek advice at an early stage.
6. Vaccination by means of a weakened form of the tubercle bacillus (Bacille Calmette-Guérin; B.C.G.) confers some immunity, and has been widely used for children and contacts of infected people. All nurses and medical students who are Mantoux negative should be given B.C.G.

SOCIAL ASPECTS OF TUBERCULOSIS

The tuberculous patient needs support and help at two stages, first when the disease is diagnosed, and later when he is trying to return to normal life and work. His family must be investigated in case they have contracted the disease, and if the patient is a child his school mates and perhaps the staff should be examined. Those who are Mantoux negative should be offered B.C.G. vaccination.

Special allowances are paid to sufferers from tuberculosis, and grants are payable for bedding to allow the patient to sleep alone. When he is fit to begin light work again, he may be able to find employment with Remploy workshops, until he is strong enough to compete on level terms in industry.

NEW GROWTHS OF LUNG

Tumours of the lung may be benign or malignant, but unfortunately the innocent ones are uncommon. Malignant tumours may be primary or secondary. Secondary growths occur when malignant cells from a tumour anywhere in the body gain access to a vein, and pass through the right side of the heart to the lungs. They are halted in the pulmonary capillaries and may begin to grow there. These secondary growths or **metastases** resemble the parent growth in structure, and sometimes bring the patient to the doctor before the primary growth produces symptoms. New growths in bone and breast are especially liable to metastasize to the lungs. Effective treatment is not possible at this stage.

Carcinoma of the bronchus is the most common malignant growth of the chest, and its incidence has been rising in an alarming way in recent years. It is especially a disease of men, and surveys show that heavy smokers are 40 times more liable to it than non-smokers. Smokers are not unnaturally unwilling to accept these findings, and blame atmospheric pollution or diesel fumes. Countries with no atmospheric problems, such as Iceland and the Channel Isles show, however, the same rise as industrial communities, and there is no doubt that a reduction in smoking would be reflected in the future in a reduction in the number of men and women affected. Prevention is important in that the results of treatment are very disappointing.

Symptoms. Cough with sputum, often bloodstreaked, is often the presenting symptom. Wheezing may be caused by bronchial obstruction, and there may be pain in the chest. Involvement of other structures in the chest may cause complications. Recurrent pneumonia is due to infection behind the obstruction. Extension to the pleura may cause pleural effusion. Obstruction to the superior vena cava causes headache, oedema of the face and arms and dilatation of superficial veins. It is one of the most distressing manifestations of cancer of the bronchus. Sometimes secondary growths in other organs, such as the brain, may be the first symptom.

Diagnosis. An X-ray of the chest and bronchoscopy are usually required, and examination of the sputum for malignant cells may establish the diagnosis. The treatment in suitable cases is surgical, but a relatively small proportion of those seen come into this category, and of those who undergo lobectomy or pneumonectomy the five-year survival rate is 20 per cent.

Radiotherapy may be successful in alleviating symptoms but does not effect a cure. It is always tried in superior vena cava obstruction, to try to relieve the patient's acute discomfort. Relief of pain, and of symptoms as they arise, is the aim of treatment.

PLEURAL EFFUSION
Fluid may accumulate in the space between the two layers of pleura for two main reasons.

1. The mechanism by which fluid is kept in the blood vessels is disturbed. Maybe the amount of protein in the blood is low, so reducing its osmotic power, or perhaps the venous pressure is raised.

The fluid produced is known as a transudate. It is clear, sterile and low in protein. Often fluid occurs in other parts of the body as well as in the pleural sac. Causes include:

a) Heart failure (page 124).
b) The nephrotic syndrome (page 225).
c) Cirrhosis of the liver.
The treatment is essentially that of the cause.
2. The pleura is irritated by inflammation, the result of infection, new growth or injury.

The fluid in this case is called an exudate. It is cloudy from the presence of blood or pus, and is high in protein. The commonest causes are:

a) Pneumonia (page 189).
b) Tuberculosis (page 205).
c) Pulmonary infarct (page 107).
d) New growth, especially of the bronchus and breast.
e) Injury such as surgical incisions and perforating wounds of the chest wall.

Fluid which is causing dyspnoea is aspirated. It may accumulate in large quantities in malignant disease, and may require frequent removal. Following aspiration, the pulse should be charted every half-hour for a few hours, and the patient inspected for cyanosis or distress suggesting pulmonary oedema. On the whole patients are much relieved following aspiration.

DUST DISEASES

The conditions caused by inhalation of dust over a long period are called **pneumoconioses.** Silicosis is due to inhaling particles of silica, and is found in miners, those who work with granite and sandstone, and in grinders. The commonest kind of pneumoconiosis in this country is found in coal miners.

Coal miners' disease in its early forms causes diffuse mottling of the lung fields on X-ray, and some shortness of breath, cough and sputum. The disease does not progress unless the patient remains exposed to coal dust.

A severe form of pneumoconiosis occurs if tuberculous infection is super-added to the lung changes. Dense fibrous tissue forms and the patient's breathing is severely impeded. Heart failure finally results.

This disease has in the past brought intense misery and death to thousands of men, especially in South Wales, but with better working conditions and more effective anti-tuberculous measures have decreased the risks. Good ventilation and damping-down of dusty working areas is practised, and coal-face workers regularly X-rayed. Those who show early changes should not be further exposed to coal-dust.

Pneumoconiosis is a prescribed disease under the National Insurance Industrial Injuries Acts. Injury, disablement and death benefits are payable to sufferers.

Asbestosis is a serious condition, which may appear years after exposure to asbestos fibres in the air, and continue to progress. There is increasing fibrosis of the lungs, with dyspnoea. Asbestosis predisposes to cancer of bronchus, pleura and peritoneum. Since there is no effective treatment prevention is very important. Asbestos is very widely used in insulation of buildings, and people who work with it should have good conditions with dust control, efficient ventilation and protective clothing. This is a condition which is causing much public concern because of the number of people who may be exposed to risk from this very common material.

Farmer's Lung

When hay is baled while still moist, as occurs not infrequently in poor summers, it becomes infected with moulds, from which clouds of spores are released. When the bale is untied for feeding to stock, farm labourers and farmers may thus be exposed to high concentrations of dust while feeding stock indoors in winter, and may become sensitized to the contained spores, especially those of the mould *Thermopolyspora polyspora*.

Once sensitization has occurred, acute attacks of cough, breathlessness with wheezing, and fever occur on exposure, and respiration becomes increasingly embarrassed unless the cause is recognized and avoided. Sometimes the condition arises insidiously, and gives rise to a state like chronic bronchitis, and is just as disabling.

Since the only treatment is that of the symptoms, the prevention of this condition by avoiding exposure to dust of mouldy hay. Improved methods of drying hay, better ventilation in byres, and the use of masks when exposure is inevitable are examples of ways in which this agricultural disease might be prevented.

Chapter 9

Diseases of the Kidney

The two kidneys lie on the posterior abdominal wall, behind the peritoneal cavity, with the aorta and the inferior vena cava running between them. From the aorta the kidneys receive a blood supply equal to a quarter of the cardiac output, which is a measure of the importance of their work.

Their function is:

a) to remove from the blood soluble waste products from protein breakdown,
b) to regulate the volume and the composition of the plasma.

In health the kidney functions very speedily and accurately, keeping the fluid that surrounds the cells constant in composition, by removing unwanted substances dissolved in water, and sending the urine thus formed down the ureter to the bladder.

The kidney unit which makes the urine is the **nephron,** a blind-ended tube of which there are about a million in each kidney. The process by which urine is made falls into two distinct phases, which take place in different parts of the nephron. The blind end is a double cup of epithelium, inside which is a cluster of capillaries; here the first process takes place, **filtration.**

A filter is a device for straining off large particles. Water and dissolved salts, waste products and foodstuffs passes through the filter from the capillary tuft or *glomerulus* and flows down the nephron. The blood proteins and cells do not pass the filter, and remain in the blood stream. The filtrate is a copious, very dilute fluid, 7200 ml. of which are produced every hour.

These remain in the blood stream	These are filtered off
Red cells	Water
White cells	Salts
Platelets	Glucose and amino-acids
Albumin	Urea
Globulin	Creatinine
Fibrinogen	

213

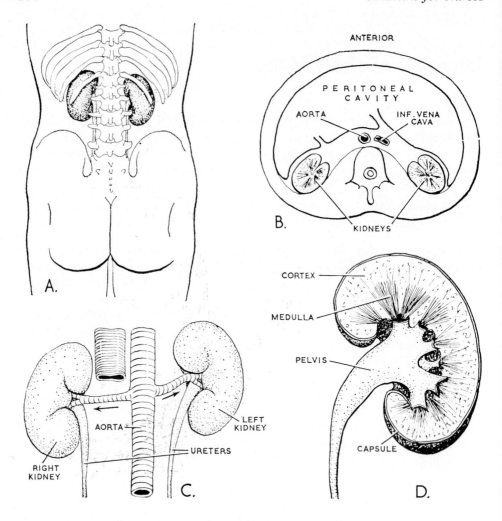

Fig. 67.

A. The kidneys lie alongside the vertebral column, with the last rib crossing the upper pole.
B. The kidneys lie outside the peritoneal cavity.
C. The right kidney lies at a slightly lower level than the left, because of the amount of space taken up by the liver.
D. In section, the kidney is seen to contain an outer layer, the cortex, and an inner, the medulla. This latter consists of the collecting tubules of the nephrons, draining urine to the pelvis of the kidney and thence to the ureters.

This filtrate is the basis from which urine is made. It passes into the next section, a tortuous tubule lined with columnar cells, which reabsorb water from the filtrate, and other substances to the extent required by the tissues. This process is one of **selective reabsorption.**

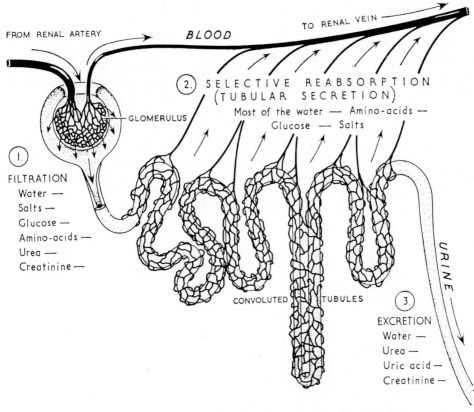

FROM RENAL ARTERY

BLOOD

TO RENAL VEIN

2. SELECTIVE REABSORPTION
(TUBULAR SECRETION)
Most of the water — Amino-acids —
Glucose — Salts

GLOMERULUS

1.

FILTRATION
Water —
Salts —
Glucose —
Amino-acids —
Urea —
Creatinine —

CONVOLUTED TUBULES

3.

EXCRETION
Water —
Urea —
Uric acid —
Creatinine —

URINE

Fig. 68. A nephron or kidney unit and a summary of its functions.

Water. The osmotic pressure of the blood influences the posterior lobe of the pituitary gland, which responds by varying its output of anti-diuretic hormone (ADH) which regulates the reabsorption of water in the tubules. If much water is lost through the skin, or by another means, the osmotic pressure of the blood rises, more ADH is secreted, and less urine is passed. This ability of the kidney to vary the concentration of the urine is a very important function, and it is only lost if kidney disease is extensive.

Foodstuffs. Amino-acids are completely re-absorbed in the tubule, and so is glucose, unless the blood sugar is more than 180 mg. per cent, a figure which is rarely reached in health.

Waste products. The urine is the vehicle for excretion of protein waste, such as urea, uric acid, and creatinine.

Salts. The most abundant salt in the urine is sodium chloride, which is usually taken in excess in the diet in temperate climates. The kidney is sensitive to the changing state of the blood in health and disease, and responds by retaining or excreting salts. For instance, if chloride is lost because acid stomach contents are vomited, the amount of chloride in the urine will diminish.

The acidity or otherwise of a fluid is described in terms of the number of hydrogen ions it contains (pH). The neutral point is pH 7; figures of more than 7 indicate alkalinity, those of less than 7 acidity. The pH of the plasma is 7·4. All the metabolic activities of the body produce acid, e.g. carbonic acid, (of which a large quantity is excreted by the lungs as carbon dioxide), and lactic acid. The slight alkalinity of the blood is kept constant because the kidney excretes these metabolic acids in the urine, which has usually a pH of about 6

THE URINE

The urine contains:
1. the products of normal metabolism, as described above. In addition, it may at times contain also:
2. products of abnormal metabolism (e.g. acetonuria, phenyl-ketonuria),
3. products of disease processes, such as inflammation, injury or new growth in the urinary tract.

Examination of the urine may therefore yield information not only about the kidney and bladder, but about the body as a whole.

Volume. The daily amount passed is usually between 500 and 3000 ml. It varies with the fluid intake, and the amount lost by the skin.

Reaction. pH. 6 (turns blue litmus red). If urine is allowed to stand, the urea in it decomposes, and ammonia is formed and the urine becomes alkaline (turns red litmus blue). Urine may be kept alkaline, if it is desirable to help the excretion of drugs that are more soluble in alkaline solutions, such as the sulphonamides, by giving sodium bicarbonate.

Appearance. The usual amber colour is due to urochrome, and normal urine is clear. Alkaline urine is sometimes opaque because urates come out of solution; a few drops of acetic acid will clear this cloud.

Specific Gravity 1000 to 1030. 40 to 60 g of solids are excreted in solution in the urine daily, and if the urine is concentrated, the specific gravity will be high. If the urine appears dilute (i.e. is pale) but the specific gravity is high, some unusual substance is dissolved in it, and this is most commonly sugar.

ABNORMALITIES

Haematuria. Blood in the urine may be obvious at a glance, or may only be sufficient to turn it smoky. Very small amounts can only be detected by microscopic examination. The blood may come from anywhere in the renal tract,

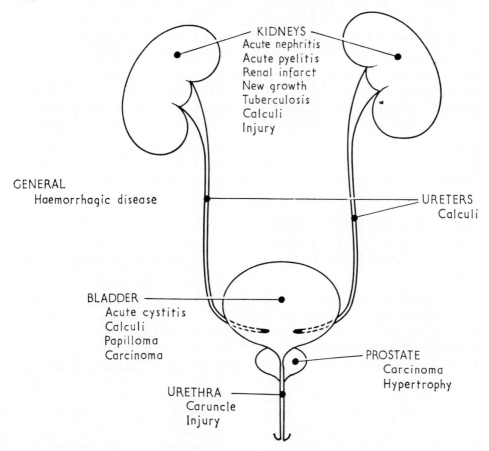

Fig. 69. The causes of haematuria and the sites from which bleeding takes place.

and it is important to notice if it is intimately mixed with the urine, or if it only appears at the end of micturition. Some causes are:

GENERAL	RENAL	URETERIC	VESICAL
Haemorrhagic disease	Acute nephritis	Calculi	Acute cystitis
	Acute pyelitis		Prostatic hypertrophy
	Renal infarct		Calculi
	New growth		Papilloma
	Tuberculosis		Carcinoma
	Calculi		
	Injury		

Pyuria. Pus turns the urine cloudy, and often imparts an offensive odour. If slight, it is only detected by finding pus cells on microscopic examination.

Proteinuria. Albumin is the blood protein with the smallest molecule, and so is the first protein to appear in the urine if the glomerular filter is damaged. The presence of albumin in the urine must always be taken seriously, but the amount of protein is not directly related to the severity of the disease process.

Casts are made of solidified material from the tubules. They may be made of amorphous material (hyaline and granular casts) or of masses of cells. Cellular casts indicate more active disease than hyaline casts, a few of which are occasionally passed by normal people.

TESTS OF RENAL FUNCTION

Production of urine has been described above as consisting of two processes, glomerular filtration and tubular secretion. Both these processes may be tested.

Tests of glomerular function. In order to test the glomerular filtration rate, the metabolism of substances excreted only by the glomeruli must be studied. The ones usually selected are urea and creatinine. **Blood-urea.** Since the kidney is the channel for excretion of urea, the blood-urea is always estimated if kidney disease is suspected. The normal level is 20 to 40 mg (2.2–6.2 mmol/l) per 100 ml, and considerable renal damage must occur before this level rises appreciably. To find the rate of **urea clearance** from the blood by the kidney, the patient is given no tea or coffee, which are diuretics, but has a glass of water in the morning. At 10 a.m. the bladder is emptied and the urine discarded; at 11 a.m. and noon specimens are collected for examination, and the blood-urea is estimated. Punctuality in collection is important, and if there is any delay the time should be marked on the specimen. The result is given as percentage of a normal figure, and if it is below 70 per cent, impaired glomerular function is indicated. The rate of creatinine clearance is another and perhaps more reliable test of glomerular function. A 24-hour specimen of urine is collected and a sample sent to the laboratory with a note of the total volume. 10 ml of blood are collected on the same day.

Tests of tubular function. The urine concentration and dilution test is the one most widely used to examine the ability of the tubules to vary the specific gravity of the urine in response to changes in the fluid balance.

Concentration. Nothing is given to eat or drink after 1800 hours, and the bladder is emptied at bedtime and the specimen discarded. Specimens are passed at 0600 and 0700 hours, and at least one of these should attain a specific gravity of 1022 or more. The test can be prolonged on the instructions of the physician.

Dilution. This part of the test is not used if the patient has oedema. One litre of water is drunk in the next half-hour and specimens are collected hourly for the next four hours. Most of the litre should have been excreted during this period, and the specific gravity of 1003 or less should be reached. Inability to vary the specific gravity of the urine is a sign of kidney failure.

Intravenous pyelogram. If an iodized oil is injected intravenously it is excreted by the kidneys, and since it is opaque to X-rays, films taken following injection will show the outline of the kidneys. It is thus a test of function, since it will show if the kidneys are working and with what efficiency. It will also show the size of the kidney, abnormalities such as stones in the pelvis of the kidney, and finally the outline of the ureters and bladder.

A renogram, a tracing of renal function can be obtained by administering hippuran, which is excreted in the urine, labelled with radioactive iodine. Counters are applied over the kidneys, and these activate writers which record the rate of excretion.

The ability to secrete an acid urine is a **tubular** function. It may be tested by giving 0·1 g of ammonium chloride per kilo body weight; urine with a pH of 5·5 or less should be passed within an hour or so.

Renal biopsy. Microscopic examination of kidney tissue obtained by needle biopsy is often necessary. After it is over, the patient is kept at rest in bed and encouraged to drink freely to keep the urine diluted. Bleeding down the ureter is common and specimens of urine should be saved to see if bleeding is decreasing or not. Colic due to clots passing through the ureter can be relieved with an analgesic.

URINARY CALCULI

Urine is a solution of substances in water, and in certain circumstances some of these substances may come out of solution and be deposited as crystals, gravel or "stone". Stones or calculi can be of calcium, oxalate, uric acid or cystine, and the circumstances that favour their formation are these:

1. **Excess calcium in the urine.** If a patient is immobilized in a long plaster cast, calcium is withdrawn from the skeleton during the period of inactivity, and if the urine volume is low, calcium stones may form in the pelvis of the kidney. This may be avoided by keeping the fluid intake high, and by turning the patient daily into the prone position for a time, to prevent stagnation of the urine in the pelvis of the kidney.

Hyperparathyroidism (page 380) and rickets (page 35) are less common causes.

2. **Kidney disease or infection** (e.g. by *Bacillus proteus*) may cause highly acid urine, in which calcium is less than normally soluble. Treatment of the infection, and the administration of alkali, such as potassium citrate, is helpful.

3. **Errors of metabolism.** Uric acid stones may form in patients who have gout. Oxalate and cystine stones occur in young people with congenital difficulty in metabolizing these substances.

RENAL COLIC

Small stones which form in the kidney pass into the ureter, and their passage to the bladder is accompanied by severe pain, known as renal or (more accurately) ureteric colic There is severe sharp pain passing from the back down the abdomen to the groin. It is spasmodic, since it is due to ureteric peristalsis, and if sharp enough is accompanied by sweating, restlessness and vomiting.

The treatment is to give an analgesic (such as pethidine) to relieve the pain; a plain muscle relaxant (such as atropine) to relax the ureteric spasm; and a high fluid intake to help wash the stone down the ureter, and to prevent deposition of more stones. The urine should be strained in order to identify the stone when it is passed. Stones which cannot be passed are treated surgically.

RENAL TUBERCULOSIS

Tuberculosis of the kidney is secondary to infection elsewhere in the body, usually in the lung, and in countries where such chest infection is becoming less common, so too is renal tuberculosis. The bacillus spreads via the blood stream.

The tuberculous process is the same in the kidney as in the lung (page 205), caseation takes place in the centre of a focus of infection, this caseous material is discharged, and an abscess cavity remains. Infection spreads from the kidney along the lymphatics of the ureter to the bladder; both kidneys are frequently involved.

The earliest symptom is usually frequency of micturition, by night as well as day. The urine contains a little albumin, and later becomes hazy with pus cells. Routine culture does not reveal an organism, since the tuberculosis bacillus takes longer to grow than others, and special culture techniques are needed. Haematuria is common, and if the bladder becomes involved micturition becomes intensely painful.

Cystoscopy is undertaken to assess the state of the bladder, and both ureters are catheterized to obtain specimens of urine from each kidney. The temperature, the weight and the erythrocyte sedimentation rate will show the activity of the disease process.

Treatment consists of the general supportive treatment and the anti-tuberculous drugs described on page 207. In unilateral cases, which do not respond to treatment, surgical excision of the kidney and ureter (nephro-ureterectomy) may effect a cure.

PYELONEPHRITIS

Pyelitis means infection of the kidney pelvis, but since the kidney tissue is usually involved as well, the condition is better described as pyelonephritis. Acute pyelonephritis is quite a common condition, and it is exceedingly important that it should be diagnosed early and thoroughly treated, since if it becomes chronic it is very difficult to cure, and may lead eventually to kidney failure.

ACUTE PYELONEPHRITIS

Acute pyelonephritis is usually an ascending infection from the bladder. It may occur at any age, and among adults is considerably more frequent in women than in men. Conditions that favour infection are:

a) Catheterization of the bladder, especially if an indwelling catheter is used. Catheterization for purely diagnostic purposes should be avoided as far as possible, and a clean specimen examined instead. Diabetic women are more prone than others to infection.
b) Trauma to the bladder or surrounding tissues, as in gynaecological operations. Pyelitis is not uncommon in the first few weeks of marriage. Stone in the kidney or bladder is usually associated with infection.

c) Obstruction to the urinary flow. Congenital abnormalities of the kidney or renal arteries, enlargement of the prostate, and urethral stricture are examples. Acute pyelonephritis in pregnancy is due to dilatation of the ureter, caused by hormone influence on its plain muscle, and perhaps pressure on it by the enlarging uterus.

Course. In a typical attack, there is a rigor, or a sudden rise of temperature with shivering, vomiting, headache and general prostration. There is pain and tenderness over one or both kidneys, and suprapubic pain, frequency and dysuria indicate the associated cystitis. The urine is hazy on inspection, and culture reveals the organism, which is commonly *Escherichia coli*, *Bacillus proteus*, or a staphylococcus. There is a raised white blood cell count (leucocytosis).

Treatment. The patient is nursed in bed, and a clean specimen of urine is sent to the laboratory for culture and antibiotic sensitivity. Pending results, treatment is commonly begun with ampicillin, tetracycline or trimethoprim-sulpha-methoxazole. Copious fluids must be taken, and if the urine is acid, an attempt is made to make it alkaline by giving sodium bicarbonate or potassium citrate. The amount passed and the frequency of micturition should be recorded. The urine should be tested for albumin, since its presence shows that the kidney substance is involved in the inflammation.

When the laboratory results are known, it may be necessary to change the antibiotic in accordance with the findings. Whatever drug is used, it is necessary to continue giving it not only until the symptoms are relieved, but until the urine is sterile. In persistent infections, this may be for weeks or months. Tetracycline is not used for pregnant women with acute pyelitis, since it discolours the teeth of the foetus.

Once the patient has recovered, an examination of the urinary system should be made to determine the cause, unless this is known. An intravenous pyelogram and perhaps cystoscopy is indicated.

CHRONIC PYELONEPHRITIS

In some patients, recurrent attacks of pyelitis follow the first one. If any precipitating causes are known, (e.g. stone in the kidney) these should be treated surgically. Treatment by an appropriate antibiotic is thorough and long-continued. Each successive attack causes more kidney damage, and increases the chances of eventual renal failure.

Prevention. The importance of avoiding catheterization except for treatment has been mentioned. If it is required, a strict aseptic routine must be used. Indwelling catheters should have the extruded part cleaned daily with cetavlon or hibitane, and the area around should be washed twice a day. Young girls and pregnant women should be taught the many beneficial results of daily vulval toilet with soap and water, and all those with any urinary symptoms should be urged to obtain medical advice without delay.

NEPHRITIS

Nephritis is a bilateral, inflammatory (but not infective) condition of the kidneys. The difficulty in describing and understanding this condition is that there are several different classifications, some based on the clinical picture, and some on the microscopic changes in the kidney, and many different types. Three varieties will be described here.

1. *Acute glomerulonephritis.*
2. *The nephrotic syndrome.*
3. *Chronic renal failure.*

ACUTE NEPHRITIS

The kidney filters are extensively damaged in acute nephritis, and it is believed that this glomerular injury is an allergic reaction to a preceding streptococcal infection. Most patients, who are usually children or young adults, have had tonsillitis or even scarlet fever two or three weeks earlier.

The symptoms are due to three causes:

1. The blood-pressure rises as a result of the kidney disease, and this causes headache and vomiting and may even lead to heart failure.
2. The kidneys are distended with blood, and inflamed, leading to fever and backache.
3. Urine secretion is inhibited, and the urinary output falls, even to the point where none is secreted. It contains blood in varying quantities, and albumin which has leaked from the damaged capillaries. The blood-urea is raised above the normal 20–40 mg (2.2–6.2 mmol/l) per cent. Oedema appears in the superficial tissues and is often noticeable in the face, lids and backs of the hands.

Course. If well cared for, most patients increase their output within a few days, and within a few weeks have completely recovered, the blood-pressure, blood-urea and urine returning to normal. In a few cases, the symptoms fail to resolve entirely, a little albuminuria or hypertension remaining, and eventually renal failure ensues.

Treatment. The conditions most favourable for resumption of kidney function and prevention of complications must be provided. The patient is nursed at rest in bed, recumbent with only one or two pillows, in order to prevent strain on the heart. Night attire and bed clothes should be warm, lest chilling of the skin should throw additional strain on the kidneys. Exposure while giving a bed bath must be avoided for the same reason. The blood-pressure is taken daily, and the temperature, pulse and respiration four hourly.

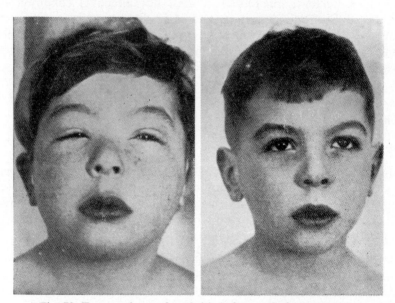

Fig. 70. Tense oedema of nephritis before and after treatment.
(*Reproduced from Textbook of Paediatrics, Fanconi and Wallgren.
William Heinemann Medical Books Ltd.*)

The urine must be measured accurately, and the amount of albumin estimated daily. Microscopic examination will reveal the presence of casts, usually of blood or epithelium in the early stages, later on becoming granular or hyaline. The blood-urea and the blood electrolyte levels must be found.

The diet must be modified in accordance with the limitation of kidney function. These are the principles on which it is constructed.

1. Water excretion is impaired, so the fluid intake is moderate until diuresis occurs. A common formula is 500 ml (the amount lost in sweat and respiration) plus the volume of the urinary output.

2. Salt in the intake leads to retention of water in the tissues, so it should be reduced to a minimum.
3. Protein in the diet is broken down to form urea, which will accumulate in the blood if the kidneys cannot excrete it. The protein intake must therefore be strictly limited.
4. If the energy value of the diet is low, wasting of muscles occurs, and this protein breakdown gives rise to urea. Joules (calories) must be supplied in the form of sugar or fat.

An ill patient may only want sweetened fruit juices at first, then fruit purees and vegetables with salt-free butter may be given. As the condition improves, salt-free bread and butter is added, then a little milk and finally a low protein diet, still with no salt. Fluid intake is increased as the output rises.

The mouth will be dry and require treatment, as will the buttocks and heels of an oedematous patient, to avert pressure sores. Drugs are not given at this stage, except for penicillin if a throat swab shows streptococci. Some physicians order penicillin in any case. Irregularity of the pulse, drowsiness and muscular twitching and breathlessness are unfavourable signs that must be reported.

In most cases, the urine output rises rapidly, blood and albumin slowly disappear from the urine, and the patient becomes convalescent. A very slow return to normal life is indicated, with weekly urine tests, and the patient must report to his doctor at once if he has a sore throat, or if urinary symptoms return.

If anuria persists, the physician must decide if the use of an artificial kidney will preserve life until diuresis begins. He may make a needle biopsy of the kidney through the loin to see how severe the renal damage is.

THE NEPHROTIC SYNDROME

This condition is one in which there is albuminuria, a low serum albumin and massive oedema. Many patients with this condition have subacute nephritis (nephrotic nephritis). In this country, a large majority of patients have had primary kidney disease. In the tropics, the nephrotic syndrome is associated with quartan malaria in more than 80 per cent of cases. It may also occur as a result of long-standing diabetes, or by mercury poisoning. The general picture is the same—the patient loses large quantities of albumin in the urine, and as a result of the fall in the plasma protein level becomes oedematous.

The symptoms usually appear gradually. The albuminuria may not be noticed until it begins to cause oedema, which starts first in the ankles, and then gradually extends to the legs and trunk. The peritoneum and other serous cavities may fill with fluid. Loss of γ globulin in the urine lowers the resistance to infections, and these used at one time to be serious, but can now usually be controlled by antibiotics.

In the early stages, the blood-urea and the blood-pressure are usually normal, and may remain so for months or years if treatment is effective, but eventually in many patients both begin to rise, and indicate the onset of chronic nephritis with renal failure.

Treatment. If the cause (such as chemical poisoning) can be found and removed, the outlook is fair. In many other people, symptoms can be improved, comfort increased, and some years of life made possible.

A stay in hospital is desirable, since the treatment used may cause disturbances of the electrolyte balance, and these must be detected and treated promptly. Rest in bed will make the oedematous patient more comfortable, though it does not by itself improve the oedema.

Throughout treatment a fluid balance chart and a record of the weight is kept. The urine is tested daily for the quantity of albumin it contains. The haemoglobin level is periodically checked, since anaemia is common.

Since the oedema is caused by the fall in the plasma proteins and the retention of sodium, a diet which is high in protein and low in sodium should be given (see page 237). Such a diet is not very appetizing, and patients need much encouragement if they are to persevere with it.

The drugs of service are:

1. Diuretics. Chlorothiazide with a potassium supplement is often prescribed. Frusemide or ethacrynic acid may be used at the beginning of treatment, but are not generally suitable for long-continued use.
2. Steroids. Prednisolone is the one most often prescribed. A course of 50 mg is given for about two weeks, and then the dose is gradually diminished. In favourable cases the amount of albumin in the urine will decrease.
3. Antibiotics must be used if infection occurs.
4. Antihypertensive drugs must be used if the blood pressure rises at all, since this is an additional strain on the damaged kidneys.

CHRONIC NEPHRITIS

Chronic nephritis usually follows either acute or subacute nephritis. This irrecoverable stage of kidney damage is signalled by a rise in the blood-urea (uraemia) and in the blood-pressure, and eventually the patient passes into uraemia (page 228).

A low protein diet is given to try to keep the blood-urea from rising too rapidly, but since a cure cannot be expected, restrictions that the patient finds difficult to tolerate should not be enforced. An adequate fluid intake is given.

If the symptoms due to the hypertension are severe, (headache, failing vision, heart failure) drugs to lower the blood-pressure may be given. Anaemia may be relieved by a transfusion of packed cells, given very slowly to avoid precipitating right heart failure by overloading the circulation. The nursing treatment for the patient in chronic renal failure is described on page 218.

RENAL FAILURE

If the kidneys cease to function, death must ensue, unless their function is taken over by an artificial kidney. Renal failure may be due to diseases of the kidney itself, and also to causes outside it. The outlook depends on the cause of the failure, and whether this cause can be effectively treated. It may arise suddenly (acute) or come on gradually (chronic).

ACUTE RENAL FAILURE OR ANURIA

Anuria is defined as a daily output of less than 250 ml.

Causes. 1. Extra renal.
   a) Prolonged periods of low blood-pressure due to shock following injury or operation.
   b) Dehydration due to haemorrhage, prolonged vomiting and diarrhoea.

The drop in the blood-pressure halts glomerular filtration.

   2. Renal.
   a) Acute nephritis and pyelonephritis.
   b) Necrosis of the kidney cortex following intra-uterine haemorrhage in toxaemia of pregnancy.
   c) Mismatched transfusion, causing blocking of the tubules with haemoglobin.
   d) Blocking of the tubules by sulphonamide crystals, which have come out of solution in the urine during the course of treatment with one of these drugs.

Prevention. It will be seen that the nurse can help in the prevention of some cases of acute failure. Regular observation of the blood-pressure following injury or operation may show the urgent need for intravenous fluids. The onset of toxaemia of pregnancy may be detected by good antenatal care, including regular urine testing, and recording of the weight and blood-pressure. Every hospital should have a strict system for checking the blood given by transfusion, and all staff should adhere to the rules. A course of sulphonamides should not last for more than ten days, the urine should be kept alkaline, and a high fluid intake kept up.

Signs and symptoms. The urine output falls suddenly, and secretion may cease altogether. The blood-urea rises, since it cannot be excreted in the urine. Acid accumulates in the blood, stimulating the respiratory centre and causing deep noisy breathing. Sodium and potassium are retained in the blood, the latter being especially dangerous because of the risk of cardiac arrest. Nausea and vomiting is usual, and if treatment is unavailing the patient lapses into unconsciousness and dies.

Treatment. This is aimed at keeping the volume and constituents of the blood as near normal as possible, so the amount of fluid given and its content is vitally important. The principles are given in the account of acute nephritis (page 223).

These requirements are met by giving a strong solution of sugar, and this cannot usually be given by mouth or intragastric tube because of nausea, but may be tolerated in the form of lactose. It cannot be put into a superficial vein, since it would cause thrombosis, so fine polythene tubing is introduced into a superficial vein, and passed along into the inferior or superior vena cava, where the blood flow is fast enough to dilute the strong solution. 500–700 ml. of a 40 per cent glucose solution is given. In order to prevent infection, penicillin is usually given, but the dosage must be low, since the kidneys will not be excreting it, and it is therefore retained in the blood.

In a favourable case, urinary output begins to rise, and large quantities of very dilute urine may be passed, because the glomeruli usually recover before the tubules. Large quantities of salts and sugar may be lost at this stage, as well as water, and very careful assessment of the blood chemistry is made daily.

If the blood urea and potassium continue to rise and diuresis does not begin, peritoneal dialysis should be performed to remove waste substances from the blood, and repeated if necessary. Since this procedure became generally available, many lives can be saved that would otherwise be lost.

CHRONIC RENAL FAILURE OR URAEMIA

The onset of uraemia is gradual, and may be due to chronic disease of the kidney itself (chronic nephritis and pyelitis); to malignant hypertension, or to increasing obstruction to the urinary outflow by an enlarged prostate gland, or a cancer of the bladder, or involvement of the ureters by new growth, as in the late stages of cancer of the cervix. As in acute failure, the blood-urea and potassium rise, acidosis develops, and disturbance of the electrolyte balance occurs.

The patient is easily fatigued, and is depressed and listless. The tongue is dry and brown, and no efforts by the nurse do more than improve it; nausea, vomiting and diarrhoea are common, due to the excretion of urea into the gut. The skin is dry and brownish in colour. The urine volume may be normal or even high, but the specific gravity is fixed and low. If the blood-pressure is raised there will be headache, and heart failure may occur. In the late stages there is deep gasping respiration because of the acidosis, muscular twitching occurs, and hiccough may be a most wearying problem.

Treatment. This is first that of the cause, and if this can be dealt with before the condition is too advanced the prognosis is not hopeless. Secondly the electrolyte balance must be maintained as near normal as possible by means of the diet, which should be low in protein.

Finally, in the last stages all means to relieve symptoms and distress must be employed. Chlorpromazine may check the vomiting and hiccough. A bed bath should be given twice daily, and the mouth treated as often as possible. Lemon juice may help to moisten the dry tongue.

In certain cases, patients whose kidneys have ceased to function may be kept alive by freeing the blood at regular intervals from the substances usually excreted by the kidneys. The process used is **dialysis,** and it may be carried out in two ways.

1. Peritoneal dialysis. This process is carried out in hospital, and the equipment used is simple. Fluid is run into the peritoneal cavity through a cannula, retained for about half an hour, then drained out again, taking with it urea and electrolytes and urea. This procedure may be life-saving in an emergency, but is not one that can be repeated indefinitely. If kidney function can never be restored, the next method must be used.

2. Haemodialysis. Polythene catheters are kept in place in an artery and vein and when necessary the blood is directed from the artery into a coiled cellophane tube in a bath of dialysing fluid, into which urea and excess salts are drawn. The blood returns to the body through the venous catheter. The process usually takes ten or twelve hours and may be performed overnight in a special unit or even at home in suitable cases.

About 7000 people die every year of chronic renal failure, and of these at least half have other disabling conditions, or are too old or too young to benefit from long term haemodialysis. Of the remainder, less than a third can at present be accepted for this treatment. The capital cost of machines is high, and so is the cost of dialysing fluids and disposables, while staff shortages imposes another kind of limitation. Neither should it be presumed that the patient can be transformed into a completely fit person, able to lead a normal life through haemodialysis. A kidney works continuously, a machine intermittently, so that the patient has a mild chronic uraemia, must accept dietetic restriction of protein and salt, and must drink only 550 ml a day. Some anaemia is always present,

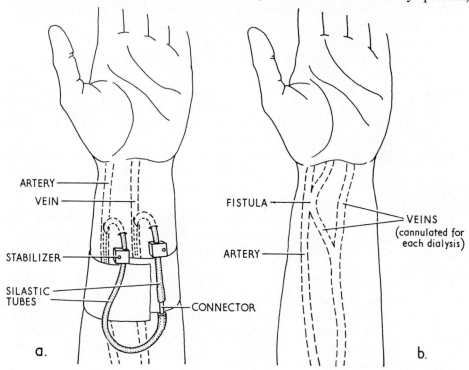

ARTERY

VEIN

STABILIZER

SILASTIC
TUBES

CONNECTOR

FISTULA

ARTERY

VEINS
(cannulated for
each dialysis)

a.

b.

Fig. 71. Two ways of permitting access to the circulation for dialysis.

the patient cannot go far from his machine, and a life of great self-discipline is necessary. Ten per cent of patients die in their first year of dialysis. There is, however, another side to this picture. Patients have been kept on dialysis for 10 years, and prospects are quite good for the intelligent determined person with the will to live.

Most troubles arise in connection with access to the circulation. An arteriovenous shunt is made at the wrist or ankle, and the two halves of this can be separated in order to pass the arterial blood into the machine, and receive it back after dialysis into a vein. Infection **and** clotting are common hazards, and most shunts requires review every few months. **An** alternative is to create an arterio-venous fistula at the wrist, and puncture one of the dilated superficial veins each time access to the blood stream is needed. This is now the preferred method.

Most physicians aim to teach their patients at a dialysis centre and to transfer them to home dialysis if conditions are favourable. Eventually it is hoped that a donor kidney will become available, and the patient will be free of his machine.

ORGAN TRANSPLANT

Apart from corneal transplants, kidney are the most successful organ transplants performed. The surgical technique required is standardized, and many first-class teams are at work. The reasons why more kidney grafts are not performed is that the body tends to reject such grafts of foreign tissue, and that donor grafts are not available in sufficient quantities.

When a patient is judged suitable for an organ transplant he is maintained in as good health as possible, and his tissues are typed so that the best match available is secured. When a kidney becomes available the patient who best matches the donor organ is summoned for surgery. After surgery, and usually indefinitely, immunosuppressive drugs are given to combat rejection. These are steroids, such as prednisone, and an anti-mitotic drug such as azothiaprine. During the first year, rejection crises occur, in which dosage must be increased, but after this the probability of rejection recedes.

Donor kidneys can be obtained from relatives of the patient who are of similar type, but most doctors are reluctant to deprive a healthy person of a kidney, especially as the pressure on him to give it may make it difficult to be sure that he is a volunteer. Kidneys may also be obtained from the very recently deceased, but these are not forthcoming in the numbers needed. All concerned with this branch of medicine agree that we hope dialysis and transplants are a temporary expedient until we can discover the cause and prevention or the successful treatment of nephritis.

SOME DIETS USED IN THE TREATMENT OF KIDNEY CONDITIONS

HIGH PROTEIN (110 g.)
LOW SALT DIET (0·7 g. Na)
BREAKFAST   Tea or coffee with milk from allowance—sugar if liked.
                   Porridge cooked without salt, puffed wheat, shredded

wheat with stewed fruit or milk from allowance, also sugar.

Egg—boiled, poached, scrambled or fried—no salt, or white fish cooked without salt.

Salt-free bread—toasted if liked.

Unsalted butter or margarine.

Marmalade, jam, honey.

MID-MORNING   Fruit drink with sugar, or coffee with milk from allowance.

DINNER   90 g meat or liver or 135 g white fish—cooked without salt—large helping.

Gravy made without salt—flour plus salt-free Marmite may be used.

Vegetables—green or root—cooked without salt.

Potatoes—cooked without salt (if roast or chipped—salt-free fat must be used).

Stewed or fresh fruit, or jelly and milk pudding, or custard with Casilan and milk from allowance.

TEA   Tea with milk from allowance—sugar.

Salt-free bread, or salt-free Ryvita, or Energen Rolls, or Matzos.

2 oz. chicken or meat unsalted.

Unsalted butter or margarine.

Jam or honey.

Salt-free shortbread, jam tart or cake.

SUPPER   90 g meat or chicken or 135 g fish—cooked without salt—large helping.

Salad or vegetables—cooked without salt.

Salt-free bread and unsalted butter or potatoes cooked without salt.

Fresh or stewed fruit and milk pudding.

BEDTIME   Remainder of milk with tea or coffee if liked, or fruit drink

DAILY   1 egg
ALLOWANCE   560 ml of milk

15 g Casilan (Glaxo) in milk puddings or drinks.

No salt to be used in cooking or added at the table.

Salt substitutes may only be used if a doctor's permission has been obtained.

To raise the Protein or reduce the Sodium a Low Sodium milk may be used in milk puddings or coffee, e.g. Edosol (Trufood).

FOODS ALLOWED AND TO BE AVOIDED AS FOR THE LOW SODIUM DIET

LOW PROTEIN DIET (40 g.)

BREAKFAST Tea or coffee with milk from allowance, sugar if liked.
Porridge or breakfast cereal with stewed fruit and sugar—no milk.
Mushrooms on fried bread or sauté potatoes and tomatoes or fruit.
Brown or white bread—toasted if liked—2 slices.
Butter or margarine.
Marmalade, honey, syrup, meat or vegetable extract.

MID-MORNING Black coffee, tea with lemon or milk from allowance or fruit juice and sugar or meat or vegetable extract.

DINNER 45 g meat, liver, chicken, ham or 60 g fish.
Potatoes, roast, chipped or boiled.
Green and/or root vegetables.
Fruit—fresh, stewed or tinned, or fruit pie, fruit crumble or jam tart.

TEA Tea with milk from allowance.
White or brown bread—2 slices.
Butter or margarine.
Jam, honey, syrup, salad, Marmite.
Shortbread, jam tart or small portion of sponge cake.

SUPPER 1 egg or 30 g cheese or 30 g meat or 45 g fish.
Salad or vegetables.
Bread—1 slice or potatoes.
Fruit as dinner.

BEDTIME Fruit juice and sugar, meat or vegetable extract or tea or coffee with milk from allowance.

DAILY $\frac{1}{4}$ pint of milk.

PROTEIN ALTERNATIVES (7 g. Protein)

     30 g   meat—ham, liver, chicken, bacon
or 45 g   fish—white fish, herring, kippers, haddock, sardines
or 30 g   cheese
or 1   egg
or 220 ml milk.

SOME LOW PROTEIN DISHES

Sweets	*Savoury*	*Breakfast*
Fruit Charlotte	Vegetable-stuffed tomato or	Savoury potato cakes
Fruit crumble	onion.	(parsley, onions, herbs, no
Fruit pie	Vegetable pie with pastry or	egg).
Jam tart	potatoes.	Tomatoes and sauté potatoes.
Fruit jelly	Spaghetti or macaroni in	Mushrooms on fried bread.
	tomato sauce.	Tomatoes and Marmite on
	Vegetables and fried rice.	toast.
	Curried vegetables.	
	Potato cakes with onions,	
	chives, parsley or mixed herbs.	
	Home made vegetable or clear	
	soups.	

Flour and water batter may be used for fruit or vegetable fritters.

FOODS MODERATELY HIGH IN PROTEIN—USE AS DIRECTED

Bread
Cereals—porridge oats, and other breakfast cereals, rice, semolina, tapioca,
      barley, flour.
Pulses—peas, lentils, beans (baked, haricot, butter).
Chocolate, Horlicks, Ovaltine, cocoa, fudge.
Ice Cream.
Nuts.

ALLOWED AS REQUIRED

Sugar, butter, cream.
Jams, marmalade, honey, syrup.
Pickles, chutneys, herbs, spices.

Small helpings of salad cream and tomato ketchup.
Boiled sweets, barley sugars, fruit gums, pastilles.
Water ices and ice lollies.

LOW SODIUM DIET (0.5 g. Na)

BREAKFAST — Tea or coffee with milk from allowance—sugar if liked.
Porridge cooked without salt, puffed wheat, shredded wheat with stewed fruit from allowance, also sugar.
Egg—boiled, poached, scrambled or fried, or white fish or herrings—cooked without salt.
Salt-free bread—toasted if liked.
Unsalted butter or margarine.
Marmalade, jam, honey.

MID-MORNING — Fruit drink with sugar, or coffee with milk from allowance.

DINNER — Meat, liver or white fish—cooked without salt.
Gravy made without salt—flour plus salt-free Marmite may be used.
Vegetables—green or root—cooked without salt.
Potatoes—cooked without salt (if roast or chipped—salt-free fat must be used).
Stewed or fresh fruit, or jelly or milk pudding made with milk from allowance.

TEA — Tea with milk from allowance—sugar.
Salt-free bread, or salt-free Ryvita, or Energen Rolls, or Matzos.
Unsalted butter or margarine.
Jam or honey.
Shortbread, jam tart or cake—using plain flour, salt-free margarine and special baking powder.

SUPPER — Meat, chicken, fish—cooked without salt.
Salad or vegetables—cooked without salt.
Salt-free bread and unsalted butter or potatoes cooked without salt.
Fresh or stewed or tinned fruit.

BEDTIME — Remainder of milk with tea or coffee if liked, or fruit drink.

DAILY   1 egg
   ALLOWANCE   280 ml of milk
                    No salt to be used in cooking or added at the table.
                    Salt substitutes may only be used if a doctor's permission
                       has been obtained as they contain potassium salts.
                    To increase Sodium to 1 g. use ordinary bread and cakes.

AVOID THE FOLLOWING FOODS

Salt.
Butter or margarine containing salt.
Bread containing salt.
Bought biscuits and cakes.
Self-raising flour.
Baking powder and soda.
Meat and vegetable extracts.
Bacon. Ham. Sausages. Tinned meat.
Cheese—unless made from sour milk and strained.
Salted and smoked fish. Tinned fish.
Tinned vegetables. Tinned soups.
Dried fruit (except prunes).
Pickles, sauces, chutneys (unless home-made without salt).
Chocolate, cocoa, malted milk drinks.
Golden syrup. Toffees.
Meat and fish pastes.
Soda water.

YOU MAY EAT THE FOLLOWING FOODS

Bread—brown or white made without salt. This can be made at home or
   sometimes local bakers will make it.
Unsalted butter or margarine.
Matzos, salt-free Ryvita, Energen Rolls.
Plain flour.
Meat pies or puddings made with plain flour or salt-free dripping or lard.
Fruit pies and tarts—pastry made with plain flour and unsalted margarine.
Fruit charlotte made with salt-free bread crumbs.
Jellies. Fruit jellies. Meringues. Cream.
Vinegar, pepper, mustard, curry powder, spices and herbs.
Boiled sweets. Sugar.
Fruit juices, fruit squashes.

SODIUM-FREE BAKING POWDER

Pot. Bicarb.	39·8 g.
Starch	28·0 g.
Acid Tartaric	7·5 g.
Pot. Bitartrate	56·1 g.

A chemist will make this up and it may be used with plain flour in place of ordinary baking powder or self-raising flour. Use 2 rounded teaspoons to 240 g plain flour. Keep in an airtight jar.

NO ADDED SALT DIET (3 g. Na)

Normal salt—no extra or excessive salt may be used in cooking.

Ordinary bread, butter, biscuits and cakes.

No salt may be added to food on the plate.

Very salty foods should be avoided—bacon, ham, cheese, salt beef, kippers, smoked haddock.

Chapter 10

Disorders of the Digestive System

Every system of the body depends on the alimentary canal for the supply of materials necessary for fuel for their normal functioning, repair and renewal. In the digestive system the many kinds of food eaten are broken down to their constituent units, absorbed and subsequently built up again into an entirely different form. Eight litres of water are poured into the canal every day from its glands, and this is largely absorbed again into the circulation. The digestive canal has a large and complicated supply of blood-vessels and nerves, and symptoms attributed by patients to their digestion may in fact originate in the nervous system.

THE MOUTH

The preliminary breakdown of the food, necessary before digestive processes can take place, is undertaken in the mouth by the action of the teeth, and of the saliva which enters the mouth from the three pairs of salivary glands; the parotid, submaxillary and sublingual. Saliva moistens the food, and contains the enzyme ptyalin which begins starch digestion. The tongue helps in mastication, in speech, and contains the nerve-endings that appreciate taste.

Teeth. An efficient set of teeth, real or artificial, is a pre-requisite for good digestion, and investigation of complaints of dyspepsia begins with examination of the teeth. Infection of the gums around the teeth is **pyorrhoea alveolaris,** in which pus forms in the pockets around the teeth. An **apical** abscess is one that forms below the root of a tooth, and the treatment of both conditions is the province of the dentist.

Extraction of an infected tooth causes the entry into the blood-vessels of the socket of bacteria, and while this is of little consequence in normal people, those with congenital or acquired disease of the heart valves should have such an extraction undertaken in hospital under cover of a course of penicillin. Organisms in the blood may settle on diseased valves, and give rise to bacterial endocarditis (page 138) unless this precaution is taken.

Salivary glands. Parotitis (inflammation of the parotid gland) can be caused by a virus (mumps, page 75), or by bacterial infection from a dry mouth in ill patients. The latter is rarely seen if such patients are given an adequate fluid

238

intake, either by mouth or intravenously, and receive regular thorough mouth toilet from the nurse. It is treated by antibiotics, and by surgical incision if necessary.

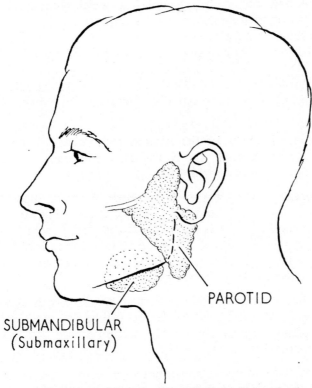

SUBMANDIBULAR
(Submaxillary)

PAROTID

Fig. 72. The parotid and submandibular salivary glands.

Stones may arise in the ducts of the salivary glands, causing painful swelling in the obstructed gland when food is taken. **Tumours** of the parotid gland sometimes occur; both conditions are treated by the surgeon.

Excessive salivation is called water-brash and is common in association with gastric ulcer, due to reflex stimulation; it will disappear when the ulcer is treated. It is not uncommon in the early stages of pregnancy, along with early morning sickness, but does not persist after the second month. Advice on having a cup of tea in the morning before rising, taking mild alkalis, avoiding fatty foods may help, and along with reassurance that the symptom will soon disappear, will help the woman until time effects a cure.

The tongue. The tongue of patients thought to be suffering from dehydration should always be inspected; if it is dry, more fluid is needed.

Inflammation of the tongue, or **glossitis,** is found in vitamin B deficiency (page 34) including pernicious anaemia, in which vitamin B_{12} is lacking (page 158). It will improve when the cause is treated.

Ulceration of the tongue may be caused by broken teeth or ill-fitting dentures; by biting of the tongue in epileptic fits; or as part of a general inflammation of the mouth. Removal or treatment of the cause is necessary, since ulceration may become chronic. In the case of chronic ulcers, biopsy should be performed to exclude cancer. In tertiary syphilis, gummata may form ulcers on the tongue.

Stomatitis, or inflammation of the mucous membranes of the mouth, often accompanies feverish illnesses, and is also caused by poor dental hygiene and excessive smoking. It should yield quickly to treatment of the cause.

Aphthous stomatitis is the term given to crops of small, superficial but very painful ulcers on the tongue and inside of the cheeks. The cause is unknown and though the condition clears fairly quickly, it often recurs. It mainly affects adults, especially young women. Attention to the general health and the local hygiene may be helpful; astringent mouth washes are often ordered. Corlan pellets placed under the tongue may be tried.

Ulcerative stomatitis is usually due to secondary infection of a sore mouth in debilitated people. It often accompanies leukaemia, and agranulocytosis (page 167). Vincent's Angina is a mouth infection caused by a spirochaete and a bacillus. Both organisms are sensitive to penicillin, which is usually prescribed.

Thrush is an infection of mucous membrane by a fungus, *Candida albicans*. It may appear in the mouths of babies who are bottle fed, and in the mouths of adults having courses of antibiotics like tetracycline. Milky-white patches appear on the tongue and the inside of the cheeks.

The mouth and tongue should be cleansed with cotton wool pledgets soaked in glycerine and attention paid to sterilization of teats if the patient is an infant. Nystatin, an antibiotic active against fungus infections, usually produces a rapid cure. Its action is a local one, and it must be held in the mouth as long as possible.

THE OESOPHAGUS

The oesophagus is the tube which takes food from the pharynx to the stomach, and is 25 cm (10 in.) long. It lies behind the trachea in the neck, passes through

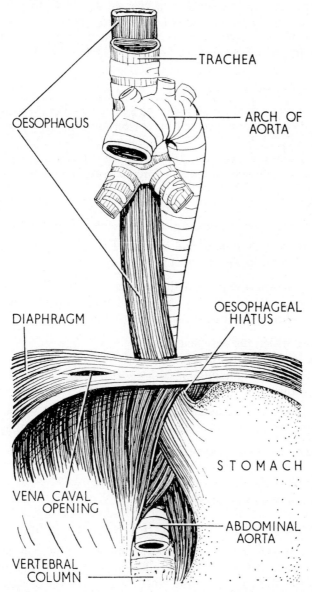

OESOPHAGUS

TRACHEA

ARCH OF
AORTA

DIAPHRAGM

OESOPHAGEAL
HIATUS

STOMACH

VENA CAVAL
OPENING

ABDOMINAL
AORTA

VERTEBRAL
COLUMN

Fig. 73. The relation of the oesophagus to the aorta, diaphragm and stomach.

the mediastinum behind the heart, and crosses the aorta to pass through the muscular part of the diaphragm to enter the cardiac end of the stomach.

Food is actively conveyed along the oesophagus by peristalsis, so that people being nursed with the head low and the foot of the bed raised have no difficulty in swallowing.

The oesophagus can be examined in two ways.

1. An X-ray taken while barium is being swallowed will show changes taking place inside the oesophagus, or if it is being subjected to pressure from other organs.

2. Oesophagoscopy allows direct inspection of this organ, and is often necessary to make a biopsy, remove a foreign body, or confirm a diagnosis.

DYSPHAGIA

Dysphagia is difficulty in swallowing, and the causes may be divided thus:

A. **Conditions of the mouth and throat.** Tonsillitis, stomatitis, and new growths of the tongue are examples.

B. **Nervous conditions,** e.g. myasthenia gravis (page 375), diphtheria (page 71), poliomyelitis (page 393) and strokes (page 385). Local anaesthetics given sometimes for investigations such as bronchography (page 199).

C. **Conditions within the oesophagus.**
Stricture, congenital or acquired.
Inflammation (oesophagitis).
New growths.

Web formation is occasionally seen in middle aged women with severe iron-deficiency anaemia, and may need removal by oesophagoscopy.

D. **Pressure on the oesophagus from outside.**
Goitre.
Carcinoma of the thyroid gland.
Enlarged mediastinal glands.

CARCINOMA OF THE OESOPHAGUS

This is the commonest cause of dysphagia coming on slowly in the middle-aged or elderly. The patient first feels that bulky solids tend to stick at some point, and gradually this difficulty increases until only fluids can be taken. Regurgitation of unaltered food or drink also occurs. Loss of weight is marked, but pain is not usually a feature.

Treatment. Oesophagectomy is advocated if the growth is an early one, but the oesophagus lies deep in the chest and presents many problems to the surgeon, while the prognosis after operation is not good. Radiotherapy is often used. Palliative treatment for the hopeless case aims at promoting comfort.

A flexible tube (e.g. Souttar's tube) may be left traversing the growth and so allowing fluids to pass. In the late stages a nourishing attractive fluid diet should be given, and the patient consulted about his likes. Thick fluid containing eggs cannot be taken towards the end, and malted milk must be used instead. Sweetened fruit juices will pass through a very small opening, and often patients express a wish for fluids with an aroma, such as coffee. If alcohol is taken, brandy or whisky with water is a help at night to sleep and relaxation.

As the disease progresses, it will become increasingly difficult to swallow the saliva, which must be expectorated or aspirated. Enough hypnotic is given to keep the patient at rest, and death is usually due to malnutrition or aspiration pneumonia, distant metastases or occasionally to erosion of the aorta. Gastrostomy to permit giving fluids below the level of an inoperable growth would not now generally be thought in the patient's best interests.

Stricture of the oesophagus is usually malignant as described above, but it may also follow injury, such as that caused by acid regurgitation in hiatus hernia, or by swallowing corrosives. This is not now very common, either accidentally or intentionally. Once stricture has occurred, regular dilatation will be necessary to keep the oesophagus patent.

Achalasia of the oesophagus is due to failure of relaxation of the cardiac end when swallowing takes place. Food is retained just above the diaphragm, and the lower end of the oesophagus may become much dilated and inflamed. No organic cause can be found.

Barium swallow will usually confirm the diagnosis, though oesophagoscopy is sometimes necessary. Regular dilatation of the cardia with a bougie weighted with mercury may be effective. It appears an unpleasant form of treatment, but many patients learn to pass it themselves without undue discomfort. If it does not produce relief, a surgeon may be asked to incise the constricted portion (Heller's operation).

HIATUS HERNIA

Laxity of the opening in the diaphragm through which the oesophagus passes to reach the stomach may allow a portion of the stomach to be drawn through this opening into the chest. This is a hiatus hernia.

Small herniae may produce no symptoms, but if the size or type of hernia is one that allows gastric juice and food to reach the lower end of the oesophagus, complaints soon occur. The patients are usually middle-aged, and most of them are women. Some are obese and others give a story of having begun to notice symptoms after heavy strainful work.

Pain of a burning kind is felt behind the sternum, made worse by bending down or straining. Often patients wake at night with regurgitation of acid.

Treatment. No treatment is necessary for symptomless herniae, and the majority of elderly patients can be kept comfortable with advice and medical treatment.

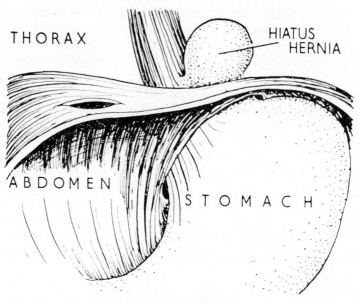

Fig. 74. Hiatus Hernia.

A bland diet should be taken, and if there is pain that shows the lower end of the oesophagus is being excoriated by gastric juice, antacids like magnesium trisilicate in fluid form or Nulacin should be taken. The last meal at night should be small and not taken too late, and sleeping with the head of the bed raised, or extra pillows, will prevent the disagreeable acid regurgitation.

THE STOMACH

The stomach is the widest part of the intestinal tract with the oesophagus entering it above, and the **pyloric sphincter** connecting it to the duodenum at its lower end. Along its two **curvatures,** the **lesser** on the right and the **greater** on the left, runs a free blood supply derived from the coeliac axis.

The functions of the stomach are:

1. to retain food while digestion takes place,
2. to act mechanically in breaking up food and mixing it with gastric juice. The contractions of the triple muscle layer are governed by the **vagus nerve,**

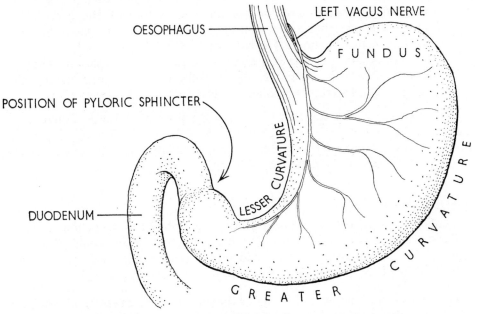

Fig. 75. The stomach.

3. to secrete the gastric juice. This secretion is also largely under the control of the vagus nerve, a fact of importance in understanding both medical and surgical treatment of stomach ulcers. Gastric juice contains two protein enzymes, pepsin and rennin; hydrochloric acid; and the **intrinsic factor,** the presence of which is necessary for the absorption of vitamin B_{12} (cyanocobalamin) an essential requirement for red blood cell formation.

INVESTIGATIONS OF GASTRIC FUNCTION

a) Barium meal. This X-ray will show not only the size, shape and position of the stomach, but on the screen its activity and rate of emptying can be seen. Craters in the mucous membrane made by ulceration may be outlined, or deformities caused by cancer may be seen.

b) Gastroscopy. Most of the interior of the stomach can be seen by passing a flexible gastroscope.

c) Biopsy. A capsule in a tube is swallowed, suction is exerted to draw a little mucous membrane into the capsule, and this scrap of tissue is cut off and withdrawn for examination.

d) Measurement of hydrochloric acid secretion. A Ryle's tube is passed into the fasting stomach, and the amount and nature of the juice can be established. The giving of test meals of gruel or alcohol has been superseded by better methods. The reaction of the stomach to an injection of histamine or of pentagastrin gives more reliable information. After the passage of the tube all gastric juice is collected for an hour, the injection is given and all secretion is collected for a further hour.

The response of the stomach to insulin injection may also be tested an increase in the volume as acidity of the aspirate being significant. 50 per cent dextrose for intravenous injection must be available in case hypoglycaemic symptoms occur, and the patient must be given a meal as soon as the test is over.

PEPTIC ULCER

Peptic ulcer is a breach in mucous membrane exposed to the action of hydrochloric acid and pepsin. Such an ulcer may be found in the stomach, the first part of the duodenum, the lower end of the oesophagus, and after surgical anastomosis of the stomach and jejunum, on the anastomosis line.

Cause. This is not known and probably there is no single cause. Evidently there is a mechanism that protects gastric mucosa from attack by the enzymes that come in contact with it, and this mechanism sometimes fails. It is at present only possible to list some of the factors that appear to make peptic ulceration more likely.

a) *Sex.* Duodenal ulcer is much less common in women than in men, though the difference is not so marked with gastric ulcer.

b) *Age.* Ulcer is very rare in childhood, unusual before 20, and reaches its peak incidence in the ages 30 to 50.

c) *Heredity.* A family history affecting successive generations is often given.

d) *Stress.* Ulcers often arise in periods of anxiety, or physical strain (e.g. after operations, or injuries such as burns). Stress is associated with a rising output of steroids from the suprarenal cortex, and patients who are being given courses of steroids are prone to develop peptic ulcers and their associated complications.

e) *Hyperacidity.* A highly motile stomach with excessive gastric acid (hyperchlorhydria) is a constant factor with a duodenal ulcer.

f) *Occupation.* Long-distance transport drivers have a high incidence of ulcers. Perhaps this is because of the constant worry of traffic conditions which induces tension.

g) *Local factors.* Alcohol, irregularly spaced and hurriedly eaten meals and heavy smoking have all been thought to encourage ulceration. Perhaps people who are tense and anxious also tend to smoke, drink and eat hurriedly, so that it is the personality pattern as a whole that is the important factor that determines the behaviour of the stomach.

Symptoms and signs

1. *Pain.* This is a constant complaint. It is localized, in the upper abdomen, in the midline or a little to the right of it; sometimes it is felt in the back. It is usually related to food, coming on immediately after a meal if the ulcer is a gastric one, later if it is duodenal. "Hunger pain" is felt when the next meal is due, and is a typical complaint of the patient with duodenal ulcer, who may say that he sleeps with milk or biscuits beside his bed in case he is wakened in the small hours by pain.

The pain is relieved in three ways; by taking food, which uses excess hydrochloric acid and pepsin; by antacids, which absorb excess acid and by vomiting, which disposes of excess acid by the quickest route.

2. *Vomiting.* This is more common with gastric than with duodenal ulcer, and is often associated with excessive salivation, or water-brash. If vomiting is persistent, weight will be lost.

The ways in which the two main symptoms affect people with gastric or duodenal ulcer is summarized thus:

	Gastric Ulcer	Duodenal Ulcer
Pain	Occurs $\frac{1}{2}$ to $1\frac{1}{2}$ hours after food Not relieved by food Usually relieved by antacids Rarely disturbs sleep	Occurs 2 to $3\frac{1}{2}$ hours after food Usually relieved by food Usually relieved by antacids Often wakes patient in night
Vomiting	Common	Unusual

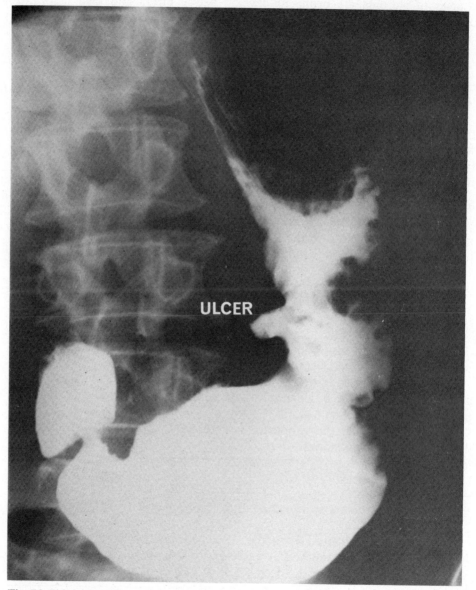

Fig. 76. This barium X-ray shows the ulcer crater in a typical position on the lesser curvature.

Diagnosis

Barium X-ray will often show the ulcer, or it may be seen under direct vision with the **gastroscope.** If the ulcer is active, there will be occult (hidden) blood in the stools, and this can be detected by Haematest.

Treatment. Most patients with peptic ulcer are not admitted to hospital, and those that nurses see in the ward are suffering from acute exacerbations, or have failed to respond to outpatient treatment, or are suffering from one of the complications of ulcer.

The patient wants to be relieved of his symptoms, and to be protected from return of his ulcer, but it is easier to do the first than the second. The basis of treatment is **rest** for the patient as a whole, since nervous tension affects the state of the stomach, and rest for the stomach.

Bed rest is necessary for a week or two, and small doses of diazepam may be given as a sedative. The food given should be bland, suitable in calorie value, and given at regular intervals. Foods which are irritating chemically or by their texture must be avoided. A suggested diet is given here.

If salads and whole fruit have to be avoided, there is a risk that vitamin C may be in short supply, and this must be made good as ascorbic acid 50 mg b.d.

Drugs. The pain of peptic ulcer can usually be relieved by giving antacids. Sodium bicarbonate reacts with acid, and will speedily relieve acute pain, but if it is taken in excess it may upset the chemical balance of the body. Neutral substances like magnesium trisilicate and aluminium hydroxide are preferable for regular use. Some preparations are laxative, while others constipate, but it is usually possible to find a mixture which does not cause intestinal upsets. Tablets like Nulacin or Gelusil can be carried for use in attacks of indigestion.

Liquorice derivatives have been shown to be effective in ulcer relief, and carbenoxolone sodium (Biogastrone) is often prescribed for gastric ulcer. Retention of salt and water may result, so this drug is not suitable for those with heart failure.

Drugs that reduce the activity of the vagus nerve include tincture of belladonna, still sometimes prescribed before meals, and propantheline.

Smoking should be discouraged, and it is inadvisable to take alcohol on an empty stomach. Moderation should be the keynote.

A patient with acute ulcer pain may be admitted to hospital for assessment and rest. He is weighed, put to bed, and a record kept of any vomiting. The stools should be observed for altered blood **(melaena)**, or tested for occult blood.

COMPLICATIONS OF PEPTIC ULCER

These are:

1. **Haemorrhage.** This is most severe from chronic ulcers with a hard fibrous tissue floor, since if an artery is opened by such an ulcer, it is difficult for the vessel to seal itself by retraction. Elderly patients with hardened arteries are also liable to continued bleeding.

2. **Perforation.** The ulcer erodes the gastric wall which gives way and allows escape of the stomach contents into the peritoneal cavity.

3. **Pyloric stenosis** may be caused by formation of fibrous tissue around the pyloric sphincter. Less frequently scar tissue around an ulcer on the lesser curvature may constrict the middle of the stomach, producing hour-glass stomach.

4. **Penetration** of a gastric ulcer into the pancreas behind the stomach causes severe pain, often felt in the back.

5. **Malignant changes** do not take place in duodenal ulcers, but may do so occasionally in gastric ulcers.

6. **Chronicity.** The ulceration-process may continue for years, with remissions and relapses.

All these complications raise the possibility of surgical treatment; in perforation, operation is usually undertaken quickly. Pyloric stenosis of any severity requires operation after medical preparation.

GASTRO-INTESTINAL HAEMORRHAGE

If blood from a gastric ulcer leaks slowly into the stomach, it is digested to a dark granular consistency before being vomited. If bleeding is more rapid, the digestive process has no time to act, and bright blood is vomited. This is called in both cases **haematemesis.** Causes include:

1. Peptic ulcer, especially gastric ulcer.
3. Oesophageal varices, i.e. varicose veins at the lower end of the oesophagus. These are caused by portal hypertension, usually due to cirrhosis of the liver (page 283) and may cause very severe haemorrhage.
3. Carcinoma of stomach.
4. Injury to the mouth or throat, e.g. tonsillectomy. Blood is swallowed and later vomited.

Blood from a duodenal ulcer may pass back into the stomach, but it is more likely to pass along the intestine. Large amounts will be passed unchanged but smaller quantities will be digested, and the stools will be black, shiny and sticky, with a smell of blood. Stools containing altered blood are termed **melaena.**

Bleeding is usually accompanied by nausea, faintness and sweating. A patient admitted following a gastro-intestinal haemorrhage is put to bed with the head low. His blood group is ascertained and morphine 15 mg is usually ordered to enable the patient to rest and relax. The blood-pressure and temperature are taken, and a half-hourly pulse chart kept. Mouth washes should be available and a vomit bowl at hand. A fluid balance chart is kept, and any stools or vomit saved for inspection. If the blood loss has not been great, the general condition will improve with rest and relaxation, and a bland gastric diet may be given. If the haemorrhage is at all severe, transfusion is necessary.

The management depends on whether bleeding is still continuing, the nurses' intelligent observations are vital. A falling blood-pressure, a pulse diminishing in volume and rising in rate, restlessness, sweating, sighing and especially yawning are signs to be reported at once to the physician. Massive transfusion may be needed, and if bleeding does not cease an emergency partial gastrectomy may have to be performed. If haemorrhage occurs on more than one occasion, surgical treatment after adequate preparation must be considered. This might be partial gastrectomy, to reduce the amount of acid-secreting mucosa, or vagotomy, i.e. interruption of the vagus nerve, to remove the nervous stimulus to acid secretion.

PYLORIC STENOSIS

Chronic ulceration near the pylorus is accompanied by scarring, oedema and muscular spasm, resulting in obstruction to the onward passage of food. The delay in emptying causes enlargement of the stomach, with nausea and a feeling of fullness, which is relieved by vomiting. The amounts brought up may be very large and may contain food eaten many hours previously, and the patient may become wasted and dehydrated, while the electrolyte balance is upset by the loss of acid in the vomit.

An X-ray will confirm the diagnosis, and the patient will be admitted to a medical ward. An initial stomach washout with normal saline may be needed, and the subsequent aim is to prevent distension of the stomach by retained food, to relax spasm and improve the nutrition. A Ryle's tube is passed last thing at night, and the stomach aspirated, the nurse may be asked to leave normal saline in the stomach. The diet should be fluid with a high calorie content, and the amount given depends on the amount of residual fluid aspirated daily. If sufficient is not absorbed, intravenous fluid is given. The levels of urea, potassium, sodium and chloride in the blood are regularly estimated.

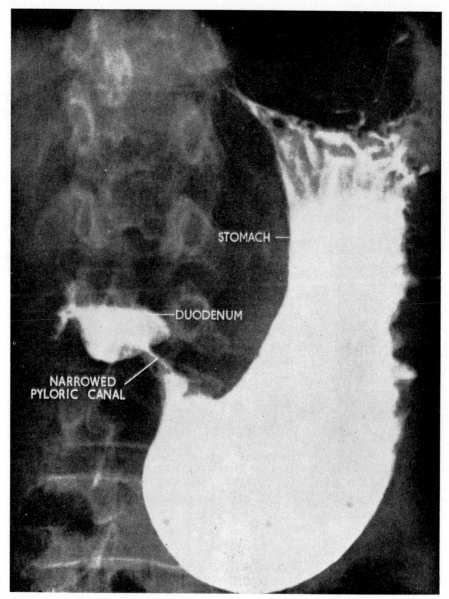

Fig. 77. Barium X-ray of stomach, showing pyloric stenosis.

Most patients improve greatly under such treatment, but if the stenosis is of any severity, surgery will be required to relieve it. If the medical treatment is in preparation for an operation, leg and breathing exercises and physiotherapy of the chest are important to avert post-operative pneumonia and venous thrombosis. Smoking is discouraged.

CONGENITAL HYPERTROPHIC PYLORIC STENOSIS

This is a disease of babies, usually boys, and often the first born, and the symptoms are caused by hypertrophy of the pyloric sphincter, delaying the onward passage of fluid and leading to vomiting and consequent loss of chloride and wasting.

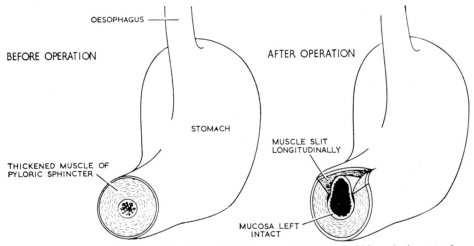

Fig. 78. Rammstedt's operation for relief of congenital hypertrophic pyloric stenosis.

The baby is normal at birth, and makes steady progress for a few weeks, and then vomiting begins; characteristically this is projectile, the stomach contents being forcibly ejected and travelling some distance. The vomit may be greater in amount than the last meal, and often contains mucus and altered blood from the congested gastric mucosa. There is progressive loss of weight, and constipation because most of the food is vomited and does not reach the intestine. The condition may be suspected from the type of vomiting, and the diagnosis is confirmed by feeling the enlarged pylorus through the abdominal wall while the baby is feeding. This lump may harden and soften as it contracts and relaxes, and sometimes waves of peristalsis can be seen passing over the stomach.

Unless the symptoms begin very early and are severe, medical treatment is usually tried first. The baby's stomach is washed out once or twice daily with normal saline to remove stale milk, mucus and blood. Atropine methonitrate (Eumydrin) 1 to 5 ml of 1 in 10,000 solution is given by mouth, and this relaxes the pyloric sphincter. Feeds must be small (30 to 60 ml) every 2 or 3 hours, and if breast milk is not available, half-cream dried milk is usually the best. Every care must be taken in the preparation of the feeds and in the nursing of the baby to prevent gastrointestinal infection, which is always extremely serious in a debilitated baby. If under this treatment the vomiting ceases and the weight begins to rise, no other form of treatment is needed.

In severe cases, or where the baby does not respond to medical measures, operation is undertaken. The abdomen is opened, and a longitudinal incision made into the hypertrophied pylorus, deep enough to allow the mucosa to bulge into the base of the incision. A careful feeding regime is begun post-operatively. Sterile saline is given first in small quantities, then diluted breast milk, and finally full strength milk. The baby must be nursed with strict precautions to prevent cross-infection. If the condition can be controlled there is no recurrence, and the child will develop normally.

PERFORATION OF A PEPTIC ULCER

Perforation of a gastric or duodenal ulcer into the peritoneal cavity is accompanied by intense pain, abdominal rigidity, sweating and tachycardia, as hydrochloric acid and stomach contents irritate the peritoneum. The usual treatment is surgical closure, but small perforations will heal if the stomach is kept empty by aspiration. The patient is nursed sitting up, morphine 10 mg is given six-hourly, fluid is given intravenously, and the mouth kept moist by adequate care. Such conservative treatment is only used if the patient is under skilled observation and any change in the pulse, temperature, abdominal condition or blood-pressure should be reported, since surgery may finally be required.

CARCINOMA OF STOMACH

Aetiology. This is a common form of cancer in the middle-aged and elderly, and affects men more often than women. Chronic gastritis appears to predispose to cancer, and patients with achlorhydria appear more prone than others.

Symptoms and signs. Loss of appetite (anorexia) is often marked. Indigestion, nausea, vomiting, and abdominal discomfort are often present. Wasting and the presence of a hard mass indicate that the growth is far advanced.

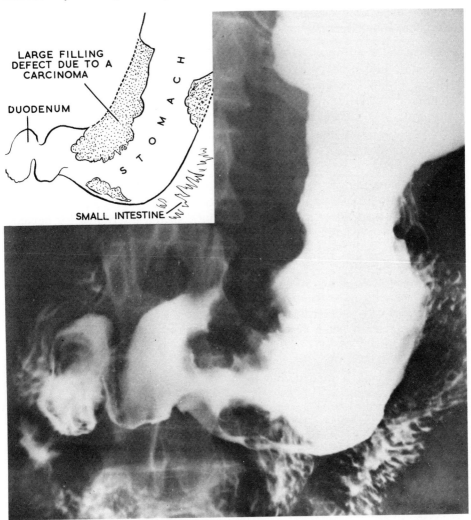

LARGE FILLING
DEFECT DUE TO A
CARCINOMA

DUODENUM

STOMACH

SMALL INTESTINE

Fig. 79. Barium X-ray of the stomach, showing a carcinoma.

Treatment. Since the only available treatment is surgical, early diagnosis is essential. Anyone who gets indigestion or anorexia for the first time in middle-age should be advised to see his doctor.

Prognosis is poor; many growths are too far advanced for excision when first seen, and even if an operation is possible, secondary deposits in the liver or peritoneum soon appear in most cases.

Treatment in the advanced case consists in giving a fluid diet which the patient can tolerate and perhaps like. Oral penicillin is sometimes useful to reduce infection in an ulcerated growth. Hiccough is sometimes a troublesome sympton, and chlorpromazine may be ordered to control it. The nursing care appropriate to a wasted, dehydrated patient with a terminal illness should be given, and analgesics in regular adequate dose should be administered.

GASTRITIS

Acute inflammation of the stomach can be caused by substances reaching it down the oesophagus, or in the blood stream. These substances may be unsuitable food or drink (e.g. excessive alcohol); chemical irritants; or bacteria or their toxins. Abdominal pain, nausea and frequent vomiting of mucus are the symptoms, and these commonly subside fairly quickly once the cause is removed. Rest, warmth, and the restriction of the intake to water are indicated until the symptoms abate, when a bland diet can be gradually resumed.

Acute **infective** gastritis is usually associated with infection of the small intestine, and will be described in the next section. **Chronic** gastritis may follow repeated attacks of acute gastritis (e.g. in alcoholics), but in some cases the cause is unknown. **Atrophy** of the gastric mucous membrane is associated with pernicious anaemia; the cause is unknown and the stomach does not recover when the anaemia is treated, but there are no gastric symptoms as long as vitamin B_{12} is given.

THE SMALL INTESTINE

The small intestine is a long muscular tube about 3 cm in diameter, in which digestion and absorption of food takes place. The duodenum, the first part, lies curved around the head of the pancreas, and receives the digestive juice from that organ, and the bile from the liver. The remaining portions, the jejunum and the ileum, are held in a fold of peritoneum, the mesentery, across which the blood vessels and lymphatics of the intestine run. The lymphatic tissue in the jejunum is gathered into large masses, **Peyer's patches,** which are the tissues especially affected in typhoid fever. The small intestine ends in the lower right part of the abdomen, and at its junction with the caecum the ileocaecal valve prevents reflux of intestinal contents.

The mucous membrane secretes intestinal juice, which is concerned with sugar and protein digestion, and absorbs the breakdown products that result

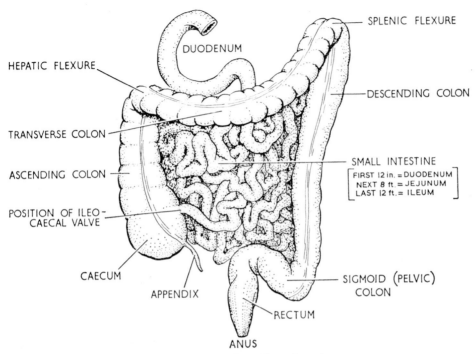

HEPATIC FLEXURE

DUODENUM

SPLENIC FLEXURE

DESCENDING COLON

TRANSVERSE COLON

ASCENDING COLON

SMALL INTESTINE
FIRST 12 in. = DUODENUM
NEXT 8 ft. = JEJUNUM
LAST 12 ft. = ILEUM

POSITION OF ILEO-CAECAL VALVE

CAECUM

APPENDIX

SIGMOID (PELVIC) COLON

RECTUM

ANUS

Fig. 80. The small and large intestine.

from digestion. The area available for absorption is increased by the many folds into which the mucosa is thrown, and by the fingerlike projections or villi which cover these folds like the pile on a crumpled piece of velvet.

Amino-acids derived from proteins, glucose from starch and sugar foods, and mineral salts are absorbed into the blood-vessels, which flow to join the portal vein and thence reach the liver. Fats are absorbed into the central lymphatic or **lacteal** in each villus, and are taken by the thoracic duct to join the circulatory system in the great veins approaching the heart.

The principal disorders of the small intestine can be classed as either:

a) infections and inflammations (gastro-enteritis, Crohn's disease),
b) failure to absorb essential nutriments.

GASTRO-ENTERITIS

Acute inflammation of the small intestine is met in typhoid fever and in chemical poisoning, but both causes are rare in England compared with "food poisoning", which remains very common. The usual infecting organisms are *Salmonella typhimurium*, which is found in the excreta of mice and rats, which may contaminate food directly, or infection may be transferred by flies or by carriers with dirty hands.

The foods most commonly infected are made-up meat dishes, soups, custard

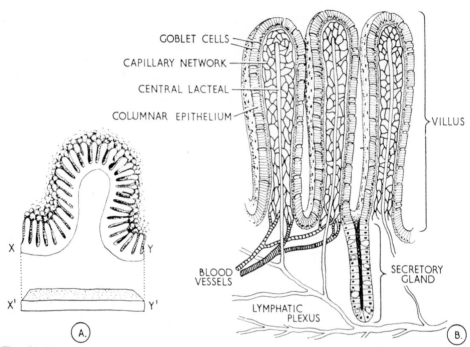

FIG. 81. The mucous membrane of the small intestine. It is deeply folded (A) to provide a large surface for absorption and secretion. (B) The villi still further increase the surface area.

and duck eggs. If such food is kept warm for some time, as in hotels or canteens, salmonellæ will multiply rapidly and the food will become heavily infected. If several people have shared the meal, all will be affected more or less at once.

Symptoms. The stomach, small intestine and sometimes the colon are inflamed, and irritated. About 12–18 hours after the meal the patient is seized with nausea, vomiting and severe colic followed by diarrhoea. Pain and fluid loss may lead to fainting and to collapse, with a cold sweating skin and pulse of poor volume.

Treatment. This is a notifiable disease and if any particular food is suspected as the cause of the outbreak, it should be saved for laboratory examination. A specimen of vomit and stool should also be collected for determination of the organism.

The patient should be put to bed in a single room, and barrier nursing instituted, with special attention to disposal of the excreta. The degree of shock is estimated by consideration of the pulse, blood-pressure, temperature and the frequency of the stools. Intravenous fluids may be needed if collapse is present or vomiting is persistent, but usually fluid can be taken by mouth, as the vomiting ceases before the diarrhoea does. Fifth-strength normal saline flavoured with fruit juice and glucose will supply water and salt as well as some calories, until the patient is able to take a more nutritious bland diet.

Antibiotics are not of great value against salmonella poisoning, except in the case of typhoid fever. Kaolin and morphine mixture may help check the diarrhoea, and codeine will not only have a similar effect but will relieve the pain of the colic. The patient is free from infection when three consecutive stool examinations are negative.

Education of food handlers in manual hygiene, and storage of cooked food in refrigerators will help to reduce the deplorably high incidence of this disease.

CROHN'S DISEASE

In this disease areas of chronic inflammation, of which the cause is unknown, appear in the intestinal tract. It occurs most commonly at the lower end of the ileum, which gave this condition its alternative names of regional or terminal ileitis. It may, however, affect the colon, rectum, any part of the small intestine, or even the stomach, and oesophagus. The patients are usually young adults, but most ages and all races can be affected. Sometimes the patient presents with an acute abdomen, or intestinal obstruction. At operation the affected areas are thickened and purplish, resembling granulation tissue, and are often separated by segments of normal intestine. Intestinal obstruction should be managed by aspirating the stomach and giving intravenous fluid, since the surgeon finds that if he resects affected portions of intestine, the peritoneum may adhere to the suture line of the gut and a faecal fistula may form through the abdominal wall. If surgery is essential in obstructed patients, a short-circuit operation is preferred.

In the chronic phase there is fever, diarrhoea, recurrent attacks of abdominal pain, and anorexia. If the disease affects the jejunum, the effects of malabsorption (see below) are shown. Fistula formation may involve the bladder or vagina, as well as the abdominal wall. Perianal fistulae and granuloma formation may be

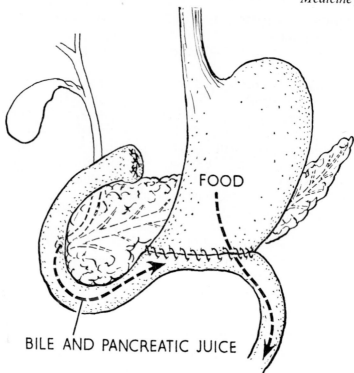

FOOD

BILE AND PANCREATIC JUICE

Fig. 82. Gastrojejunostomy.

the first signs of Crohn's disease. Septic ulcers on the legs (pyoderma) may appear, as in ulcerative colitis, and skin lesions can occur, though not commonly, anywhere where skin surfaces are in contact.

Medical treatment includes rest in bed with a low residue diet and added vitamins. Sulphonamides like salicylazosulphapyridine are often useful, and steroids are often prescribed in acute attacks. Some doctors use azathioprine, in the belief that it is an auto-immune disease. For perianal lesions, a non-adherent bland dressing is applied. Anaemia must be corrected. The course of the disease is long and relapses are frequent; since the cause is unknown there is no specific cure.

MALABSORPTION SYNDROME
If nutrition is to be normal:
   a) adequate protein, fat, carbohydrate, mineral salts and vitamins must be taken in the diet;

b) these substances must be broken down into their component parts by the digestive juice;

c) they must be absorbed.

If any of these are wanting, signs of malabsorption will appear. Iron deficiency causes anaemia, calcium deficiency may cause tetany (page 308), lack of vitamins gives rise to specific signs, failure to absorb sufficient joules causes loss of weight. Since fat is the most difficult food to digest and absorb, fat often appears undigested in the stools, which are bulky and offensive.

Failure to digest foods adequately may be due to obstruction to the entry of bile and pancreatic juice into the intestine, or to lack of mixing of food and digestive juices. For instance, after gastric operations the food leaves the stomach by the newly-fashioned opening, and may not thoroughly mingle with the bile and pancreatic juice.

Failure to absorb foodstuffs may be due to insufficient absorbing surface, as after a resection of part of the small intestine; or it may be caused by excessively rapid passage of food through the small intestine, which does not allow time for absorption; or by sensitivity to wheat protein.

Investigations will include examination of the stools, a weight record, haemoglobin, and estimation of the blood calcium. Signs of vitamin deficiencies (Chapter 3) will be looked for. Mineral and vitamin lack must be made good, and the diet corrected where necessary, paying special attention to the protein intake. Patients who have had partial gastrectomy or gastro-jejunostomy are especially vulnerable to malabsorption, and should be carefully supervised after operation, to ensure that anaemia does not occur.

COELIAC DISEASE

This is a form of the malabsorption syndrome found in children who are sensitive to the protein (gluten) found in wheat and other cereals. The villi in the small intestine becomes flattened, the absorbing surface of the gut is reduced in area, and many substances needed for normal nutrition are lost in the stools instead of being absorbed into the blood.

Symptoms begin when the child starts to receive solid food. He loses his appetite, fails to grow, and passes large, bulky and offensive stools. Wasting of the limbs is marked, while the abdomen becomes distended, and the contrast between the protuberant abdomen and the wasted buttocks gives a typical picture. Growth is slow, the child is irritable and miserable and parents find him very difficult to deal with. Anaemia and rickets, due to failure to absorb iron and calcium, may both occur.

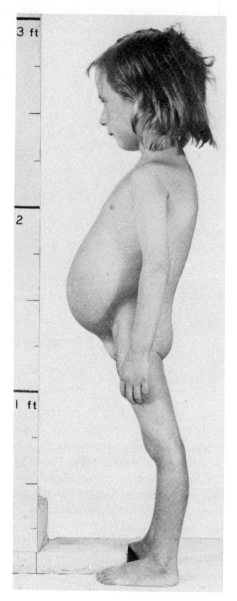

Fig 83. Coeliac Disease. The distended abdomen and the wasted gluteal muscles are characteristic.

Treatment. The diet must be gluten-free, which means excluding all food containing flour, bread, cakes, biscuits, and soups thickened with flour. Multivite tablets should be given to make good vitamin deficiency, and iron is usually required. An astonishing improvement takes place mentally and physically, and though it is necessary to maintain a gluten-free diet for some years, eventually a normal diet can be taken.

Idiopathic steatorrhoea is a related disease of adults, usually beginning between the ages 40 to 50, who are sensitive to gluten. About a third had coeliac disease in childhood. These people usually complain of diarrhoea, the stools are large, offensive and fatty. Anaemia, due to lack or iron and of folic acid, is common. Loss of weight and lassitude are the result of the failure to digest fat and the anaemia. Biopsy of the jejunal mucous membrane by a Crosby capsule shows that the villi are flattened or blunted. If xylose, which is usually absorbed by the jejunum, is given by mouth, it should be excreted in adequate amounts in the urine within 5 hours; adult coeliac patients have a low output due to failure to absorb the test dose.

Treatment is basically dietetic; as in children with coeliac disease gluten-containing foods must be omitted. The diet is fairly easy to manage at home, unless the patient has other food idiosyncrasies, but is difficult for people who eat out, as flour is used in so many dishes. Calcium and vitamin deficiencies must be made good, and anaemia corrected.

THE COLON

The small intestine enters the large at the ileo-caecal valve, which allows onward passage of the intestinal contents, but prevents reflux from the colon. The first part of the colon is the caecum, a dilated pouch lying in the right iliac fossa, with the appendix opening from its lower end. From here the colon ascends the right side of the abdomen to the lower border of the liver, crosses in a loop to the left side, and turns downwards at the spleen. From the splenic flexure the descending colon runs down the left side to the brim of the pelvis. The next part is the coiled sigmoid or pelvic colon which is continuous with the rectum. This lies in the curve of the sacrum, and is closed at its lower end by the anal sphincter. The only freely mobile parts are the transverse and sigmoid colons, each of which is held in a fold of peritoneum.

FUNCTIONS

a) Absorption. The intestinal contents are fluid at the caecum, semi-solid at the rectum, and this indicates the amount of water that has been absorbed. Salts such as sodium chloride can be absorbed as can glucose, but the comparatively simple internal structure of the colonic lining indicates that absorption is limited in its scope.

b) Excretion. The unwanted residues of digestion are collected in the rectum and expelled thence. The colon abounds in bacteria, some of which are responsible for synthesizing vitamin K and some of the vitamin B complex. These bacteria are therefore of importance to the body, and their destruction by wide-spectrum antibiotics may require the prescription of vitamins.

The entry of food into the stomach sets up reflex contractions in the colon, which may lead to defaecation. This gastro-colic reflex is a physiological fact of importance in the treatment of constipation, and in the management of a colostomy.

DIVERTICULOSIS

Diverticula are small pouches, which may occur anywhere in the intestine, but are only common in the large intestine, especially in the transverse and sigmoid colons. Small herniae of mucous membrane protrude through weak places in the muscular wall. They are present in a fair number of middle-aged people, especially those with poor muscle tone, and give rise to no symptoms unless they become inflamed.

Such inflammation is called **diverticulitis.** In mild cases it gives rise to abdominal pain and tenderness, with bouts of constipation and sometimes diarrhoea. Occasionally there is rectal bleeding, which may be severe.

Cause and prevention of diverticulosis. Diverticulosis is unknown among races that take a high residue diet, until they begin to eat Western-type food. It is now widely held that this condition only became common when millers began to remove the bran from the outside of wheat, and that it is a consequence of straining to pass a low-residue stool, thus raising the intracolonic pressure. Those with diverticulosis (and those who wish to avoid it) should eat whole wheat bread, salads and fruit, and enough bran daily to ensure the passage of a soft formed stool once or twice a day. Bran can be used as a breakfeast cereal, used to thicken soups, or make scones.

Diagnosis. A barium enema will show the diverticula, but the physician always bears in mind the possibility of cancer of the colon, which has similar symptoms.

Treatment. During an attack of diverticulitis, the patient should rest in bed and be given a low residue diet. A course of tetracycline will help to limit the inflammation and prevent complications. Propantheline will relieve spasm of the colon.

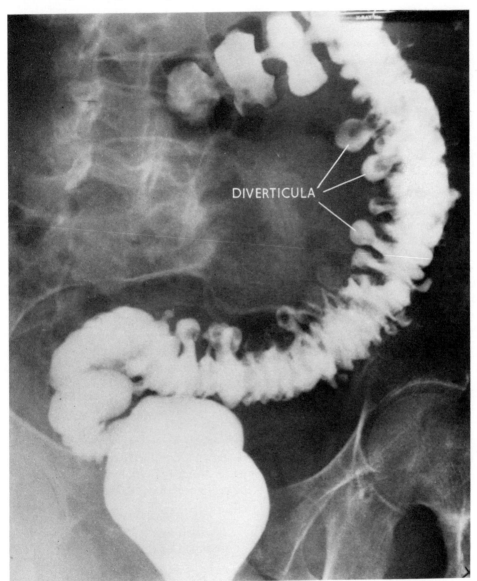

Fig. 84. Barium enema, showing diverticulosis of the descending colon.

Complications. If the bowel inflammation associated with diverticulitis is severe enough, intestinal obstruction may be caused, or perforation of the bowel can occur. The treatment of these is surgical. Vomiting, sudden acute pain, distension and a rising pulse rate are all signs that should be reported immediately.

ULCERATIVE COLITIS

In this disease there is inflammation and ulceration of the colon, but no special organism has been found to account for it. It is principally a disease of young people, which typically runs a long course, periods of improvement being followed by relapses.

Symptoms. The leading symptom is diarrhoea; in the course of the day dozens of stools may be passed, containing blood, mucus and pus, during an acute attack. The other symptoms are due to the diarrhoea; there may be anaemia due to the blood loss, exhaustion and depression, loss of weight, fever and tachycardia. Abdominal pain and anal soreness are often present, and signs of vitamin B shortage (page 34) may appear.

Aetiology. Not only are we unable to detect an organism as the cause of ulcerative colitis, but no other factor is consistently connected with the onset of the disease or the relapses. Many physicians believe that there is a psychological reason, and some patients feel that this is true. There are, however, no mental signs common to all patients. Tension and depression are often found, but this is not unnatural in view of the symptoms. Emotional stress and dietetic indiscretion can cause relapse, but these can cause diarrhoea in normal people.

Course of the disease. The inflammation usually begins in the rectum and sigmoid colon, and in less severe cases may be confined to this area. Often, however, the inflammation process spreads along the whole colon, sometimes at a rapid speed, which may threaten the patient with death from toxaemia and exhaustion.

Investigations. Sigmoidoscopy will show the state of the rectum and sigmoid colon, and a barium enema will reveal how much of the colon is affected, and to what extent.

Medical treatment of the acute phase. If the patient is well enough to use a commode, he may be nursed in a single room, but if he is confined to bed, this must be somewhere where the nurse can provide him quickly with a bedpan.

For this reason and because the stools are offensive, it is best to choose a bed near the sanitary offices.

On admission the patient is weighed, and his nutritional state assessed. The temperature, pulse and respiration rate are taken four-hourly, the number of stools must be recorded, and fluid balance chart kept. The urine is tested, and a stool saved daily for inspection. If the patient is very thin, a pad of wool on the edge of the bedpan will protect the sacrum from pressure. Soft absorbent tissue is supplied for anal toilet, and a barrier cream applied to the perianal area.

The biggest contribution that the nurse can make to the patient's peace of mind is to bring a bedpan with the same prompt courtesy the twentieth time as she does the first. Patients may be glad of the use of an aerosol deodorant around the bed after defaecation.

The fluid intake must be kept high to make up for the fluid loss, and if the patient is very dehydrated, intravenous fluid may be necessary, and blood transfusion is often required for anaemia.

The diet is an important part of the treatment. It should be bland, low in residue and high in protein and calorie value. The patient's views should be consulted, since he often knows what foods disagree with him. Scrambled, poached or boiled eggs, milk and cream, pounded fish and meat, cream cheese, strained cereals and fruit purées may be given. Chocolate and malted milk drinks are useful extras, and Casilan may be given with sweets or drinks to supply added protein.

Drugs. Codeine is useful for abdominal pain and helps check diarrhoea. Vitamin supplements will be given, and a sedative such as diazepam or chlordiazepoxide is often prescribed. Steroids are often given during an acute attack; prednisone or prednisolone by mouth or as a retention enema are often used. Steroids reduce the inflammation in the bowel, and increase the appetite. Antibiotics are of little use in the normal course of the disease, though invaluable in dealing with the infective complications.

The chronic nature of the disease is borne in mind when prescribing drugs. Tincture of opium, for instance, is excellent for relieving pain and checking diarrhoea, but its long term use carries a real risk of addiction.

Complications. The inflamed colon may adhere to neighbouring structures and **fistulae** may develop (e.g. between sigmoid colon and bladder). **Perforation** of the colon into the peritoneal cavity can occur. **Stricture formation** and **malignant change** are not uncommon after years of inflammation. Septic ulcers (**pyoderma**) may appear on the legs. **Arthritis** may develop.

Surgical treatment. Acute fulminating disease that threatens life, perforation, fistula formation and cancer are treated surgically. If the disease is localized it may be possible to excise a portion of the colon and establish an anastomosis, but it is often necessary to perform total colectomy, bring the terminal portion of the ileum to the surface to discharge the intestinal contents, i.e. to establish an **ileostomy.** An ileostomy may be performed also in the hope of allowing the inflamed colon to rest, and reunite the ileum to the colon later. This hope is not often fulfilled, and most surgeons who undertake this type of surgery believe that an ileostomy should be permanent.

Patients naturally regard an ileostomy with abhorrence when the idea is first suggested, but even in the early days the relief from the abdominal pain and diarrhoea is welcomed. Its owner need suffer few restrictions because of it; with a modern appliance, swimming and quite energetic sports can be undertaken. There are three important differences between the action of a colostomy and an ileostomy. These are:

1. The efflux from an ileostomy contains digestive enzymes, and must not be allowed to come into contact with the abdominal wall or the skin will be excoriated.
2. The efflux is fluid, and will act without the patient's volition every hour or two, and always following a meal, though with the passage of time the faeces become thicker in consistency.
3. The ileostomy patient loses a great deal of fluid in this way, and his fluid intake must therefore be higher than other peoples.

For details of appliances, a surgical textbook should be consulted. All consist of a ring which is fixed to the abdominal wall with adhesive, and a bag which can be emptied by a tap, or by detaching it from the ring. The patient will need detailed practical instruction in:

a) Skin care and the management of the appliance. Powdered Indian tragacanth may be dusted around the ileostomy before applying the adhesive.
b) Diet. The diet should be full and varied, which will ensure good health. The only foods to avoid are those which evolve gas, or are difficult to digest by normal people.
c) Social aspects. The Ileostomy Association may be a great help, especially in the early stages. The example of others and contact with instrument makers will enable the patient to make the best of his condition and minimize its handicaps.

CARCINOMA OF COLON

Cancer of the colon is treated surgically, and is only mentioned here because the nurse is sometimes consulted about bowel irregularity by patients in the cancer age-group, and should always urge medical examination to someone who in middle life experiences for the first time constipation, diarrhoea or bleeding. The outlook for the patient treated early is good. The nurse who meets many of these patients will be struck by the frequency with which they "feel" that something serious is wrong, even though the symptoms seem slight.

DYSENTERY

In ulcerative colitis, no specific organism can be found as the cause. Dysentery is the term used for inflammation of the colon and rectum due to infection either by bacilli, or by a protozoon.

BACILLARY DYSENTERY

Shigellae are a class of bacilli which cause dysentery all over the world. There are three groups of Shigella responsible, named Shiga, Flexner, and Sonne. Almost all the cases of infection in England are Sonne dysentery.

Method of spread. The organism is excreted in the stools, so dysentery, like typhoid, is most common in crowded conditions with bad sanitation. Outbreaks in this country often arise in connection with infected food in canteens or institutions.

Signs and symptoms. These may be slight, or severe enough to cause death. Typically there is diarrhoea, often with blood and mucus in the stools, fever, headache and muscular pain. In severe cases, there is shock and prostration from loss of fluid and salts. The diagnosis is made by finding the organism in the stools, or from a rectal swab.

Treatment. The patient should be admitted to hospital even if not very ill, so that he can be isolated to prevent spread to others. Barrier nursing is used, and the stools dealt with on the lines suggested in Chapter 5. If dehydration and shock are present, intravenous saline is given, and it may be necessary to examine the blood chemistry to see if potassium is required. The diet should be fluid, or low residue, according to the symptoms.

One of the insoluble sulphonamides, which will remain in the intestine and exert is action there, is usually prescribed. Phthalylsulphathiazole and succinyl-sulphathiazole four-hourly are the most useful, or tetracycline is effective.

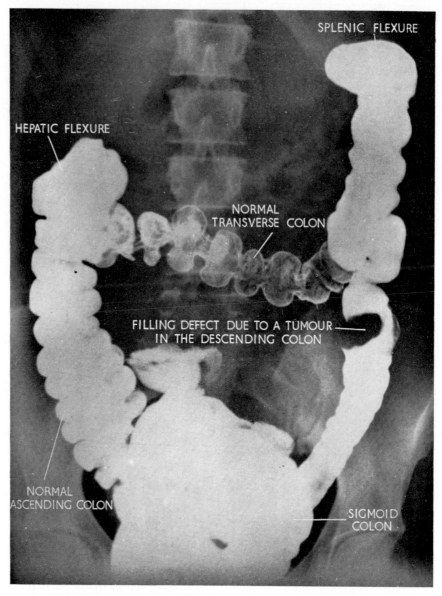

Fig. 85. Barium enema, revealing a tumour in the descending colon.

Codeine phosphate or tincture of opium can be given for pain. The test of cure is three negative stools or rectal swabs.

Prevention. Food hygiene and sanitation are obvious methods of reducing the incidence of dysentery.

AMOEBIC DYSENTERY

Amoebic dysentery is caused by *Entamoeba histolytica*, and is a chronic disease usually acquired from infected food in tropical countries.

The amoeba is found in two forms: a) the active or vegetative form, which lives in the mucous membrane of the colon and causes ulceration; b) the inactive or cystic form, which corresponds to the spore stage of some bacilli. This form may persist in the stools for long periods, and may infect others.

Signs and Symptoms. These are often slight, and may not arise for some months after the patient has been infected. There is diarrhoea, often slight, with episodes of constipation interposed. The stools are usually offensive and contain mucus or occasionally blood. Acute episodes with bleeding may occur. The most important complication occurs when amoebae reach the liver via the portal vein, and cause hepatitis or amoebic abscess.

Investigation. The amoeba or its cysts may be found in the stools, if a fresh specimen is examined. Sigmoidoscopy with biopsy of the mucous membrane is often necessary.

Treatment. The specific cure is emetine, and this is usually given by hypodermic injection for three or four days. It is usually necessary to effect a cure to follow this by emetine bismuth iodide daily in capsule form. Unfortunately, as its name indicates, this drug causes vomiting, and every effort must be made to avert this. The patient should be given a hypnotic (e.g. amylobarbitone 0·2 g) on retiring, and an hour later is given the capsule and a glass of water to dissolve the capsule and dilute its contents.

Diloxanide furoate (Furamide) is a newer and less toxic drug. Amoebic hepatitis is usually treated with chloroquine, but if an abscess has formed, this usually requires surgical drainage.

CONSTIPATION

Constipation is failure or delay in emptying the bowel by defaecation. Acute constipation occurs in intestinal obstruction, either mechanical or because of cessation of peristalsis (paralytic ileus); its treatment, if the cause is mechanical, is surgical.

Apart from this, constipation is always caused in the colon. In a few cases, this is organic, and the condition is known as **megacolon.** The colon is dilated, and its walls hypertrophy.

HIRSCHSPRUNG'S DISEASE

A barium examination in this uncommon disease will show a greatly dilated colon, with a narrow empty segment. This segment has no ganglion cells in its walls and so obstructs the onward peristaltic wave. The part of the colon above it dilates and thickens in an effort to overcome the obstruction. Symptoms may develop soon after birth, with constipation and increasing abdominal distension.

It must be realized that the distended part is the normal one, and if biopsy of the narrow section shows no ganglion cells, resection of this part will usually cure the condition.

If no narrow segment can be shown, the disease must be classed as idiopathic (page 12), and surgery is not indicated. A diet high in roughage, and the use of aperients or washouts will usually keep the symptoms under control.

COLONIC CONSTIPATION

Food enters the caecum in a liquid form, and as water is progressively absorbed from it, it moves more slowly. We have already seen that an ileostomy discharges every hour or two; an opening in the transverse colon acts about four-hourly.

A sigmoid colostomy when well established acts once or twice a day. The contents of the sigmoid colon pass into the rectum once or twice a day, and the distension of the rectum is the stimulus to defaecation. If this is postponed, the rectum adapts itself to the burden and retains the faeces often until the sigmoid colon passes more into it.

Causes of constipation include the following:

1. *Starvation.* If there is no food entering the colon, there is no residue to be expelled. This is well recognized in post-operative patients.

2. *Low residue diets.* The unabsorbed cellulose in the diet is a stimulus to peristalsis. Some people take low residue diets for medical reasons, others may take them because of indigestion.

3. *Poor muscle tone.* This is often so in the ill and old.

4. *Depression.* Patients may be too wretched to eat unless urged, and muscle tone is slack.

5. *Misuse of aperients.* Advertisements promise glowing health in return for taking aperients, or praise inner cleanliness, and a large quantity of aperients

is taken for insufficient reason. The rectum has no opportunity to fill in the usual way, and the normal rhythm is lost.

6. *Faecal impaction.* Faeces accumulate in the rectum, water is absorbed, and a large hard mass forms. If an aperient is taken, a liquid stool may be passed, but the faecal impaction remains.

This condition is most common in the aged, but may occur in younger people in hip spicas, or with a leg on traction, who find their unusual position inhibits defaecation. The nurse who records bowel actions must be sure that the stool is adequate. A knowledge of the bowel actions of geriatric patients is important; faecal incontinence may be the result of undiagnosed faecal impaction. Manual removal, usually with an anaesthetic, is often required, and adequate supervision should ensure that it does not recur.

7. *Dyschezia* means failure of rectal emptying, and is used about the commonest kind of constipation, which is due to lack of habit. The rectum dilates and loses tone because of its distension.

Children should be trained to empty the rectum after breakfast, and their programme should allow time for this.

Treatment. The treatment of constipation is that of its cause. Normal bowel physiology should be explained, and advice given on diet and exercise if necessary. At the outset of the treatment it may be necessary to use some additional means of emptying the rectum.

1. *Enemata.* A litre or less of warm water or saline is run into the rectum and sigmoid colon, and its distension stimulates reflex contraction, with expulsion of the faeces. Small quantities of sodium phosphate are put up in disposable containers with a nozzle, and these form a convenient and labour-saving substitute for the traditional enema. Rectal PLC 3 stimulates contraction of the colon and is often used in emptying the colon prior to X-ray examination. It is only used per rectum, and the recommended strength must not be exceeded.

2. *Suppositories.* Glycerin suppositories are hygroscopic and when they melt lubricate the rectum and its contents. Bisacodyl ("Dulcolax") suppositories are usually effective in securing bowel action in 15 minutes.

3. *Aperients.* A very large number of opening medicines are available, and some of these are classified below and their uses indicated.

   a) Those adding bulk to the stools, e.g. agar, methyl cellulose. These substances swell when they absorb water.
   b) Saline purgatives, which are hygroscopic. Magnesium salts are the most effective, sodium sulphate rather less so. "Health" salts all have magnesium

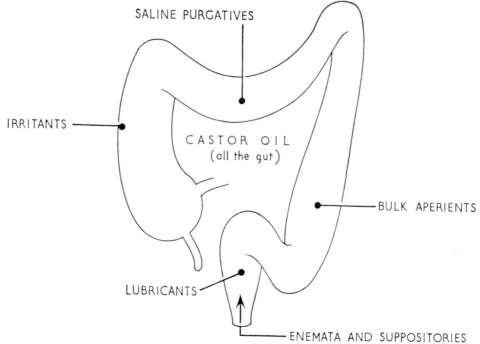

Fig. 86. Site of action of aperients and suppositories.

or sodium sulphate as their active ingredient, with some effervescent agent added. Salts should be taken before breakfast, well diluted.

c) Lubricants, e.g. liquid paraffin. This is given in divided doses, otherwise it tends to leak through the anal sphincter. Its long-continued use is not recommended by rectal surgeons, who think it interferes with vitamin absorption, and is not good for the nutrition of the rectal mucosa.

d) Irritants. These may be mineral (e.g. phenolphthalein), or vegetable (e.g. castor oil). Castor oil is now little used since it irritates the whole gut, when only the rectum may be at fault. Rhubarb, senna, cascara and figs all provide preparations which act on the colon, and are safe and widely used.

VOMITING

Vomiting is the reflex emptying of the stomach by way of the oesophagus and the mouth. Though it is often associated with gastro-intestinal disease, there are many other causes. Vomiting is usually preceded by nausea, salivation, and often yawning. The oesophagus and the fundus of the stomach relax, and the pyloric portion contracts. The diaphragm and the abdominal wall contract and compress the stomach, expelling its contents via the oesophagus and mouth. The larynx rises and is pressed against the epiglottis, to protect the airway from entry of vomitus, while the soft palate shuts off the nasopharynx.

Causes of vomiting. These may arise in the brain as well as in the digestive system, and may be classified according to the site.

A. *THE BRAIN*

The digestive reflexes—swallowing and vomiting—are centred in the medulla. The vomiting centre can be stimulated as follows:

1. *By drugs.* These include **morphine,** to which many people are sensitive; another alkaloid of opium, **apomorphine,** which has a specific stimulating action on the vomiting centre; **sulpha** drugs; **digitalis, sodium salicylate** and many new drugs.

2. *By raised intracranial pressure.* **Intracranial tumours, oedema, bleeding** or **hypertension** may raise the pressure inside the skull and stimulate the vomiting centre.

3. *By changes in the blood,* e.g. acidosis or alkalosis, or toxaemia.

4. *By cerebral influence.* **Horrifying sights** or even thoughts or memories; **conflicting sensory stimuli** (as in motion sickness); **recovery from unconsciousness** as after an anaesthetic or concussion.

B. *THE DIGESTIVE TRACT*

1. *The stomach.* This can be stimulated by overeating; by irritants like **alcohol, blood** or **irritant poisons;** by bacterial infections, as in food. In **uraemia,** urea is excreted into the saliva and gastric juice, and causes troublesome vomiting. Early morning sickness of **pregnancy** is probably gastric in origin.

2. *Intestinal obstruction.* This always causes vomiting. Large amounts of fluid are normally poured into the intestine from the digestive glands, most of it being reabsorbed in the colon. If obstruction occurs, whether **mechanical** or **paralytic,** this fluid as well as what is drunk, is vomited, and very severe dehydration ensues, especially if the obstruction is in the small intestine. Vomiting by a newborn baby may be a sign of congenital obstruction.

Treatment. Vomiting is not a disease but a symptom, and the cause must be sought and treated, either by medical or surgical means. The observations of the nurse may be of prime importance in making a diagnosis, and the questions she should ask herself are these:

1. Is nausea present? Vomiting without previous nausea is often associated with raised intracranial pressure.
2. What is the total amount lost?
3. Was this lost all at once, or was vomiting repeated?
4. Does the vomiting follow meals, or taking drugs?
5. What is the material vomited? e.g. food, bile-stained mucus, opaque intestinal contents, fresh or altered blood?
6. What is the relation between intake and the amount vomited?
7. If vomiting is severe, what has been the effect on the pulse?
8. Is the normal amount of chloride present in the urine? Vomiting entails loss of electrolytes as well as water, and the kidneys may conserve salt by decreasing excretion in the urine.

Assistance. A patient who vomits during semi-consciousness must be turned into the semi-prone position to ensure that the airway is not obstructed. A clean receiver and paper towels are provided for anyone who is nauseated, and the patient may sit up or turn on his side. Support to the forehead is always appreciated. The vomitus is measured and charted before discarding it, or saving it for inspection and a clean receiver replaced. A mouth wash should then be given.

THE LIVER

The liver is the largest organ in the body (1·5 kg., or 3 lb. in weight) and fills from front to back the space between the ribs and the diaphragm on the right side of the abdomen. It performs a very large number of functions, and life cannot be sustained without it. Its importance in metabolism is shown by the fact that the venous blood from the digestive canal, pancreas and spleen does not return directly to the venous circulation, but is diverted through the liver by means of the **portal vein.**

Liver cells are arranged in small masses or **lobules,** all similar in their arrangement. Two channels **enter** each lobule:

a) a branch of the hepatic artery, bringing oxygen,
b) a branch of the portal vein, bringing the products of digestion. The blood from these two sources mingles in the lobule.

Two channels **leave** each lobule:

a) a branch of the hepatic vein, by which the liver returns blood from both sources to the inferior vena cava,

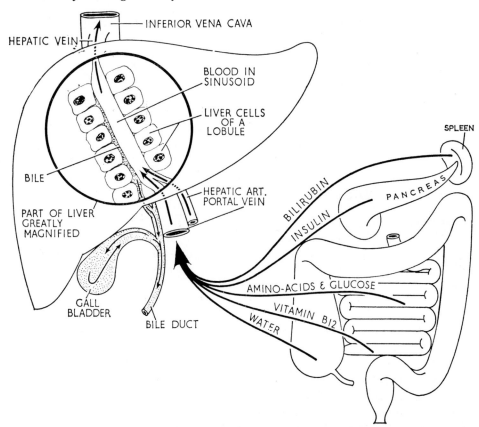

Fig. 87. The portal vein brings blood to the liver from the stomach, spleen, pancreas, small intestine and colon. Each organ sends some substance necessary for the liver functions. The intrinsic factor contributed by the stomach is shown in Fig. 47.

b) a bile vessel. These small ducts unite and bile finally leaves the liver on its lower surface by one of the two hepatic ducts. The common hepatic duct formed by the union of these two is joined by the cystic duct coming from the gall bladder. The common **bile duct** thus formed enters the duodenum along with the pancreatic duct.

The main functions of the liver can be grouped as follows.

A. **Manufacture. Prothrombin,** an essential factor in blood clotting; **heparin,** which prevents clotting of blood within the vessels, and the blood proteins fibrinogen and albumin are made here.

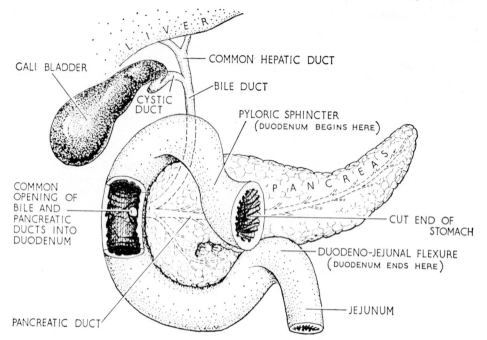

Fig. 88. The biliary and pancreatic ducts.

B. Excretion. The bile excreted by the liver is essential for fat digestion. The fat enzymes in the intestine cannot act adequately unless the fat has been broken up into tiny globules by bile, which has an action similar to soap or detergent in the washing-up water.

Cholesterol, a substance of importance in arterial disease (chapter 6) is excreted in bile. **Bilirubin** (page 159) gives bile its colour.

C. Metabolism and storage.

1. *Carbohydrate* metabolism. Sugar is stored in the liver as glycogen.

2. *Protein* metabolism. Amino-acids not required for use have the nitrogen-containing portion broken off and made into **urea,** which is excreted by the kidney in the urine.

3. *Vitamin* metabolism. Vitamins A, D and B_{12} (see chapter 4) are stored in the liver. Vitamin K is used in making prothrombin. The role of bile in fat digestion has been mentioned, and if bile is not present in the intestine, absorption of the vitamins soluble in fat (A, D and K) will be interrupted.

D. **Detoxication.** This means "making harmless". Toxic or unusual chemical substances are broken down or changed chemically, and either destroyed or excreted, often in the urine. Some iodine-containing substances are excreted in the bile, and use is made of this function by the radiologist, who can give a radio-opaque substance by mouth, and obtain an X-ray that will show the bile ducts and gall bladder (if they are functioning correctly) filled with the dye. Many drugs and anaesthetics are acted on by the liver.

JAUNDICE

The process by which the haemoglobin from broken-down red cells is excreted was described on page 150, and should be re-read now. In summary, the pigment ("blood" bilirubin) from these cells is changed by the liver into a water-soluble form ("liver" bilirubin) and excreted in the bile. This pigment is oxidized by bacteria in the colon to stercobilinogen, some of which is re-absorbed into the blood, and appears in the urine when it is called urobilinogen.

The amount of bilirubin normally present in blood is small (0·2 to 0·8 mg per cent). If it rises much above 1·5 mg per cent, it imparts a yellow colour to the tissues, known as **jaundice.** This varies from a faint tinge only seen in the whites of the eyes, to a deep yellow-brown of the whole skin.

The causes of jaundice are two.

1. Excessive production of bilirubin. This type, **haemolytic jaundice,** has been described on page 161.
2. Interference with the excretion of bilirubin. This causes **obstructive jaundice.** The obstruction may be **outside** the liver (*extrahepatic*), in which case the treatment if feasible is surgical; or **inside** the liver (*intrahepatic*), a group that includes all the medical causes of obstructive jaundice. Extrahepatic causes include stones in the common bile duct; carcinoma of the head of the pancreas, and secondary malignant growths in glands below the liver. Common medical causes of obstructive jaundice are described later.

Signs and symptoms associated with jaundice. All patients with jaundice show certain signs in common, apart from those associated with the specific condition.

The yellow is first noticed in the sclera of the eyes, and as it deepens the skin becomes increasingly yellow. If bile is not entering the intestine, the **stools** are pale, and if a normal diet is being taken, will be bulky and offensive because of undigested fat. The **appetite** is usually poor, and **vomiting** is common.

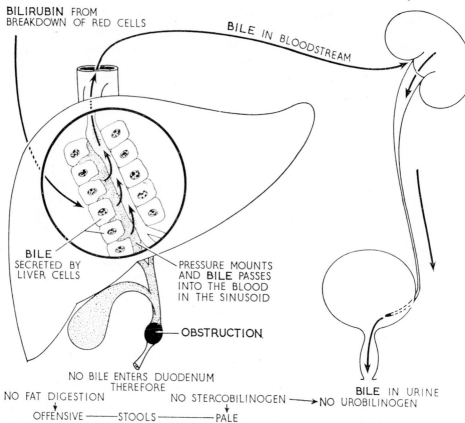

BILIRUBIN FROM BREAKDOWN OF RED CELLS

BILE IN BLOODSTREAM

BILE SECRETED BY LIVER CELLS

PRESSURE MOUNTS AND **BILE** PASSES INTO THE BLOOD IN THE SINUSOID

OBSTRUCTION

NO BILE ENTERS DUODENUM THEREFORE

NO FAT DIGESTION

NO STERCOBILINOGEN ⟶ NO UROBILINOGEN

BILE IN URINE

OFFENSIVE ——— STOOLS ——— PALE

Fig. 89. Interference with the excretion of bile causes obstructive jaundice.

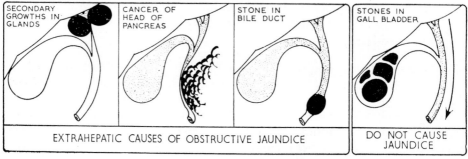

SECONDARY GROWTHS IN GLANDS

CANCER OF HEAD OF PANCREAS

STONE IN BILE DUCT

STONES IN GALL BLADDER

EXTRAHEPATIC CAUSES OF OBSTRUCTIVE JAUNDICE

DO NOT CAUSE JAUNDICE

Fig. 90. Some causes of obstructive jaundice.

"Liver" bilirubin is reabsorbed into the blood, and since this form is water soluble, it appears in the **urine** which may be deeply coloured. Irritation of the **skin ("pruritus")** is common in obstructive jaundice, the pulse is often slow, and **depression** may be marked. Because fat absorption is poor, vitamin K is not absorbed and the prothrombin level in the blood falls, bringing a risk of haemorrhage. If the cause cannot be effectively treated, hepatic coma and death will ensue.

It may be useful to compare some of the findings in haemolytic and obstructive jaundice.

Haemolytic Jaundice	Obstructive Jaundice
Anaemia always present.	Anaemia not necessarily present.
Stools contain stercobilin++	Stools pale.
Urine contains urobilinogen++, but not bilirubin.	Urine contains bilirubin, but urobilinogen may be reduced.
Appetite normal.	Appetite often poor.
No pruritus.	Pruritus may be present.

Nursing. Apart from the treatment appropriate to the cause, certain points are common to the nursing of all jaundiced patients in medical wards. A specimen of urine and a stool are saved daily for testing and inspection. A fluid balance chart should be kept. If a special diet is ordered, this is given, but if not, patients will usually tolerate best a diet low in fat (especially cooked fat), adequate in carbohydrate. Common sense should be used; jaundiced patients do not want liver, and often dislike yellow foods like scrambled eggs. A good fluid intake is essential.

Bile stains linen badly, and if nightclothes and bedlinen are contaminated with urine or vomit, they should be changed at once. Though the pruritus cannot be rationally treated by applications to the skin, a bed bath, or treatment of pressure areas, or use of talcum powder or calamine lotion may be helpful.

TESTS OF LIVER FUNCTION

The physician examines the **blood,** to find if the level of substances made in the liver is normal (serum proteins, prothrombin), or if substances which the liver excretes or modifies are present in normal amounts (serum bilirubin, alkaline phosphatase). The **urine** is tested for bilirubin and urobilinogen, and the **stools** for undigested fat and pigment.

Biopsy of the liver may be undertaken with a special instrument. Haemorrhage is the most important complication following biopsy, and the pulse should be taken every 15 minutes and the blood-pressure hourly for the next four hours. Pallor, sweating, yawning, restlessness or abdominal or pleuritic pain should be reported.

Many sophisticated tests of liver function may be used, and the nurse who wants to know about these should consult a handbook of medicine.

INTRAHEPATIC CAUSES OF JAUNDICE

Disease within the liver may be acute or chronic. **Acute hepatitis** is caused by **infections** (e.g. virus hepatitis, or a spirochaetal infection, Weil's disease), or by **toxins** such as the cleaning agent, carbon tetrachloride; chloroform; many drugs, including chlorpromazine (Largactil) and its allies, and para-amino salicylic acid (PAS). **Chronic hepatitis** is characterized by fibrous tissue formation in the liver causing hardness or **cirrhosis.**

ACUTE DISEASE
INFECTIVE HEPATITIS

This common disease is caused by a virus which is present in the stools of patients and carriers. Most patients are children or young people. The incubation period is two to four weeks, and the majority recover completely.

The onset is with fever, headache and very marked anorexia. Pain in the upper abdomen is due to stretching of its capsule by the swelling liver. Jaundice appears a day or two later, and as the bile channels become compressed by the inflamed liver, the stools become pale and bile appears in the urine. It may be up to six weeks before all signs have disappeared.

Treatment. There is no specific treatment. The patient must be cared for with all the means that will prevent further liver damage and promote his comfort. He should be nursed in bed, and precautions taken in dealing with the stools to prevent cross-infection. While nausea and anorexia persist, a good fluid intake with plenty of sugar should be given. As soon as possible, a diet of good calorie value is ordered. If vomiting is severe, intravenous fluid should be given, and potassium may be needed to restore the electrolyte balance. Drugs are best avoided until recovery is in sight; sleeping drugs like the barbiturates are particularly dangerous as they are broken down in the liver, and may increase the liver damage. Alcohol is banned.

Serum hepatitis is a form of infective hepatitis, transmitted by unsterile syringes and needles, by blood products (as in transfusion), and possibly by biting insects such as mosquitoes. It is common among drug addicts who almost always use non-sterile injection equipment. The incubation period is longer than in the usual form or viral hepatitis (up to 24 weeks). The presence of Australia antigen in the blood confirms the diagnosis.

Treatment is as for infectious hepatitis. Prevention is by adequate sterilization of syringes and needles, and by screening of blood from donors for the Australia antigen.

WEIL'S DISEASE

This condition is due to infection of the liver and kidneys by a spirochaete which is harboured by rats and excreted in their urine. It is an occupational disease, mainly seen in this country in sewer workers. It is a more severe disease then infective hepatitis, with some fatal cases. Bleeding into the skin or from the nose is common at the onset, and renal failure is the most feared complication. A specific anti-serum exists, but is only effective in very early cases when diagnosis is difficult. Large doses of penicillin are effective.

Protection of the skin in sewage workers, and campaigns to reduce rat infestation are important.

ACUTE YELLOW ATROPHY

This uncommon condition, in which necrosis of the liver occurs, may complicate infective hepatitis (rarely) or Weil's disease, and sometimes is due to drugs. Intense jaundice, a tendency to haemorrhage, fever and prostration lead on to coma and in many cases to death. Those who recover may later show the signs of cirrhosis. There is no curative treatment, and symptoms must be relieved as far as possible as they arise. Careful attention is paid to the blood chemistry.

CHRONIC HEPATITIS

CIRRHOSIS OF THE LIVER

Chronic fibrosis of the liver may follow acute disease, and there are other known predisposing factors, including the following.

1. **Alcohol.** This is the factor of which the general public is most conscious, but although alcohol is metabolized in the liver, it is not by itself a cause of cirrhosis. Most serious drinkers take a diet grossly deficient in energy value, since they do not have the appetite or the money for food. Vitamin B deficiency may be important.

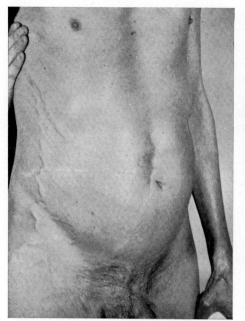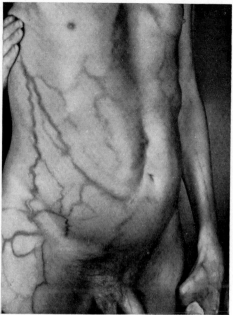

Fig. 91. Cirrhosis of the liver. Ascites is present, and the vessels of the abdominal wall have dilated to form a collateral circulation around the liver. This is well shown in the infra red photograph on the right.

2. **Poor diets.** Cirrhosis is common in countries with a low dietetic standard. Lack of protein appears a possible cause, but people who have insufficient food are short of many factors.

3. **Chronic heart failure.** Long-standing cardiac inefficiency may cause cirrhosis because the liver receives insufficient oxygen.

4. **Acute hepatitis** may in a few cases result in chronic disease.

Signs and symptoms. Men suffer more often from cirrhosis than women do. The onset is insidious, and the course may be slow and mild. Some or all of the following may occur.

a) Portal hypertension. The portal vein is obstructed and its tributaries dilate. Varicose veins appear at the junction of the systemic and portal circulation, i.e. the lower end of the oesophagus and the anus. Haematemesis from ruptured oesophageal varices is a much-feared complication that is sometimes fatal. Dilated veins appear round the umbilicus. Anaemia is common. Ascites and oedema of the legs occurs in many cases.

b) Hepatic failure. Jaundice is usually mild, and occurs rather late in the disease. A tendency to bleeding because of a low prothrombin level may occur. Mental derangement and hepatic coma are often precipitated by bleeding from the oesophagus, and are thought to be due to the protein absorbed from the blood, which the damaged liver cannot deal with.

c) Gynaecomastia means enlargement of the male breasts and is sometimes seen in men with advanced liver disease, when the liver is no longer able to inactivate oestrogen, which is produced by men in small quantities. Gynaecomastia is also seen in men who are receiving oestrogen therapy for carcinoma of the prostate gland.

Treatment. Alcohol must be forbidden, and advice given on the diet, which should be high in joules and contain adequate protein, unless liver damage is severe. Vitamin B should be taken as Marmite or Bemax. If ascites or oedema is present, the diet should be low in salt. If fat cannot be tolerated, the fat soluble vitamins A, D and K must be prescribed.

Any predisposing condition, such as infection in the bile passages, should if possible be treated. Diuretics such as chlorothiazide or frusemide are often effective in keeping ascites in check, but paracentesis of the abdomen is sometimes required.

Haemorrhage will necessitate admission to hospital, and massive transfusion may be needed. The Sengstaken tube, which compresses bleeding oesophageal varices with an inflatable balloon, may be required.

In a proportion of cases of portal hypertension, surgery may be helpful. The portal vein is anastomosed to the inferior vena cava in order to lower the portal pressure. Surgery is most successful when liver function is fairly well preserved.

CARCINOMA OF THE LIVER

Primary cancer of the liver is not common in Europe, but occurs more frequently in Asia and Africa, especially in elderly men who have cirrhosis. Secondary growths from cancer of the stomach, colon, bronchus or breast. Effective treatment is not possible, and symptoms should be relieved as they arise.

STONES IN THE BILIARY TRACT

Formation of gall-stones (cholelithiasis) is caused by the deposition from solution of some of the substances dissolved in the bile. Because the bile is concentrated in the gall-bladder for storage, it is here that stones most frequently form. They may be classified as follows:

a) Pigment stones. These are small dark stones made of bile pigment, and they are usually found in patients with haemolytic disease, who excrete large amounts of bilirubin because of the excessive breakdown of red cells. They are the least common type.

b) Cholesterol stones. These are often single and may fill the fundus of the gall-bladder without producing obvious signs or symptoms.

c) Mixed stones, of cholesterol, calcium and pigment. Very large numbers of small mixed stones can occur, and give rise to acute symptoms if they travel down the ducts.

Gall-stones occur more often in women than in men, and are most frequent in the middle-aged and obese patient who has had several children. As long as the stones remain in the gall-bladder, they may give rise to no complaints, though flatulent indigestion is common in such patients. If a stone moves into the cystic or common bile duct, it gives rise to biliary colic.

Biliary colic causes severe pain, spasmodic and sickening in nature, in the right upper abdomen or in the back. Patients may roll about in agony, and vomiting during an attack is usual. The pain may last for several hours, and if the stone is in the common bile duct, jaundice often occurs and bile appears in the urine. Jaundice is seldom very marked, and fluctuates in intensity.

The pain should be treated with morphine or pethidine. Since morphine causes spasm of the sphincter at the entrance of the common bile duct into the duodenum, propantheline may be given as well to relax this spasm, and possibly allow the stone to pass into the duodenum. When the acute attack has subsided, the biliary system is examined by an X-ray. Some stones are opaque, and will be shown by a plain X-ray. Others can only be shown by outlining them with a radio-opaque dye, i.e. by performing a cholecystogram. In the evening after a light, fat-free supper, an iodine compound is given by mouth, and the patient fasts until after the X-ray next day. The dye is absorbed from the intestine and excreted by the liver into the bile. If the gall-bladder is functioning normally, it should concentrate the dye and will be seen with any stones outlined. A high-fat meal (e.g. milk and well-buttered toast) will cause the gall-bladder to contract and empty via the common bile duct into the duodenum, and a further X-ray is taken.

Failure to take the dye, vomiting the dye, or breaking the fast before the X-ray is taken will of course render the X-ray useless. The most common cause of difficulty is gas in the colon, to which such patients are prone. If possible, they must walk about before going to the X-ray department in order to help the expulsion of flatus.

PANCREATIC DISORDERS
FIBROCYSTIC DISEASE OF THE PANCREAS

This is a hereditary disease due to a recessive gene, and it affects not only the pancreas, but all mucus-secreting glands in the body. Ducts become blocked with thick secretion, and this causes atrophy and cyst formation in the gland drained by the duct. Babies with severe forms of the disease may have intestinal obstruction soon after birth because of the thickening of the meconium that fills the intestine of the newborn (meconium ileus).

The structures chiefly affected are the pancreas, the intestinal glands, the lungs, and the sweat glands. In infancy, the symptoms are chiefly abdominal but if the child survives, changes in the lungs lead to bronchiectasis, and broncho pneumonia is often fatal. The amount of salt in the sweat is greatly increased and this is a useful test to distinguish fibrocystic disease from coeliac disease

Absence of pancreatic enzymes causes loss of fat in the stools, with diarrhoea and abdominal distension. Although the appetite is good, wasting is severe.

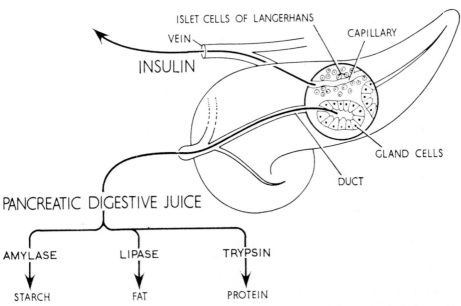

Fig. 92. The functions of the pancreas are *digestive* and endocrine. The enlarged part in the circle shows the gland cells that make digestive juice and the islet cells that pass *insulin* into the blood.

Treatment. The prognosis is poor, but some children survive to grow up. The diet should be low in fat, and high in protein and carbohydrate. If protein digests can be tolerated, they can be added to the feeds. Infection of the cystic lungs can sometimes be prevented by antibiotic treatment.

ACUTE PANCREATITIS

The pancreas secretes enzymes which act on protein, fat and carbohydrate. These powerful enzymes normally only become active when they meet with enterokinase in the duodenum. Acute pancreatitis is caused by activation within the pancreas of these enzymes, which start to digest the pancreatic tissue. Perhaps intestinal juice gains entry to the pancreatic duct through a lax sphincter of Oddi. In many cases there is disease of the gall bladder, and pancreatitis is relatively more common in alcoholics and morphine addicts than in other people.

The onset is sudden, with severe and persistent pain in the upper abdomen and back. Nausea, vomiting and abdominal rigidity are usual, the temperature is low and the pulse thin and rapid. These signs suggest an abdominal catastrophe, and laparotomy is often performed.

If the condition is recognized, perhaps by the raised level of amylase in the blood, operation is not usually performed. The patient is nursed sitting up, with all nursing measures to keep him at complete rest. Pethidine 100 mg is given to relieve the pain, and repeated at intervals. A nasal tube is passed into the stomach, and continuous suction begun. Intravenous fluid or blood is given, and the electrolyte balance of the blood maintained. Antibiotics are ordered to prevent pneumonia.

CHRONIC PANCREATITIS

In this condition, fibrous or scar tissue is laid down in the pancreas. It most often affects middle-aged or elderly men, and is sometimes associated with disease of the liver or biliary system. Both the endocrine and the exocrine functions of the pancreas are disturbed, as shown by a raised blood sugar, and excess fat in the stools.

Surgical treatment of biliary disease may halt the progress of the pancreatitis. Insulin is given if the blood sugar is high. A low fat diet is prescribed, which means that the fat-soluble vitamins must be given if deficiency is to be avoided. Pancreatic enzymes are given by mouth, and abdominal pain is relieved by suitable analgesics.

SOME DIETS USED IN THE TREATMENT OF DISORDERS OF THE DIGESTIVE TRACT

LOW RESIDUE DIET

BREAKFAST
Tea or coffee with milk and sugar if desired.
Cornflakes, rice krispies or strained porridge with milk and sugar.
Egg, boiled, poached or scrambled, or crisp grilled bacon, ham or fish.
White bread, toasted if liked.
Butter or margarine.
Jelly marmalade, honey, meat or vegetable extract.

MID-MORNING
Coffee or other beverage with milk, fruit juice, meat or vegetable extract.
Plain biscuit or sandwich.

DINNER
Tender meat, fish, poultry, offal or eggs.
Sieved vegetables or flower of cauliflower, marrow or tomatoes without skins or pips.
Mashed potatoes with milk and margarine.
Milk pudding, junket, milk jelly, baked custards, yoghourt (without fruit), ice cream, sponge pudding and custard.
Fruit puree, jelly or cheese and biscuits.

TEA
Tea with milk and sugar if liked.
White bread and butter or margarine with jelly jam, syrup or sandwich with filling of egg, cream or grated cheese or meat.
Plain biscuits or sponge cake with jelly jam.

SUPPER
Tender meat, fish, chicken, offal, ham or egg, or cheese dish.
Mashed potatoes or bread and butter.
Vegetables—as dinner.
Sweet dish—as dinner.

BEDTIME
Milk drink flavoured with cocoa, Horlicks or Ovaltine.
Plain biscuits and sandwich.

AVOID THE FOLLOWING FOODS

New bread, wholemeal bread, coarse cereals and wholemeal biscuits, fruit
  cake.
Raw fruit, dried fruit unless well soaked, stewed and sieved.
Peas, beans, onions, leeks, celery, cucumber, radishes, cress, parsley.
Roast and chipped potatoes, skins of potatoes.
Skins and pips in jam and marmalade. Nuts.
Pickles, chutney, vinegar, spices, curry powder, sauces, mustard, pepper.
Kippers, herrings, sardines.
Goose, pork, duck, sausages, tinned spiced meats.
Very strong tea or coffee.
Very hot drinks.
Fried foods, pastry, suet and batter puddings.

LIGHT DIET ALSO SUITABLE AS A CONVALESCENT AND PREVENTIVE DIET FOR PEPTIC ULCERS

BREAKFAST — Weak tea or coffee with milk.
Cornflakes, rice krispies, fine porridge, groats.
Egg, lightly boiled, poached or scrambled, crisply grilled bacon, cold ham, grilled or steamed white fish.
White bread (one day old) or crisp toast (buttered cold).
Butter or margarine.

MID-MORNING — Milk flavoured as desired.
Plain biscuits, sandwich or plain cake.

DINNER — Baked, boiled, steamed or grilled fish, chicken, rabbit, tender cold lamb, veal or ham, stewed tripe or brains, or eggs.
Gradually include minced beef, liver, hot tender roast meat.
Small helping of well-mashed potatoes, crisp toast or bread.
Small helping soft parts well-cooked vegetables—avoid skins, pips and stalks.
Milk pudding, egg custard, junket, milk jelly, fruit fool or stewed fruit and custard, or lightly steamed sponge and custard.
Fresh orange juice, strained and diluted.

TEA	Weak tea with milk.
	Bread (not new) or toast (buttered cold) with butter or margarine.
	Plain sponge cake or plain biscuit.
SUPPER	Grilled, steamed or boiled fish, or egg scrambled, boiled or poached, grated or cream cheese, or chicken.
	Pudding as at dinner.
BEDTIME	Milk flavoured as desired.
	Plain biscuits.

SANDWICHES. The following are suitable fillings if you take sandwiches to work:

Cold ham, lamb or tongue. Minced meat, tinned salmon.
Cheese—cream or grated, mixed with fresh tomato purée if liked.
Scrambled egg or hard-boiled egg, sieved and mixed with fresh tomato purée.

SOME GENERAL ADVICE

1. Take your meals regularly. Large meals are bad, you should take small frequent meals. Have something every 2–3 hours. If you are cold and tired when you get home from work, have a small cup of weak tea (half milk) with a plain biscuit and postpone your evening meal until you are warm and rested.

2. Chew your meals thoroughly and avoid hurrying them. Have a short rest after your main meal.

3. Should you wake hungry with a pain, or are restless during the night, keep a tin of plain biscuits near by and place a thermos of warm milk by the bed each night. If you do not require the milk it may be used in cooking the next day.

4. Smoking makes your symptoms worse. If you *must* smoke, it should be after a meal, never on an empty stomach.

5. Be careful to keep the bowels acting properly. Only use laxatives prescribed by the doctor. A glass of hot water first thing will help.

AVOID THE FOLLOWING FOODS

New bread and rolls, hot toast, crumpets, doughy buns.
Coarse biscuits—Ryvita, Vita Wheat or wholemeal biscuits (Digestive).
Fruit cake.
Pastry, suet puddings, batter puddings.
Fried foods, twice cooked meat, pork, sausages, curry.
Shell fish, kippers, herrings, bloaters, sardines.
Pickles, spices, vinegar, pepper, mustard.
Raw vegetables, peas, beans, onions, herbs, parsley.
Hard unripe fruit, tough skins, fruit and jam with pips (gooseberries and raspberries), marmalade with peel.
Currants, raisins, nuts.
Very hot, strong stewed tea or coffee.
You should not take excessive quantities of sugar, sweets, milk, honey, syrup, jelly jam or jelly marmalade.
You may find that one or two other foods disagree with you, if so, avoid them.

HIGH PROTEIN SEMI-SOLID DIET

BREAKFAST
0800 hrs.

Tea or coffee with milk and sugar.
Strained porridge or thin groats with sugar and milk mixture.
Egg in milk or fruit juice, or softly boiled or scrambled.

MID-MORNING
1000 hrs.

Coffee, cocoa or malted drink made with milk mixture and sugar.

LUNCH
Noon

Strained soup with milk mixture.
Pureed meat, chicken, ham, liver, fish (no bones), soft smooth cheese or egg dish.
Pureed potatoes and vegetables.
Baked custard, junkets, milk jelly, ice cream, fruit puree and thin custard, fruit fools, thin smooth milk puddings, (cornflour blancmange, semolina, ground rice, sago). All made with milk mixture.

AFTERNOON
1400 hrs.

Milk mixture, flavoured as liked.

PROTEIN VARIATIONS

	← — Low — →				← — Normal — →		High
Protein	12 g	20 g	30 g	40 g	50 g	60 g	80 g	100 g
Breakfast								
Tea or coffee, milk from allowance	√	√	√	√	√	√	√	√
Oats or L.P. dish	15 g	15 g	15 g	15 g	15 g	15 g	cereal	——→
Bread, white, brown or toasted	30 g	60 g	60 g	60 g	60 g	60 g	60 g	60 g
Butter and marmalade	√	√	√	√	√	√	√	√
Fruit juice and sugar	√	√	√	√	√	—	—	—
30 g bacon or 1 egg or 45 g fish	—	—	—	—	—	× 1	× 1	× 2
Mid-morning	Black coffee or tea with lemon or milk from allowance Fruit juice or Bovril, Oxo or Marmite							
Dinner								
Meat or alternative	Thick gravy	15 g	30 g	45 g	45 g	60 g	75 g	105 g
Potatoes, boiled, roast or chips	90 g	120 g	120 g	120 g	120 g	120 g	180 g	180 g
Vegetables—green or root	++	++	++	++	++	++	++	√
Fruit—fresh, stewed or tinned	Fruit	Fruit	LP sweet	LP sweet	LP	LP	LP	LP
Tea								
Tea, milk from allowance	√	√	√	√	√	√	√	√
Bread	30 g	30 g	30 g	60 g	60 g	60 g	60 g	60 g
Butter and jam, honey	√	√	√	√	√	√	√	√
	Salad	Salad	Salad	Shortbread, jam tart or cake				
Supper								
Meat or alternative	Thick gravy	LP dish	LP dish	30 g	45 g	45 g	60 g	75 g
Potatoes	90 g	90 g	90 g	90 g	120 g	120 g	120 g	120 g
Salad or vegetables	++	++	++	++	++	++	++	√
Sweet	Fruit	Fruit	Fruit	Fruit	Fruit	Fruit	Milk pudding	
Bedtime	← — As mid-morning — →						Cocoa Horlicks Ovaltine etc. with milk from allowance	
Daily milk	Lemon	60 ml	150 ml	150 ml	300 ml	300 ml	450 ml	600 ml

TEA	Tea with milk and sugar.
1600 hrs.	Junket, milk jelly, jelly and cream, jelly whip, mousse, baked custard, ice cream, yoghourt.
EVENING MEAL	Strained soup made with milk mixture.
1800 hrs.	Main course as at midday.
	Sweet as at lunch.
DURING	Milk mixture with egg or other flavouring.
EVENING	
2000 hrs.	
BEDTIME	Milk mixture flavoured with cocoa or malted milk drink.

TO INCREASE MILK MIXTURE, PROTEIN AND CALORIES. 1½ pts. milk and 60 g skim milk powder, or 60 g Complan (Glaxo). An egg may be added to milk puddings and porridge.

TO PUREE foods use either a sieve or liquidizer. If these are not available meat may be minced three times and plenty of thickened gravy added. Mashed potatoes and cooked vegetables may be pushed through a sieve and then re-heated. A sieve with a 10–12 cm diameter is most convenient. In an emergency, tins of strained baby foods may be used.

LOW FAT DIET (35 g)

BREAKFAST	Grapefruit or fruit juice with sugar.
	Cereals or porridge with skimmed milk from allowance and sugar.
	Lean bacon, ham, fish or egg.
	White or brown bread with scraping of butter from allowance.
	Marmalade, honey, syrup, meat or vegetable extract.
	Tea or coffee with skimmed milk from allowance.
MID-MORNING	Tea or coffee with skimmed milk from allowance.
	Fruit juices or meat and vegetable extract.
LUNCH	Lean meat or fish—see list.
	Green, root vegetables or salads.
	Boiled potatoes, or baked in the jacket.
	Fruit, jelly or milk pudding made with skimmed milk.
	Tea or coffee made with skimmed milk from allowance.

TEA White or brown bread with scraping of butter from allowance.
Jam, honey or syrup, meat or vegetable extract.
Salad and/or lean meat if desired.
Tea or coffee with skimmed milk from allowance.

EVENING MEAL Lean meat or fish—see list.
Green, root vegetables or salad.
Boiled potatoes or bread and scraping of butter from allowance.
Fruit or pudding as lunch.
Tea or coffee with skimmed milk from allowance.

LATE SUPPER Tea or coffee with skimmed milk from allowance.
Fruit juices, meat or vegetable extract.

DAILY 1 pt. separated milk or powdered skim milk.
15 g butter or margarine. (120 g to last 8 days).

YOU MAY HAVE

Milk—Skimmed or dried skimmed milk.
Meats—Grilled, steamed, boiled or roast lean beef, lamb, veal, ham, bacon, chicken, corned beef—all without fat.
Offal—Kidney, liver, hearts, tripe, sweetbreads.
Poultry—Chicken, turkey, rabbit.
Fish—White fish, smoked haddock, shell fish, soft roes.
Egg—Egg whites, whole eggs, not more than one a day.
Cheese—Made from skimmed milk.
Vegetables—Boiled, green or root vegetables. Potatoes may be boiled, or baked in their jackets.
Fruit—All fruit—fresh, canned, stewed or dried, fruit juices.
Pudding—Jellies, skimmed milk puddings, fat free yoghourt.
Preserves—Jams, marmalade, honey, syrup, meat and vegetable extracts.
Beverages—Tea, coffee, black with lemon or skimmed milk from allowance, water, fruit squash.
Sweets—Boiled sweets, jellies, pastilles, liquorice, sugar and glucose.
Sauces—Made with skimmed milk and no added fat.

YOU MAY NOT HAVE

Fried foods, cream, dripping, oil, salad cream, mayonnaise.

Pork, luncheon meats, tongue, sausages, goose, duck and all fat meat.

Herrings, eels, salmon, bloaters, cheese, cream cheese, savoury tinned products.

Fried and roast potatoes and vegetables, Yorkshire puddings, fritters, potato crisps.

All puddings, pastries and cakes.

Rich sweet biscuits, cream crackers and shortbread.

Chocolates, toffees, butterscotch and marzipan, nuts, cocoa and malted milk drinks.

Milk except as stated, tinned milk, yoghourt, ice cream.

Lemon curd, peanut butter, meat and fish pastes, chocolate spreads.

Extra butter or margarine.

Chapter 11

Diseases of the Endocrine Glands

There are two systems in the body concerned with communication; the nervous system, which is able to register action and reaction with great rapidity, and the **Endocrine system.** Most glands are exocrine ones and discharge their secretion down a duct onto the surface of the skin, or onto the mucous membranes lining one of its systems. The secretions of the endocrine glands, called **hormones,** pass directly into the blood vessels with which such glands are richly supplied, and so can exert their effect on widely separated structures in the body. The organs that make such hormones include:—

1. The pituitary gland.
2. The thyroid.
3. The parathyroids.
4. The islets of Langerhans in the pancreas.
5. The suprarenal glands.
6. The sex glands, male and female.

The widespread and complex functions of these glands do not attract notice when they are proceeding normally, but excessive (hyper-) secretion, and diminished (hypo-) secretion both occur and cause disease-states. Hyper-secretion is usually treated by surgery, or using drugs or radiotherapy to depress the gland's action. Undersecretion can often be rationally and satis-factorily treated by giving the missing hormone, or a man-made substance resembling it.

THE PITUITARY GLAND

This little gland (2 cm across) is attached to the lower surface of the brain by the hypothalamus, and lies in a hollow of the sphenoid bone in the base of the skull called the pituitary fossa. Immediately in front of it is the crossing (chiasma) of the optic nerves. The hypothalamus and pituitary gland are closely connected physiologically as well as in anatomy, and pituitary output is controlled in the hypothalamus. The anterior lobe secretes hormones controlling the endocrine output of the thyroid, the sex glands and the suprarenal cortex, and one regu-

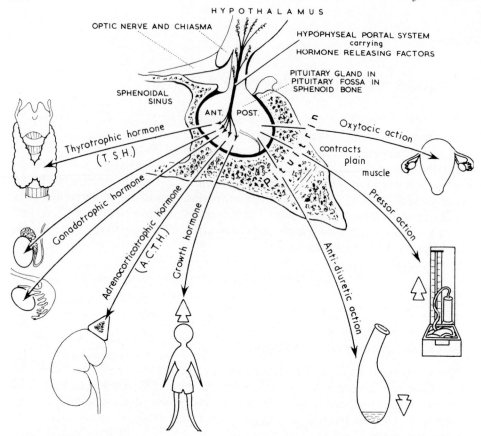

Fig. 93. A diagram to show the relations of the pituitary gland or a summary of its functions.

lating growth. The posterior lobe secretion contracts plain muscle, raises the blood-pressure, and decreases the amount of urine secreted.

OVER-SECRETION

Overproduction of the growth hormone in youth causes gigantism by excessive bone growth. In adults it causes **acromegaly,** in which the overgrowth is confined to the bones and tissues of the face and extremities. These gradually increase in size, and the large feet, spade-shaped hands and massive jaw are characteristic. Patients are sensitive about their changed appearance, and often suffer from

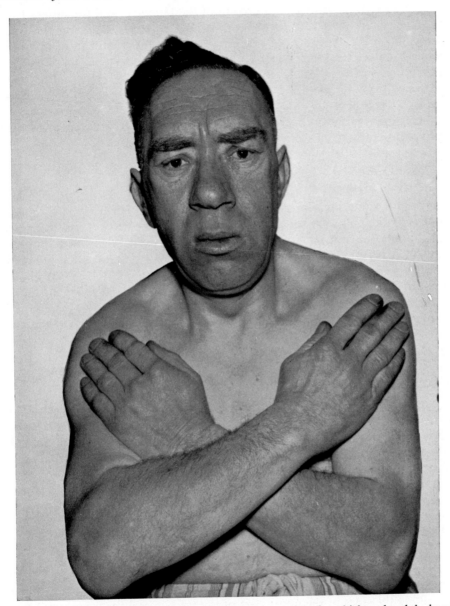

Fig. 94. Acromegaly. The skull is enlarged, the soft tissues of the face thickened and the hands spade-shaped.

very severe headache if there is a growth of the pituitary, and sometimes from interference with sight due to pressure of the enlarged gland on the optic chiasma. Bromocriptine, a drug first developed for the treatment of infertility in women, can control the excessive output of growth hormone, and if changes in the face and extremities are not too advanced will reverse them. Drug treatment seems likely to supersede radiotherapy and surgical removal of the gland as forms of treatment

Oversecretion of the cortical stimulating hormone (ACTH) causes symptoms due to excess suprarenal secretion, and is described on page 321.

UNDER-SECRETION by the ANTERIOR LOBE
SIMMONDS' DISEASE

Atrophy of the anterior lobe of the pituitary will cause its hormones to disappear from the blood, and since these hormones stimulate the thyroid and the suprarenals, to put out their secretion, the effect may be a very widespread hormone failure. It is usually due to thrombosis of the pituitary artery, often following childbirth, or sometimes destruction by a tumour.

Loss of body hair, pallor, weakness, low blood sugar, and low temperature are among the many signs that may occur.

Treatment. A tumour may be treated by surgery or radiotherapy. If the condition is due to thrombosis it cannot be cured, and substitute hormone therapy will be necessary for life.

UNDER-SECRETION by the POSTERIOR LOBE

Lack of the pituitary water-balancing hormone may follow surgical destruction of the pituitary gland in the treatment of malignant disease, or may arise without a known cause. The condition produced is *diabetes insipidus,* and the leading symptom is the passage of very large quantities of dilute urine and a correspondingly severe thirst.

The hormone can be supplied in the form of intramuscular pitressin tannate in oil, or as a snuff, which is inhaled and absorbed from the nasal mucous membrane. The symptoms in some cases tend to grow less severe as time passes, and the other water-balancing mechanisms of the body come into action.

THE THYROID GLAND

The thyroid is a gland which has a large blood supply, and consists of two lobes lying along the sides of the upper part of the trachea and the larynx, and these are joined in the middle by a bridge of tissue, the isthmus. Behind it lie the two recurrent laryngeal nerves on their way to the larynx, and the four parathyroid glands. All these relations are of great importance to the physician and the surgeon who treat diseases of the thyroid.

Iodine is necessary for the formation of thyroxine, the principal hormone of the thyroid gland. It must be taken in the food in adequate amounts if health is to be maintained. Iodine is found in sea fish, in water near the sea, and in foods to which it is often added, such as table salt. Thyroxine acts on most tissues in the body, and governs their rate of metabolism. Normal secretion of thryoxine is

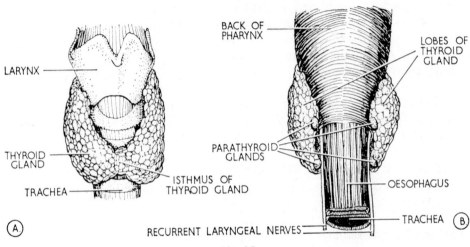

Fig. 95.

A. The thyroid gland, larynx and trachea, anterior view.

B. Posterior view, showing the relation of the parathyroids to the thyroid gland. Notice the position of the recurrent laryngeal nerves.

necessary for physical and mental activity. Calcitonin is a hormone that lowers the blood calcium level. It is produced not only in the thyroid but in the parathyroid and thymus glands.

The way in which the amount of thyroid hormone in the blood is regulated is the same as that of many other hormones, and it must be known if one is to understand the details of treatment of those patients who have hormonal disturbances. The pituitary secretes a thyroid-stimulating hormone (TSH) which causes increased output of thyroxine; as the level of thyroxine in the blood rises this acts on the pituitary and decreases the secretion of TSH. This is like the use of the accelerator when driving a car. Pressure on the accelerator raises the engine speed; as this rises to the desired level the pressure is slackened, until the speed falls and causes the driver once more to press down the accelerator.

A goitre is a swelling of the thyroid gland, and is found in people who are secreting too little thyroxine, as well as too much. The following varieties may be met.

1. **Endemic goitre.** This is due to lack of iodine, and is not uncommon in areas distant from the sea, such as Switzerland, or even Derbyshire. It can be prevented and also cured by the administration of iodine.

2. **Puberty goitre.** Swelling of the thyroid in girls at puberty may be due to excessive stimulation of the thyroid by the pituitary. Often the swelling is slight and rights itself without treatment.

3. **Hypothyroid goitre.** Goitre can be caused by under-secretion; this condition is discussed on page 306.

4. **Toxic goitre.** Over-secretion of thyroxine can be associated with diffuse or with nodular enlargement of the gland, or with the presence of an adenoma.

5. **Cancer of the thyroid** is not uncommon.

OVER-SECRETION; THYROTOXICOSIS or TOXIC GOITRE

Incidence. Women are affected eight times more often than men, and children only occasionally suffer from thyrotoxicosis.

Signs and Symptoms. The patient often complains of "nerves", and says that though her appetite is good, she is losing weight. Exophthalmos, or prominence of the eyes, is most common in younger patients, and lid retraction may expose the white of the eye all round the iris, giving a startled expression. The pulse is rapid, the skin warm and moist, and a fine tremor may be seen in the outstretched fingers. Frequently the thyroid gland is enlarged, and this may cause a change in the voice and a slight cough. In older women, the complaints may be of breathlessness and swollen ankles, and the pulse is irregular. These signs show that the heart is beginning to fail. The nurse finds the thyrotoxic patient restless and jumpy, knocking over articles on her locker or dropping them on the floor; she is prone to marked swings of mood, and needs tactful and calm kindliness.

Investigations. The pulse is taken four-hourly, and if it is irregular the apex as well as the radial rate must be taken, as atrial fibrillation (page 122) is not uncommon. A record of the pulse rate during sleep is made, because a pulse

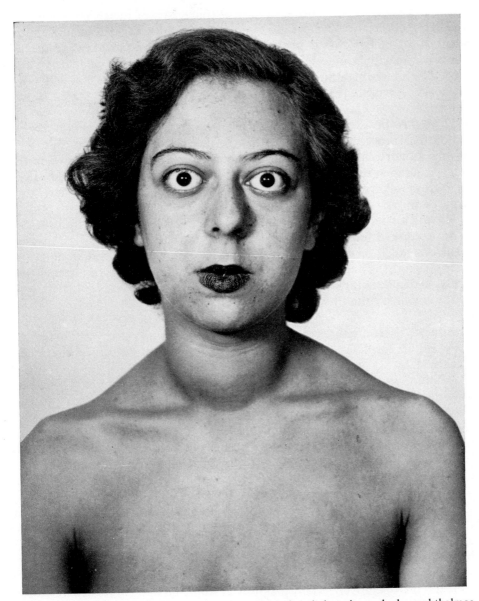

Fig. 96. Thyrotoxicosis. The thyroid gland is enlarged and there is marked exophthalmos.

rate that remains raised during sleep is characteristic of hyperthyroidism. The weight is recorded weekly, an intake and output chart kept, and the urine tested. Sugar is sometimes passed in the urine until the thyrotoxicosis is controlled. The basic metabolic rate is estimated by finding the rate at which oxygen is used. This simple breathing test is not a very discriminating test and better ones now exist. For instance, the amount of thyroxine in the blood can be directly estimated.

The iodine uptake test depends on the fact that the thyroid gland takes up radioactive iodine, whose presence can be detected by the Geiger counter, as readily as normal iodine. The patient must omit medicines and foods that contain iodine (such as sea-fish) from the diet, and should not have had an X-ray involving taking radio-opaque substances within the last three months.

Thyroid scanning (scintillography) is carried out following the administration of an isotope of technetium rather than of radioactive iodine (I^{131}) because it involves a much smaller dose of radiation. The scan is performed an hour after after giving the isotope, and is useful in showing the presence of a retrosternal goitre, and in deciding whether nodules in the gland are active.

The amount of thyrotoxine in the blood can be directly estimated.

Treatment. There are three methods of reducing the over-activity of the thyroid, each suitable for different types of patient. These are drugs, surgery and radio-active iodine.

a) Anti-thyroid drugs. These inhibit the production of thyroxine, and are suitable for most young patients. Carbimazole, beginning with a dose of 10–20 mg t.d.s., is the most widely used, but methyl thiouracil can be tried if carbimazole is not well tolerated. All these drugs can depress the bone marrow, and can on rare occasions cause a dangerous decrease in the white blood cells. Patients should be warned to report a sore throat at once, and should be given penicillin to protect them against infection until the leucocyte count becomes normal. Jaundice, skin rashes and fever are other undesirable side-effects.

b) Partial thyroidectomy. Middle-aged women with atrial fibrillation; those with a much-enlarged gland; those with nodular goitres; and patients who are not prepared to submit to a medical regime that may last a year, may be treated by surgery. Careful medical preparation is essential, and Lugol's iodine 0·6 ml t.d.s. in milk, or tablets of potassium iodide, is given for a fortnight pre-operatively. Many people who would be suitably treated by surgery are now often given the next kind of treatment.

c) Radioactive iodine. This treatment is generally used for those of middle

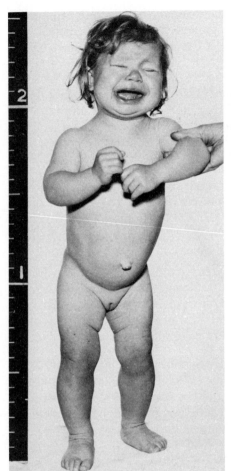 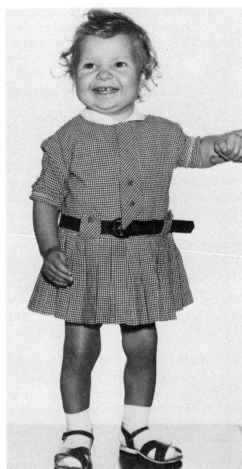

Fig. 97. This little girl is a cretin. The effect of six months' treatment with thyroxine is seen on the right.

age and over, since there is a possibility that cancer may be produced at a later date. A larger dose of radioactive iodine is given by mouth, taken up by the thyroid gland, and irradiates and destroys the secretory tissue.

Nursing. The patient having treatment in hospital requires a bed in a quiet position, with neighbours who will not arouse anxiety. Blankets should be few, as thyrotoxic patients feel the heat, and there should be adequate supporting pillows. Rest should be encouraged—the patient should remain in bed, and should be washed by her nurse. Sweating is free, and a daily blanket bath is given.

The diet should be generous if the weight is low. Protein is given freely and sugar is useful and can be given as sweet malted milk or chocolate drinks jams and jellies, while cream on desserts is a useful generous addition. The nurse should notice if the lids fail to cover the eyes when the patient is asleep and should report this, since failure to do this can lead to ulceration of the cornea and even blindness.

Treatment. Sedation by diazepam in regular small doses is valuable for all thryrotoxic patients, and if atrial fibrillation is present, digitalis (page 126) is given until the heart beat is controlled.

HYPOTHYROIDISM

A baby with congenital inability of the thyroid gland to secrete thyroxine is a **cretin.** When the signs are fully developed, the condition is easy to recognize. The baby is usually heavy at birth, often more than 9 lb., with a distended abdomen and an umbilical hernia. Physical and mental development is slow, the skin is dry, and the enlarged tongue may protrude from the mouth.

Treatment. Thyroxine by mouth will improve the physical symptoms markedly, and the mental deficiency to an extent that depends on when treatment is begun. Thyroxine must be taken throughout life, and the nurse should impress on the mother of a cretin how dependent he is on regular administration of his medicine for development, since without it he will be mentally subnormal.

ACQUIRED HYPOTHYROIDISM

This is called **myxoedema.** Though it can occur at any age or in either sex, it is most common in women of post-menopausal age. It may arise apparently spontaneously, or follow thyroidectomy or treatment with radioactive iodine.

Signs. These are those of lowered metabolic rate. The patient becomes slow mentally and physically, puts on weight, and feels the cold. The face seems swollen with an opaque skin and a flush on the cheeks, while the hair is thin and dull. The pulse is slow, anaemia is common, and thought and speech are slow. Mental derangement with delusion and attacks of depression are sometimes seen. The basal metabolic rate is low.

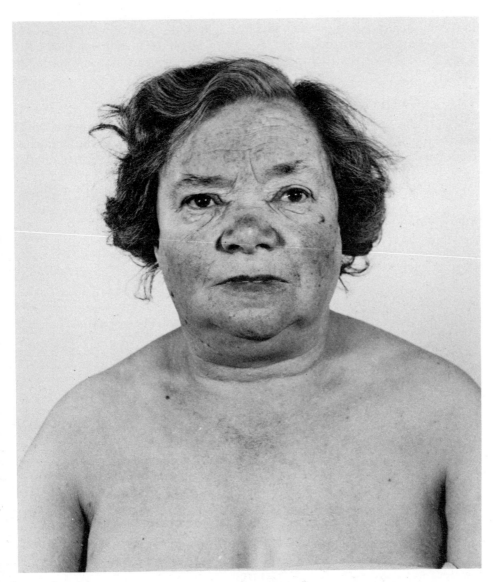

Fig. 98. Myxoedema.

Treatment. Thyroxine 0·1 mg is given as a starting dose, and may be increased to 0·2 mg if response is not seen in a fortnight. Improvement will be shown by a rising pulse and metabolic rate. A diet of about 1000 calories (4200 kJ) is given if obesity persists after treatment, and the patient encouraged to persevere with it.

THE PARATHYROID GLANDS

The hormone secreted by the four parathyroid glands is parathormone, which has the function of raising the level of calcium in the blood by releasing calcium from bone, and controls the reabsorption of phosphorus in the kidney tubules.

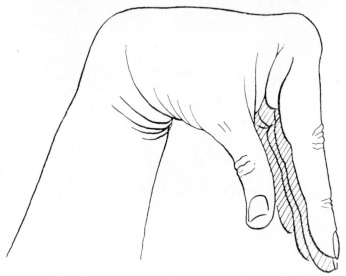

Fig. 99. The position of the wrist and fingers in tetany.

Oversecretion of parathormone is usually due to a tumour in a parathyroid gland, and it causes a rise in the amount of calcium in the blood. This produces muscle weakness, anorexia and constipation. The increased amount of calcium and phosphorus in the urine leads to polyuria, which causes thirst, and some times stones in the renal tract. The withdrawal of calcium from the bones may produce cysts and spontaneous fractures.

The treatment of the tumour is surgical removal.

Hyposecretion, or lack of parathormone, is mostly seen when the parathyroids have been accidentally removed during the surgical removal of the thyroid to which they are closely attached. This causes a fall in the calcium level of the blood, and this gives rise to **tetany.**

The patient experiences numbness and cramp in the feet and hands, which eventually pass into a fixed and painful spasm. The feet are plantar flexed, and the hands adopt the position shown in the picture, with wrists bent and fingers straight. Spasm of the larynx causes whistling respiration, or *stridor*, and convulsions may occur.

The most effective treatment is giving calcium gluconate, up to 1 g (i.e. 20 ml of a 10 per cent solution) by intravenous injection. This will rapidly relieve the painful spasms, and calcium by mouth can then be prescribed.

About 1 g of calcium is needed daily by an average adult; the pregnant woman whose baby's bones are being formed needs more. It is obtained from milk, cheese, fish, beans and nuts, and for its absorption vitamin D is required. This in its turn is either taken in the food in liver oils or summer dairy produce, or is made in the skin when sunlight falls on it. The absorption and utilization of calcium is therefore quite intricate.

Tetany is caused in two ways:

A. By a low blood calcium. This can arise not only through parathyroid deficiency, but also in rickets (page 35). Failure to absorb calcium because of lack of vitamin D may lead to tetany in children with this deficiency disease.

B. By alkalosis or relative excess of alkali in the tissues. The cause of this can be *metabolic* (e.g. through loss of acid in excessive vomiting) or *respiratory*. Over breathing will wash carbonic acid out of the blood, and if persisted in will result in tetany. This hyperventilation is quite often seen in people with anxiety states and youngsters in emotional upsets. The condition will disappear if the breathing can be quietened, and cure can be hastened by holding a paper bag over the nose and mouth for a minute or two, so ensuring re-breathing of carbon dioxide until it reaches its normal level in the blood again.

CARBOHYDRATE METABOLISM

Starches and sugars are digested in the small intestine, are absorbed from there, and appear in the blood as glucose. Before breakfast, the amount of glucose in the blood is about 80 mg per 100 ml (3 mmol/l). After food is taken, the level rises to about 120 mg (5 mmol/l). Just as the body temperature must be kept within narrow limits in health, so must the blood sugar be maintained around the figures quoted by constant physiological adjustments. There are many factors that influence the blood sugar; the principal ones are hormones, especially those secreted by the pancreas.

Most of the pancreas consists of the tissue that makes the pancreatic juice, which passes through ducts to the duodenum; but scattered throughout the pancreas are patches or islands of a different nature. These are the islets of Langerhans, which produce hormones from two distinct kinds of cells. Three quarters of the islets consist of β cells, which produce insulin which lowers the blood sugar by increasing the storage of glucose as glycogen in the liver and muscles. The remainder (the α cells) produce glucagon, which raises the blood sugar. Both hormones pass directly into the pancreatic blood stream, and so to the liver by the portal vein.

There are several substances in the body which raise the blood sugar (e.g. the suprarenal and pituitary hormones, insulin antagonists in the tissues, the glucagon just mentioned). This is because it is so vital to the body to be able to keep up the blood sugar when temporarily short of food. Insulin, however, appears to be the only substance that lowers the blood sugar, probably by making possible the entry of glucose into the cells that need it. Should the blood sugar level rise above 180 mg, glucose begins to appear in the urine, and glycosuria will continue until the blood sugar has fallen below this threshold level.

DIABETES MELLITUS

Diabetes mellitus is a disease in which this process is deranged. It is not simply that the diabetic does not manufacture insulin, since in many the islets of Langerhans appear to be normal. It is perhaps better to say that in the diabetic insulin is not available in quantities enough to enable the liver to store glycogen; the blood sugar rises and sugar appears in the urine. The kidney requires more water in which to dissolve this sugar, so that there is **polyuria** as well as **glycosuria.** The patient must increase his fluid intake to make good this loss, so complains of **thirst.** Body proteins are oxidized in excess, so **loss of weight** is another symptom. Fat metabolism is also disordered if sugar metabolism is not normal, and acid substances such as diacetic acid and **acetone** appear in the blood. These acids belong to a class known as **ketones.** The number of people in any community thought to have diabetes depends on how strict are the standards adopted. If a diagnostic drive is undertaken in any area, many will be detected who display no symptoms. Besides these, there will be a number with some abnormality of glucose tolerance, who may be though of as pre-diabetic, and as the average age of the population rises, so will the number of diabetics.

Prevalence. Diabetes affects 2 to 3 per cent of most populations, but the course of this condition and of its complications varies from country to country. In the United Kingdom arterial disease is common; coronary occlusion and cerebral thrombosis affect twice as many diabetics as non-diabetics; diabetic retinal disease is the commonest cause of blindness registration in those under 65 and diabetic nephritis afflicts many. In Japan the atheroslerosis that underlies all these complications is very much less frequent, both in diabetics and others.

The most important factor in causation of diabetes seems to be heredity; half of all young diabetics have a family history of this disease. The other is obesity, especially, in the middle-aged. It is not common in children under 5, and the highest incidence is in women of 45 to 60; otherwise the sexes are equally prone. It is convenient to consider two kinds of diabetes, which we can call mild, since it occurs with few symptoms, and severe, the form which most young people show.

MILD (INSULIN-RESISTANT) DIABETES

Many middle-aged people discover they have diabetes only on routine examination of the urine, or because they have one of the complications (page 315) of diabetes. There are certainly a large number of people who have this condition and are not aware of it.

In this group are many middle-aged obese women. These suffer only from a relative lack of insulin, and if the weight can by a suitable low calorie diet be reduced to normal, the blood sugar may also fall and the glycosuria disappears.

SEVERE (INSULIN-SENSITIVE) DIABETES

This group includes all the young people, as well as some older ones, and the onset is often sudden. They complain of thirst, polyuria and loss of weight, and sometimes of muscular cramp, blurred vision, numbness or tingling in the hands and feet. Irritation (pruritus) of the vulva is common in women. The most important fact about severe diabetes is the tendency to form **ketones,** mentioned above. The accumulation of these acids in the body leads to **diabetic coma,** and unless the condition is diagnosed and treated, all patients with severe diabetes will end in this way. It was the final result of all diabetics before the discovery of insulin, but can be prevented by good care, and usually successfully treated if it should arise.

Diagnosis. 1. Examination of the urine. This is usually pale because it is dilute, but of high specific gravity because of the sugar it contains. In mild cases sugar may only be present after meals. The presence of ketones in the urine is an important finding.

2. Blood sugar. About 0·2 ml of capillary blood is collected in a fluoride

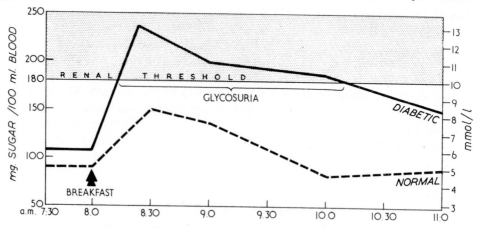

Fig. 100. Normal and diabetic glucose tolerance curves.

tube. It is possible to make a fairly reliable estimate directly by means of impregnated paper strips (e.g. Dextristix).

3. Glucose tolerance curve. In this test the blood and the urine are examined before and after taking 50 G of glucose. Normally this amount does not raise the blood sugar above 180 mg (10 mmol/l), so that no sugar appears in the urine, but in the diabetic hyperglycaemia (high blood sugar) and glycosuria follow. This test is used to distinguish doubtful cases.

Treatment. The patient with severe diabetes will receive a diet of known carbohydrate content, and injections of insulin adequate to balance this carbohydrate. Some physicians believe that if a patient has stable eating habits there is no need to impose any dietetic restrictions other than that sugar should be omitted, and that a dose of insulin can be prescribed to cover any normal intake. Most would, however, construct a diet on the following lines.

The diet must be one that will keep the patient at his ideal weight, and must be suited to his circumstances. He must be asked what his work is, what he normally eats, when he takes his main meal, whether a milk drink or tea can be obtained at work. It is useless to order soup, meat and vegetables for the evening meal of a man who usually has a high tea of boiled eggs or kipper.

The carbohydrate intake should be moderate, perhaps 150 g or 200 g a day, and should be taken mostly as starch, since this is bulkier and more satisfying than sugar. He is given a list of such foods, and it is convenient to use the idea of a "portion" or "helping" of carbohydrate, consisting perhaps of 10 g of carbohydrate. The patient is given a sheet of instructions, and is told how many "portions" of carbohydrate are to be taken at each meal. It will probably be thought necessary for him to weigh or measure his "portions" until he is experienced in judging them. With a little experience he will learn to exchange one "portion" for another equivalent.

Protein such as meat, fish and eggs can be taken in average amounts without weighing. Cheese contains a fair amount of fat, and eating too much may lead to undesirable weight gain. The same applies to such fats as butter, cream, olive oil and meat fat.

High-residue vegetables such as greens, celery and salads may be taken without restriction. Tea and coffee without milk can be freely drunk. "Diabetic" foods should not be taken except with permission, since many of them contain slowly-absorbed carbohydrate that will raise the weight.

The growing belief that a diet containing saturated fats from meat and dairy produce is a cause of atherosclerosis has had its influence on the construction of diabetic diets. Some feel that the traditional diabetic diet, rather low in carbohydrate and high in saturated fat may have been to some degree responsible for the prevalence of arterial disease in diabetics. Some clinics would prefer to raise the carbohydrate allowance and lower the fat intake. The substitution of polyunsaturated margarine for butter would also be advised. Children must be given a diet with enough protein to allow for growth.

Patients' food intake should be regularly reviewed. They tend to drift from the prescribed pattern if it becomes too expensive with changing food prices, or too complex for them to tolerate. All diets require adjustment as time passes, and patients' work or domestic arrangements change.

Insulin. Soluble insulin resembles in its action the normal pancreatic secretion. It is made in strengths of 20, 40 and 80 units per ml. All other insulins contain substances to prolong their action, which may enable the doctor to prescribe only one injection in 24 hours. They are made in strengths of 40 and 80 units per ml. The duration of action is summarized below.

The type prescribed depends on how the patient's blood sugar is best controlled. New insulins coming into use are highly purified ("monocomponent") preparations, and when less expensive may supersede older varieties.

Insulin should be given from a standard insulin syringe and a sharp hypodermic needle. Most patients learn to give their own, and must be taught to draw up the correct amount. It is probably better to give them a card showing the number of "marks" given from phials of different strength, rather than to

Type	*Average length of action*
1. Soluble	6 to 8 hours
2. Globin insulin	8 to 16 hours
3. Insulin zinc suspension amorphous (Semilente)	8 to 16 hours
4. Insulin zinc suspension crystalline	16 to 20 hours
5. Insulin zinc suspension (Lente; a mixture of 3 and 4)	16 to 24 hours
6. Protamine Zinc	16 to 24 hours
7. Isophane insulin injection	6 to 8 hours
8. Neutral insulin injection e.g. Actrapid	8 to 16 hours

attempt to teach the very simple arithmetic involved.

The syringe and needle may be kept in spirit, and boiled once a week. The process of assembling the syringe, drawing up the insulin, cleaning the skin and giving the injection must be taught in meticulous detail. The site chosen can be the anterior abdominal wall, either thigh or upper arm. Too-superficial injection into the skin will cause sore places or even ulceration. Once the insulin has been given (or the oral hypoglycaemic tablets described below) food must be taken within fifteen minutes, or an undersirable fall in the blood sugar will occur.

The patient should test the urine daily for sugar with clinitest, and occasionally for acetone. He should attend a diabetic clinic for weighing, estimation of the blood sugar and general advice. Some may like to join the Diabetic Association.

Treatment of mild diabetes. The obese middle-aged diabetic must be encouraged to regain the normal weight by means of a reducing diet, as on page 27, and will in most cases not need insulin.

Those with mild diabetics and normal weight may often have the blood sugar controlled by means of an oral hypoglycaemic. These drugs are not suitable for anyone under 40, or any diabetic liable to ketosis, but are invaluable for the elderly who cannot see well to fill a syringe. Among those currently in use are tolbutamide and chlorpropamide. Tolbutamide is rapidly converted to an inert form in the body, and is excreted by the kidneys. It must normally be taken three times a day; patients taking it may show a deposit in the urine if acid is added to it when testing for proteinuria. Chlorpropamide has a longer-lasting action, and need only be given once a day. It takes ten to fourteen days

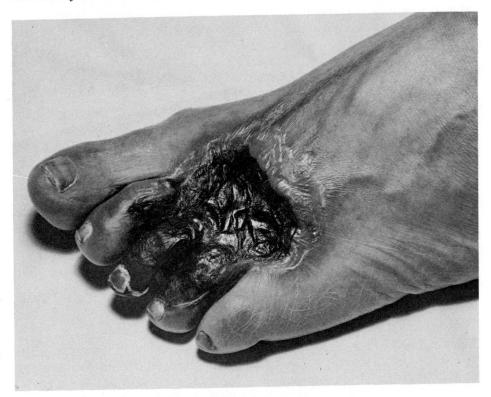

Fig. 101. Diabetic Gangrene.

to eliminate from the body after administration ceases, and if hypoglycaemia occurs it is quite difficult to control. Phenformin and metformin are hypoglycaemics of a different chemical class. Side effects with all these drugs include anorexia, nausea, vomiting and diarrhoea. Later preparations include glibenciamide, glypizide and glymidine, and more new ones are appearing.

Complications of diabetes. These affect nearly every system. **Infections,** such as tuberculosis, are more common in the diabetic, while sepsis such as **urinary infection** and **boils** is very common when the blood sugar is high. *See* arteriosclerotic gangrene p. 115.

Circulatory. Atherosis leads to coronary disease and to gangrene of the toes and feet, and may require amputation. Attention to the cleanliness of the feet, care over nails and corns, well fitting socks and shoes are very important to the elderly diabetic.

Nervous. Loss of sensation in hands or feet occurs.

Ocular. Cataract and retinitis may interfere with sight. Diabetic retinopathy is a not uncommon cause of failing sight and blindness. Arteries, veins and capillaries are all involved in the changes that occur. Photocoagulation is the best available treatment for the new vessels that appear in the retina. Light from a xenon arc or an argon laser is absorbed by the retina and turned to heat which coagulates the unwanted vessels. The treatment may be required monthly for long periods.

Renal. Kidney failure with hypertension leading to death from uraemia is not infrequently the end of a long diabetic life.

It is at this time impossible to say if the complications are an inevitable part of the diabetic process, or if with better control we may hope to avert them.

HYPOGLYCAEMIA

Diabetics having insulin are liable at times to a fall in the blood sugar below the normal level. This may be because they have delayed or omitted a meal, or the bed time drink, or taken unusually vigorous exercise which has used up sugar, or because they have accidentally received an overdose of insulin. The early symptoms—pallor, sweating, fast pulse and tremor—are similar to those of excitement of the sympathetic nervous system, and are an example of the body's admirable self-righting mechanisms. The low blood sugar causes production of adrenaline, which stimulates the liver to convert glycogen to glucose and so raise the blood sugar.

The nurse often notices as well a glassy look in the eyes, incoherence or an unusual emotional attitude. The patient often feels faint and giddy, or ravenously hungry. If untreated he becomes unconscious with muscle tremor that sometimes leads onlookers to think he is having a fit.

Treatment. If the patient is a diabetic having insulin, he usually carries sugar to eat in such an emergency. A sweet drink, such as fruit juice or even milk can be given. If he is unable to swallow, an injection of 0·6 ml of adrenaline may revive him sufficiently to take sugar by mouth. An intravenous injection of glucose, 20 ml of a 60% solution, is immediately effective. In an emergency sweet fluids may be given into the stomach by Ryle's tube. After recovery the patient should be given his next meal, and carefully observed for further symptoms, since relapse into hypoglycaemia is not uncommon, especially after long-acting insulins.

KETOSIS or PRE-COMA

The presence of ketones in the urine of the diabetic is serious, since if it is not corrected the patient will pass into coma, as described in the next section. Whenever there is a marked amount of sugar in the urine, a test for acetone should be performed by putting a drop of urine onto an "Acetest" tablet, and watching for the appearance of a purple colour. The causes of ketosis are:

1. Inadequate control of the diabetes, requiring adjustment of the insulin dose, or the times at which it is given.

2. Carelessness by the patient over taking his insulin or adhering to the diet.

3. Acute infections. Gastroenteritis is especially important, as the patient cannot take his diet, and feels he ought therefore to omit his insulin. Septic infection, as by skin or urinary infections, usually cause ketosis.

Signs and symptoms. In addition to ketonuria, acetone may be excreted in the breath, and has a sickly-sweet smell like fruit-drops. These acids stimulate the respiratory centre so that the respiration is deep and sighing. Nausea, vomiting and giddiness are common, and drowsiness indicates that coma is near.

Treatment. The diabetic must be warned of the danger of leaving off his insulin. Should he not feel well enough to take his food, he should take the carbohydrate portions as milk, or orange juice, or glucose water, give himself his insulin, and send for his doctor. All infections, even trivial ones, must be treated seriously and cured as quickly as possible.

DIABETIC COMA

Ketosis, if left untreated, will result in coma, a serious medical emergency. It is never sudden in onset, and the signs are due to two conditions, acidosis and shock due to fluid loss. Both these must be corrected. It has already been noticed that this is not the only cause of unconsciousness in a diabetic, and since the nurse may in some circumstances be able to supply information that will lead to the correct diagnosis, the conditions are described side by side.

	Diabetic Coma	Hypoglycaemia
History	Missing insulin injection. An infection.	Missing a meal. Unusual exercise. Insulin overdose.
Onset	Felt unwell for a few days.	Sudden.
Pulse	Rapid and feeble.	Often full.
Respiration	Sighing, air hunger, smell of acetone.	Shallow.
Blood-pressure	Low.	Normal.
Skin	Dry, inelastic, often flushed.	Sweating, pale.
Tongue	Dry, furred.	Moist.
Blood sugar	High.	Low.
Urine	Sugar and ketones present.	No ketones, perhaps a little sugar if bladder not recently emptied.
Vomiting	Usual.	Unusual.

The patient is laid on his side in bed, and the foot of the bed raised in order to raise the blood-pressure and prevent inhalation of fluid from the stomach. If the patient is unconscious, a naso gastric tube should be passed. Blood is taken to estimate the blood sugar, and an intravenous infusion of normal saline begun at once to correct the dehydration and the loss of chloride through vomiting. Soluble insulin 80 units is given at once, and subsequent dosage of insulin is regulated by the blood sugar level.

Most physicians would think there was a risk of bladder infection involved in catheterization, and would omit examination of the urine until the patient regained consciousness. The nurse will keep the records of temperature, pulse, respiration, blood-pressure and fluid balance, and would treat the dry mouth frequently.

When consciousness returns, a specimen of all urine passed is put up for examination, and the slow return to normal diet and insulin injections is begun. The events that led to the coma should be discussed with the patient, in the hope of avoiding such accidents in the future.

THE DIABETIC IN THE COMMUNITY

Diabetes lasts throughout life, so that time spent on careful teaching on insulin, diet and general management is never wasted. The diabetic should carry a card stating his complaint, and the name of his doctor or clinic, and a few lumps of sugar. He should know the symptoms of hypoglycaemia and what to do about them.

Questions that often arise include these:

1. Is it hereditary? The answer is yes, to a certain extent, and if there is a history of diabetes on both sides of the family the risk is increased.

2. Can the diabetic drive a car? If he is subject to hypoglycaemic attacks the answer is obviously no, since he would be a danger to others as well as to himself. If he has no such reactions, he may conscientiously do so.

3. Is pregnancy dangerous to the diabetic? There is little increased risk to the mother, provided she is well cared for, but the risk to the baby is above average, though this is becoming less high.

4. What general advice is valuable? The diabetic should follow intelligently his doctor's advice on diet and injections. He must never omit his insulin, even when he cannot take his full diet. He must not allow his weight to increase, and must seek advice over infections, even minor ones. He should take good care of his feet in middle-age, and may hope to lead a long and healthy life.

SPONTANEOUS HYPOGLYCAEMIA

People with insulin-producing tumours of the pancreas sometimes suffer from attacks of hypoglycaemia, with symptoms like those of the kind described on page 316. If the diagnosis is confirmed by finding that the blood sugar is low during one of these "fainting" fits, and that sugar revives the patient, laparotomy is undertaken in the hope that a tumour can be identified in the pancreas, and removed.

THE SUPRARENAL GLANDS

The suprarenal or adrenal glands lie one above each kidney, as their name implies, with a big artery from the aorta supplying each. The outer layer of the gland is the **cortex,** the inner the **medulla**; each is an endocrine organ, and the two differ widely in their nature and actions. The medulla is derived from the same cells as the sympathetic nervous system, the outer cortex from cells similar to those of the sex glands.

MEDULLA

The secretion of the suprarenal medulla is adrenaline, which has the same action as the sympathetic nervous system. It constricts the blood vessels, raises the blood-pressure and the blood sugar, increases the pulse rate, and dilates the bronchioles. All these uses are of value in medicine, and adrenaline is given in the following circumstances:

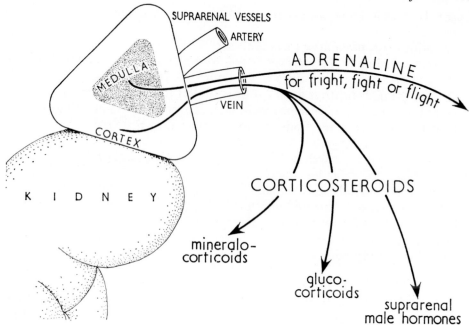

SUPRARENAL VESSELS

ARTERY

MEDULLA

ADRENALINE
for fright, fight or flight

VEIN

CORTEX

CORTICOSTEROIDS

K I D N E Y

mineralo-
corticoids

gluco-
corticoids

suprarenal
male hormones

Fig. 102. The medulla and the cortex at the suprarenal gland have separate endocrine functions.

1. To allay capillary bleeding, e.g. as a gauze pack soaked in 1 : 1000 adrenaline for epistaxis.

2. With local anaesthetic; it diminishes oozing, and by constricting the blood vessels keeps the anaesthetic longer in the operation area.

3. To raise the blood sugar. A patient in hypoglycaemic coma (page 316) may be restored to consciousness by a hypodermic injection of 0·5 ml of 1 : 1000 adrenaline.

4. To dilate the bronchioles of the patient having an asthmatic attack.

5. To cure allergic rashes.

Oversecretion of adrenaline is sometimes seen in people with tumours of the suprarenal medulla. These from time to time pour an excess of their hormone into the blood, causing attacks of hypertension, with severe headache, sweating, tachycardia and a high blood sugar. The condition can be cured by excision of the tumour; the blood-pressure tends to rise while the tumour is being handled, and hypotensive drugs will be needed. After it has been removed, the blood-pressure will fall, and during the post-operative period must be maintained at normal by injections of nor-adrenaline.

THE SUPRARENAL CORTEX

Steroids are a group of substances with a similar chemical structure. Vitamin D is a steroid, and so are all the sex hormones, male and female. The hormones of the suprarenal cortex belong to this group, and are a numerous and complex set called **corticosteroids.** The following is a simple version of this hormone group; they can be considered in three classes.

a) *Mineralocorticoids.* They raise the blood-pressure by causing retention of salt and water in the body.

b) *Glucocorticoids.* These break up protein from muscle and bone and turn it into sugar, and they increase the amount of glycogen in the liver; they suppress the inflammatory and allergic reactions.

c) *Suprarenal male hormones.* These are responsible for the distribution of body hair, and encourage laying down of protein in muscles.

OVERACTION OF THE SUPRARENAL CORTEX

Excessive secretion by the suprarenal cortex may be due to a tumour in the cortex, or to a growth of the pituitary causing excess output from the cortex. Whichever the cause, the symptoms are the same, and produce the clinical picture of **Cushing's disease.**

Signs. The appearance is characteristic; fat is laid down in a pad on the shoulders and on the abdomen, and the cheeks are distended with fat so that the ears are hidden from the front view, and the mouth looks tiny. The cheeks are red because the skin is thin, and in women there is usually hair in the beard area. The blood-pressure is high, causing headaches, and the urine often contains sugar.

Investigations. The nurse will be required to keep a chart of the intake and output, to test the urine daily for sugar and perhaps to collect a twenty-four hour specimen of urine for estimation of steroid excretion and to record the blood-pressure daily. The weight is regularly estimated.

Treatment. If a tumour of pituitary or suprarenal gland can be identified, it is removed, or the pituitary gland is treated by radiotherapy. Alternatively, bilateral adrenalectomy may be performed, and the patient is kept on a maintenance dose of cortisone.

UNDER-SECRETION BY THE SUPRARENAL CORTEX

The suprarenals may be removed by adrenalectomy, may be destroyed by tuberculosis or tumours; they may atrophy, or may cease to secrete because their stimulus from the pituitary stops. In every case, a condition develops, named (from the physician who first described it) **Addison's disease.**

Signs and symptoms. The patient has lost weight, and is easily fatigued. Most notice brown patches inside the mouth, in the flexures and in body creases, and the whole skin may be darker than usual. Lack of appetite and vomiting or diarrhoea occur from time to time, and may lead to acute attacks known as Addisonian crises. The blood-pressure is always low, and the levels of sodium and of chloride in the blood are reduced. The amount of 17-ketosteroids in the urine is below normal, especially in women, in whom the suprarenal cortex is the source of most of these substances.

Treatment. The missing hormone is supplied, usually as cortisone 10–40 mg. a day by mouth. Usually cortisone is supplemented with fludrocortisone a mineralocorticoid as well. The importance of continuing this maintenance dose must be stressed to the patient who must also be told to avoid infections as far as possible, and to consult his doctor at once if he contracts one. He should be seen regularly at a clinic, where his blood-pressure is recorded and the weight also in case salt and water are being retained by the tissues.

If the patient is admitted in a "crisis", intravenous dextrose saline should be given to raise the sodium and chloride levels in the blood, and hydro-cortisone is also given intravenously. The pulse and blood-pressure must be recorded hourly, a fluid balance chart kept, and the urine tested. If the crisis has been caused by an infection, this must be treated.

CORTICOSTEROID TREATMENT

This term is used about treatment by means of the steroid hormones of the suprarenal cortex and by the man-made drugs with similar actions (e.g. prednisone, prednisolone, fludrocortisone, triamcinolone). The most easily understood use for the steroids is for people who are deficient in these substances, either because of Addison's disease or pituitary disease (page 300).

Steroids are however given to many people with normal suprarenal glands, and below is a list of some of the actions of these hormones, with instances of the way they are used.

1. Steroids suppress the inflammatory reaction. This reaction is a normal part of the body's resistance to infection, but sometimes it is excessive, e.g. in rheumatoid arthritis, where joint movement is limited by inflammation. Steroids are used in small continuous doses for some patients.

2. Steroids reduce allergic reactions, and can therefore be used in asthma, drug sensitivity reactions and allergic skin diseases.
3. Steroids reduce lymphatic enlargement, and may be helpful in lympho-sarcoma or lymphatic leukaemia (page 168).
4. Steroids given in large amounts restrict the ability of the pituitary gland to secrete the cortico-stimulating hormone ACTH. In times of stress (e.g. in illnesses or after operation), when more corticosteroids ought to be produced, these are not forthcoming, and patients may die of adrenal failure unless this state is foreseen. This is the reason why patients' notes often contain a special section for the record of these drugs.

Such powerful substances have important side effects and complications. These are:

1. Acute infections may arise with few signs.
2. Haemorrhage may occur from peptic ulcers.
3. Mental symptoms amounting to psychoses can arise.
4. The blood-pressure may rise.
5. Muscle weakness and bone-thinning.
6. Weight gain, water retention, and hair on the face in women.

These are serious, but so are the conditions for which the steroids are used. The prescription must never be stopped abruptly since this may precipitate adrenal failure, and nurses who learn that new patients have been having steroids must report this at once.

SOME DIETS USED IN THE TREATMENT OF DIABETES

CHO	150 grams
PROTEIN	71 grams approx.
FAT	85 grams approx.
CALORIES	1660 approx. (6800 kJ)
INSULIN	Soluble bd.

CHO-gram

EARLY
  MORNING   Tea with milk, 2 teaspoons if desired

BREAKFAST	Tea or coffee with milk 7 oz. (210 ml)	10
	½ oz. (15 g) cereal or (15 g) ½ oz. oats	10
	Egg, bacon, ham, fish or cheese	
	Grapefruit, tomatoes or mushroom if desired	
	1 oz. (30 g) bread. Toasted if liked	15
	Butter or margarine	
		35

MID-MORNING	Coffee with milk 3½ oz. (105 g)	5
	2 plain biscuits (½ oz.) (15 g)	10
		15

MIDDAY MEAL	Clear soup if desired	
	Meat, fish, liver or chicken	
	Unthickened gravy	
	Green vegetables or salad	
	3 oz. (90 g) potatoes or 1 oz. (30 g) bread	15
	Fruit. 2 portions from Food Tables	
	2 oz. (60 g) bread as sandwich + 3½ oz.	
	(105 ml) in coffee	
	or 2 cream crackers (⅔ oz.) (20 g) and cheese	
	or ½ oz. (15 g) cereal + 7 oz. (210 ml) milk	
	as milk pudding	20
	Black coffee	
		35

TEA	Tea with milk 3½ oz. (105 ml)	5
	Bread or 2 plain biscuits (½ oz.) (15 g)	10
		15

EVENING MEAL	Cheese, egg, meat or fish	
	Salad or green vegetables	
	2 oz. (60 g) bread or 6 oz. (180 g) potatoes	30
	Butter or margarine from allowance	
	Fruit. 2 portions	
	or 2 cream crackers (⅔ oz.) (20 g) and cheese	10
		40

BEDTIME	Milk 3½ oz. (105 ml) Tea or coffee	5
	1 plain biscuit (¼ oz.) (8 g)	5
		10

Saccharin may be used for sweetening

If you are unwell and cannot eat your diet take the following amounts of sugar or glucose dissolved in water, tea or fruit squash in place of your meals. Continue to take your normal dose of insulin at the usual time.

CHO gram		rounded teaspoons *or* large lumps sugar
35	Breakfast	7
15	Mid-Morning	3
35	Midday	7
15	Tea	3
40	Evening	8
10	Bedtime	2

Alternative CHO replacement drinks

10 g CHO
1. 7 oz. (210 ml) milk.

2. 4 oz. (120 ml) fresh orange juice.

20 g CHO
1. 7 oz. (210 ml) milk
   + 2 level teaspoons Ovaltine, Horlicks or Benger's.

2. 4 oz. (120 ml) fresh orange juice
   + 2 rounded teaspoons sugar or glucose dissolved
   + few drops of lemon juice if desired.

1 rounded teaspoon sugar or glucose = 5 g CHO

This may be used to increase the CHO content of these drinks to the amount you require.

IF YOU CANNOT TOLERATE THESE DRINKS TAKE HALF YOUR USUAL DOSE OF INSULIN AND CONSULT YOUR DOCTOR

CHO	200 grams
PROTEIN	89 grams approx.
FAT	89 grams approx.
CALORIES	2050 approx. (8400 kJ approx.)
INSULIN	Lente

Suitable for a 10-year-old child

		CHO-gram
BREAKFAST	Tea or coffee with milk 7 oz. (210 ml)	10
	1 oz. ceral (30 g) or 1 oz. (30 g) oats	20
	Egg, bacon, ham, fish or cheese	
	Grapefruit, tomatoes or mushroom if desired	
	1 oz. (30 g) bread. Toasted if liked	15
	Butter or margarine	
		45
MID-MORNING	(School milk) milk 7 oz. (210 ml)	10
	2 plain biscuits (½ oz.) (15 g)	10
		20
MIDDAY MEAL	Clear soup if desired	
	Meat, fish, liver or chicken	
	Unthickened gravy	
	Green vegetables or salad	
	6 oz. (180 g) potatoes or 2 oz. (60 g) bread	30
	Fruit. 2 portions from Food Tables	
	+ 2 cream crackers (⅔ oz.) (20 g) and cheese	
	or ½ oz. (15 g) cereal + 7 oz. (210 ml) milk	20
	as milk pudding	
		50

TEA	Tea with milk 3½ oz. (105 ml)	5
	1 oz. (30 g) bread + 2 plain biscuits	
	(½ oz.) (15 g)	15
	Butter or margarine	10
	Salad if desired	
	Cheese	
		30

EVENING MEAL	Cheese, egg, meat or fish	
	Salad or green vegetables	
	2 oz. (60 g) bread or 1 oz. bread (30 g)	
	+ 3 oz. (90 g) potatoes	30
	Butter or margarine	
	Fruit. 2 portions	10
	or 2 cream crackers (⅔ oz.) (20 g) and cheese	
		40

BEDTIME	Milk 7 oz. (210 ml)	10
	1 plain biscuit (¼ oz.) (8 g)	
	or ¼ oz. (8 g) Ovaltine or Horlicks	5
		15

Saccharin may be used for sweetening

If you are unwell and cannot eat your diet take the following amounts of sugar or glucose dissolved in water, tea or fruit squash in place of your meals. Continue to take your normal dose of insulin at the usual time.

CHO grams		rounded teaspoons *or* large lumps sugar
45	Breakfast	9
20	Mid-Morning	4
50	Midday	10
30	Tea	6
40	Evening	8
18	Bedtime	3

Alternative CHO replacement drinks

10 g CHO	20 g CHO
1. 7 oz. (210 ml) milk	1. 7 oz. (210 ml) milk + 2 level teaspoons Ovaltine, Horlicks or Benger's.
2. 4 oz. (120 ml) fresh orange juice	2. 4 oz. (120 ml) fresh orange juice + 2 rounded teaspoons sugar or glucose dissolved + few drops of lemon juice if desired.

1 rounded teaspoon sugar or glucose = 5 g CHO

This may be used to increase the CHO content of these drinks to the amount you require.

IF YOU CANNOT TOLERATE THESE DRINKS TAKE HALF YOUR USUAL DOSE OF INSULIN AND CONSULT YOUR DOCTOR

FOOD TABLES FOR USE WITH DIABETIC DIETS
EXTRAS

Vegetables

Artichokes, green
Asparagus
Avocado Pear
Beans, french
  „   runner
Broccoli
Brussels Sprouts
Cabbage
Cauliflower
Celery
Marrow
Mushrooms
Onions
Scarlet runners
Seakale
Spinach
Tomatoes

Salads

Cucumber
Lettuce

Salads

Mustard and Cress
Radishes
Watercress

Beverages and Soups

Tea and Coffee (ground or instant)
Water and soda water
Clear meat or chicken soup
Oxo, Bovril, Marmite
Dietetic Squash, Low Calorie Squash

Fruits

Gooseberries, stewing
Grapefruit
Rhubarb

Condiments, etc.

Salt, Pepper, Mustard
Vinegar, Salad oil
Saccharin, Gelatine, Rennet
Lemon juice, Herbs, Vanilla essence

PROTEIN FOODS

You may eat average helpings of the following foods, but if you are to lose weight, take care with the foods in the left-hand column.

Cheese—not cream cheese
Grilled lean bacon
Lean ham
Lean mutton chop
Duck—small portion
Goose—small portion
Lean roast beef ⎫
Lean roast lamb ⎬ inside
Lean roast mutton ⎪ cut
Lean roast pork ⎭
Sardines—drain off the oil

Egg
Corned beef
Boiled beef
Liver
Chicken
Grouse
Kidney
Herring

Crab meat
Bloaters
Fish roes
Salmon—fresh, smoked and
  tinned
Rabbit
Tripe
White fish
Kipper
Smoked haddock

FAT FOODS

If you have been told to lose weight do not eat more of the following foods than is stated on your diet sheet. You should also avoid fried foods.

Butter	Dripping
Margarine	Olive oil
Cooking fat	Cream

SUPPLEMENTS

You may take one tablespoon of any one food from this list once a day if you wish.

Vegetables	*Fruit*
Artichokes—Jerusalem	Blackberries
Carrots	Blackcurrants
Leeks	Loganberries
Swedes	Redcurrants
Turnips	Whitecurrants

CARBOHYDRATE FOODS

To be weighed

Each given weight contains about 10 grams of Carbohydrate

VEGETABLES

	oz.	
Beans, baked, tinned	2	(60 g)
„ broad, boiled	5	(150 g)
„ butter, boiled	2	(60 g)
Beetroot, boiled	4	(120 g)
Corn on the Cob	3	(90 g)
Sweet corn, tinned	1½	(45 g)
Sweet potato	1¼	(38 g)
Lentils, boiled	2	(60 g)
Onions, fried	4	(120 g)
Parsnips, boiled	3	(90 g)
Peas, fresh or frozen, boiled . . .	4	(120 g)
„ tinned	2	(60 g)

		oz.	
Potatoes, boiled	. . . . .	2	(60 g)
„ chips	. . . . .	1	(30 g)
„ roast	. . . . .	1½	(22 g)
Yam	. . . . . .	1½	(22 g)

CEREAL FOODS

		oz.	
Allbran	. . . .	½	(15 g)
Biscuits, Cream crackers (2)	. . .	⅔	(20 g)
„ most plain kinds (2)	. . .	½	(15 g)
Bread	. . . . .	⅔	(20 g)
Chappatis, made from ½ oz. wheat flour	.		(15 g)
Cornflour	. . . . . .	½	(15 g)
Custard powder	. . . . .	½	(15 g)
Flour, white	. . . . . .	½	(15 g)
Macaroni, Spaghetti, etc., raw	. . .	¼	(8 g)
Breakfast cereals	. . . . .	½	(15 g)
Oatmeal	. . . . .	½	(15 g)
Rice, sago, semolina, tapioca, raw	. . .	½	(15 g)
Ryvita, Vitawheat, Matzos, etc	. . .	½	(15 g)

BEVERAGES

		oz.	
Bengers Food, powder	. . . .	½	(15 g)
Bournvita, Ovaltine powder	. . .	½	(15 g)
Cocoa powder	. . . . .	1	(30 g)
Malted milk (Horlicks) powder	. . .	½	(15 g)

MILK

		oz.	
Fresh, whole or skimmed	. . .	7	(210 g)
Unsweetened, condensed	. . . .	3	(90 g)

FRUITS

Stewed fruits should be cooked without sugar and weighed

oz.

Apples, raw with skin and core	4	(120 g)
,, stewed	5	(150 g)
,, baked with skin	4	(120 g)
Apricots, fresh, with stones, or stewed	6	(180 g)
Apricots, dried, raw	1	(30 g)
,, dried, stewed	2	(60 g)
Bananas, no skin	2	(60 g)
Cherries, raw with stones	4	(120 g)
Cherries, stewed with stones	4	(120 g)
Damsons, stewed with stones	5	(150 g)
Dates, with stones	$\frac{2}{3}$	(20 g)
,, without stones	$\frac{1}{2}$	(15 g)
Figs. green, raw	4	(120 g)
Figs, dried, raw	$\frac{2}{3}$	(20 g)
,, ,, stewed	$\frac{2}{3}$	(20 g)
,, ,,	$1\frac{1}{2}$	(45 g)
Gooseberries, dessert, raw	4	(120 g)
Grapes, whole fruit	2	(60 g)
Greengages, raw, with stones	3	(90 g)
,, stewed with stones	4	(120 g)
Melon, no pips	7	(210 g)
Orange, no skin	4	(120 g)
,, juice	4	(120 g)
Peaches, fresh with stones	4	(120 g)
Peaches, dried, before cooking	$\frac{2}{3}$	(20 g)
,, dried, stewed	2	(60 g)
Pears, raw, with skin and core	4	(120 g)
,, stewed	5	(150 g)
Pineapple, fresh, edible part	3	(90 g)
,, juice, unsweetened	3	(90 ml)
Plums, any dessert variety, raw with stones	4	(120 g)
,, stewed with stones	8	(240 g)
Prunes, dry, raw, with stones	1	(30 g)
,, stewed, with stones	2	(60 g)
Raisins, dried	$\frac{1}{2}$	(15 g)

	oz.	
Raspberries, raw or stewed . . .	6	(180 g)
Strawberries, fresh, ripe	6	(180 g)
Sultanas, dried	½	(15 g)
Tangerines, weighed with peel and pips .	6	(180 g)

MISCELLANEOUS FOODS

	oz.	
Jam, marmalade, honey, syrup and treacle	½	(15 g)
Sugar, Glucose	⅓	(10 g)
Jelly in packet as purchased . . .	½	(15 g)
Ice cream ,plain	2	(60 g)
Sausages (2)	3	(90 g)

NUTS

Each given weigh contains 10 g CHO Carbohydrate. Weighed without shells.

	oz.	
Almonds	8	(240 0)
Barcelona Nuts	7	(210 g)
Brazil Nuts	8	(240 g)
Chestnuts	1	(30 g)
Cobnuts.	5	(150 g)
Desiccated Coconut	6	(180 g)
Peanuts	4	(120 g)
Walnuts	7	(210 g)

BEER CONTAINING 10 g CARBOHYDRATE

Brown Ale	½ pt.
Draught Ale—bitter	¾ pt.
Draught Ale—mild	1 pt.
Pale Ale—bottle	1 pt.
Stout—	½ pt.
Stout extra	1 pt.
Strong Ale	¼ pt.

Chapter 12

Diseases of Bones and Joints

Bone gives strength and shape to the body, and gives attachment to muscles, enabling them to perform work and movement effectively and quickly. Bone shelters vulnerable structures, such as the brain and spinal cord, heart and lungs, and within it are made all the red blood cells and most of the white. Bones contain the greater part of the calcium and phosphorus of the body, and some of the disorders that arise in connection with its metabolism and endocrine control are described in chapters 3 and 11.

Where bones meet, they form joints. The structure of these varies according to the work they have to do. There are three basic patterns.

A. Fibrous joints. Such joints are built not for movement, but for stability. Fibrous joints are found between the bones of the vault of the skull, and uniting the lower ends of the tibia and fibula that hold the ankle bone.

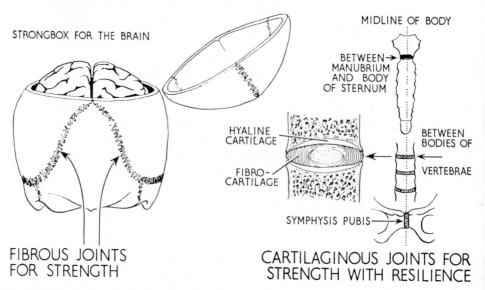

FIBROUS JOINTS
FOR STRENGTH

CARTILAGINOUS JOINTS FOR
STRENGTH WITH RESILIENCE

Fig. 103. The flat bones of the vault of the skull are joined by fibrous tissue. These immovable joints are called sutures. Cartilaginous joints allow a little movement.

B. Cartilaginous joints. These joints are found only in the midline of the body. The two pubic bones join at the symphisis by a pad of fibro-cartilage, and the bodies of the vertebrae are joined in the same way.

C. Synovial joints. This kind of joint connects the limb bones to each other and to the trunk. The articulating bones are held in position by a cuff of fibrous tissue, the joint capsule; the bone surfaces that are in contact with each other are covered with a smooth layer of hyaline cartilage; the rest of the interior of the joint is lined with synovial membrane, which secretes into the joint asticky lubricating fluid.

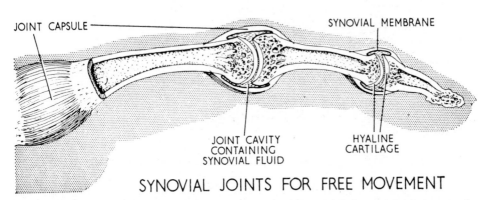

Fig. 104. The synovial hinge joints of the finger. On the left is seen the intact joint in its capsule. The others are drawn in section to show the internal structure of a synovial joint.

The stoutness of the capsule, the fit of the bones, and the amount of muscle surrounding the joint varies in different situations, allowing for mobility or for strength according to the function of the particular joint. In the shoulder joint, for instance, a very free range of movement is required. The hip joint carries the weight of the trunk, and stability is of prime importance.

Instances of all the causes of disease classified in chapter 1 can be found in the diseases of joints and bone, and in addition unrelated conditions may affect them. For instance, the haemophiliac may be severely affected as a result of bleeding into his joints.

Congenital. Achondroplasia is a hereditary abnormality of those bones formed in cartilage, and is one of the cases of dwarfism. In severe forms, death occurs in utero. The trunk length is more or less normal, but the limbs are drastically shortened, and in an adult the body height is not usually more than 1.25 m.

Osteogenesis imperfecta is a hereditary disorder of bone-forming cells, which results in repeated fractures from very minor stresses. This is however a rare disease, and infants who are brought to hospital or the doctor's surgery with repeated or multiple injuries are more likely to be victims of the battered baby syndrome. The parents who bring such a child are making an indirect appeal for help, and they as well as the baby need this help. Among the nurses involved, the health visitor is important.

Inflammatory. Joints may be the site of acute pyogenic infections, or of chronic conditions like tuberculosis. Joint involvement can occur in the two important venereal diseases, syphilis and gonorrhoea. Less dramatic and more common are the painful joints that are associated with conditions like influenza and acute bronchitis.

Traumatic. This section would include fractures, and also some of the occupational conditions like writer's cramp and tennis elbow.

Neoplastic. Malignant secondary deposits frequently arise in bone from such primary sites as the breast and prostate gland. Primary sarcoma of bone is not common.

Nutritional. Rickets and scurvy are good examples of this cause.

Metabolic. e.g. gout.

Degenerative. Osteoarthritis is one of the commonest of the degenerative disorders.

ARTHRITIS

Arthritis means inflammation of a joint. The interior of a joint is sterile and, if organisms gain entry to it, either from a wound or from the blood stream (as in tuberculosis), an infective arthritis will result, the management of which is surgical, and need not be considered here.

There are other cases in which the inflammation is due to wear and tear, or to causes as yet unknown, and give rise to common and important diseases.

RHEUMATOID ARTHRITIS

Rheumatoid arthritis is a condition characterized by inflammation which especially affects the small joints of the hands and feet, but which may extend to the larger ones. It runs a prolonged course, with remissions and relapses, and it is accompanied by general signs and symptoms which indicate that this is not merely a joint disease.

Aetiology. No one cause is known. It is usually a disease of adults, but children can be affected, and rheumatoid arthritis in children is called Still's disease (page 340). More than twice as many women are affected as men. It is most common in countries with a cool, moist climate, such as Britain. The fact that corticosteroids will produce an improvement has led workers to search for an endocrine cause, but their action seems only to be anti-inflammatory. The most widely held view now is that there is an abnormal immunological effect, pro-

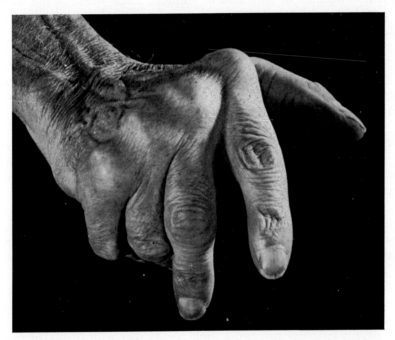

Fig. 105. Rheumatoid arthritis involving the metacarpophalangeal joints.

voked, by an agent such as infection. A *rheumatoid factor* can be identified in the blood and joint effusions of many sufferers from the disease.

Course. In most cases the disease is gradual in its onset, though sometimes it is sudden and severe in its effects. The joints first affected are usually those of the fingers, toes, wrists and ankles, and swelling of the synovial membrane occurs first, with enlargement of the joints and pain. The joints are often kept flexed in an attempt to relieve the pain. Granulation tissue forms, limiting movement and eventually attacking the articular cartilage. Lack of movement causes muscle atrophy, so that the joints appear even more swollen than they really are. In time the acute inflammation settles, but if it has been severe the joints may be locked by fibrous adhesions resulting in deformity and loss of activity. In the hand, the typical effect is flexion and ulnar deviation of the fingers at their junction with the hands.

The joint changes are accompanied by slight fever, anaemia and a raised sedimentation rate, suggesting that this is a general rather than a local disease. The patient complains of pain and of stiffness, often worst in the mornings, so that getting dressed is laborious and slow. Loss of weight is common in the acute stage.

The general tendency of rheumatoid arthritis is to run a prolonged course, with ups and downs which alternately encourage and depress the patient. About half the patients will, with effective treatment, be able to lead a normal or only moderately restricted life. The less fortunate suffer medium to severe disability, and about 10 per cent will eventually be crippled by their disease.

Treatment. The broad aims of treatment are to rest the patient and her joints by support and relief of pain in the acute stage, and to minimize disability by active measures once the acute stage is over. This must be explained to patients, who are often puzzled by these apparently contradictory policies, and feel that doctors and nurses have not really made up their minds what is best.

The patient with acute joint inflammation is put to bed on a firm mattress, with a cradle over the feet and a footrest to keep the feet dorsiflexed. The wrists and hands are supported in a good position with plastic splints. The patient may sit up with a back rest and foam air ring, but must lie down at night in case flexion deformity of the hips develops. The temperature is charted while fever lasts, the haemoglobin level is ascertained, and the blood sedimentation rate assessed at intervals.

If the weight is below normal, a high energy diet with plenty of protein is given, and milk is desirable in order to supply calcium, which is always lost from the bones during times of immobility. The fluid intake must be high, since calcium is lost in the urine, and may come out of solution to form stones if the urine is concentrated. Movement of unaffected joints and breathing exercises will help maintain the physical condition.

Splints are removed daily and the skin washed. Patients like to put the hands and feet in a bowl of warm water. After washing the skin is well dried, especially where skin surfaces are in contact between fingers and toes, and powder applied.

When the acute stage is over, as shown by the disappearance of pain, and by a normal temperature and sedimentation rate, the splints are removed by day for active exercises and treatment of hands and feet by wax baths or radiant heat. If damage to the joints has been slight, the patient has a good chance of return to normal life. The almoner and health visitor will co-operate in adjusting home circumstances if necessary, perhaps with the provision of a home help at first. The patient must remain in touch with her doctor, since relapses may occur and slow deterioration may follow without treatment.

Drugs. The effects desired are relief of pain, inflammation, depression and anaemia. Aspirin is the most useful pain-reliever and is given in large doses at first, and is best tolerated in the soluble form. Dihydrocodeine and paracetamol may also be helpful. Iron is given if anaemia is present. Phenylbutazone is a powerful analgesic, and would be more widely used for rheumatoid arthritis, were it not that about 25 per cent of patients suffer from its toxic effects— nausea, fluid retention, rashes, gastric bleeding and leucopenia. People taking phenylbutazone should be regularly supervised by their doctor while having this drug, which is usually only prescribed when safer analgesics are ineffective. Azothiaprine may be tried, in the hope that its immunosuppressive action may be helpful in what may prove to be an auto-immune disease.

In severe or progressive cases more powerful drugs than simple analgesics may be required. Corticosteroids will usually improve the stiffness, but the dangerous side effects of these drugs (page 322) limit their usefulness in chronic conditions, and if they have to be abandoned because of such complications, there is usually a marked deterioration in the condition of the joints. Steroids can be given by injection into joints.

A course of gold injections may cause improvement, but gold is toxic like all the heavy metals and must be used with caution. Soluble gold salts (e.g. Myocrisin) are given weekly by intramuscular injections of up to 50 mg until a total of 1 g has been given. The side effects are dermatitis, nephritis, and a fall in the white cell count (leucopenia). Before injection the urine is tested for albumin, and the patient is asked if there have been any rashes. The white count is regularly checked. Improvement is slow, and the patient must be encouraged to persevere, even though weeks pass with no apparent relief.

Home care. A great deal can be done to help the arthritic maintain a reasonable life. Rehousing in a ground floor flat may be possible. Installation of ramps instead of steps, raised toilet seats, a chain and pulley over the bed, a shower instead of a bath may be undertaken by the Local Authority. An occupational therapist can suggest many gadgets to make eating, the toilet and housework easier, and safer. The Red Cross have an equipment loan service, organizations such as Task Force may help with shopping, the health visitor will know how to mobilize aid from many sources.

The lot of the breadwinner, especially the manual worker, is harder than that of the housewife. Getting on and off buses is very difficult, and at times when unemployment is high, it is difficult for the arthritic to compete. The younger man or woman finds it very hard to accept unemployment which may be permanent, and efforts must be made to provide social contacts.

Surgical treatment. Chronic disability may often be improved by the orthopaedic surgeon by such measures as manipulation and plaster; traction; tenotomy and arthrodesis. Synovectomy (removal of redundant synovial membrane) of the knee and finger joints is being increasingly performed in early cases, before severe joint damage has occurred.

Chronic rheumatoid arthritis does not threaten life, but may cause long years of disability. A hopeful outlook must be maintained by doctors, nurse, physiotherapist and social workers. Symptoms must be treated as they arise, and a change of drug or new treatment may often benefit the patient, even when the joint changes are permanent.

STILL'S DISEASE

This is the name given to rheumatoid arthritis in children, who show all the signs found in adults, and also have as a rule enlarged lymph glands and spleen. It commonly runs a severe course, and joint movement may be greatly limited. Growth of bones is often affected, so that when the disease has run its course, the child is small and much handicapped by stiffened joints. The treatment is along the lines described for adults.

OSTEOARTHRITIS

Osteoarthritis is a degenerative disease affecting the articular cartilage of joints and eventually causing outgrowths of new bone around the margins of the joints attacked.

Aetiology. Normal wear and tear of joints ages them, and osteoarthritis is an exaggeration of this process. It naturally occurs in the elderly, and chiefly in those joints which carry weight and take strains. The hips, knees and spine are most affected, especially if the owner is engaged in heavy work or is overweight. Joints which have suffered injury or disease may be affected early by osteoarthritis.

Course. Slowly increasing stiffness and pain are the leading symptoms. The pain is a dull ache, appearing after exercise and relieved by rest. As time passes, pain becomes more severe and constant, and may keep the patient awake at night. The range of movement becomes restricted by pain and muscle wasting. If outgrowths of new bone (osteophytes) appear in the inflamed joint, grating may be felt on movement, and deformity and locking eventually occur.

The worst effects of osteoarthritis are seen when one or both hip joints are affected. This is most common in those who are overweight and put much strain on the hips. The hip joint becomes increasingly flexed and adducted, until pain and deformity may make walking difficult or impossible. Unless the patient decreases his intake to match his limited activity, his weight will rise still further, and useful treatment will be hard to find.

Treatment. Since osteoarthritis is a degenerative process, a return to normal cannot be expected. It is wrong, however, to think that old people must expect increasing pain and stiffness, and learn to live with them, since there are many ways of relieving symptoms.

Reduction of weight is the most useful measure for obese patients whose hips and knees are affected. Detailed practical advice and encouragement on the diet must be given. Analgesics like aspirin, paracetamol or codeine are prescribed. Periods of rest are helpful, and if the hips and knees are affected, these should be taken lying down, rather than sitting in a chair with the joints flexed.

Warmth is comforting, and since movements are more easily performed under water when weight is less, gentle exercises in a warm bath should be performed. Sleep in a warm bed will help prevent painful spasm, but if the patient is old, he must know how to use a hot water bottle or electric blanket with safety. Bottles should have a flannel cover, and blankets should be kept in good order, and should not be moved without being switched off.

Surgical treatment for arthritic hips may relieve pain and disability in selected persons. The post-operative period is arduous, and the patient must be of good general health, not obese, and determined to adhere to the regime of exercises and physiotherapy that must be followed. The operation may be an arthoplasty, in which the joint is refashioned perhaps with the insertion of an acrylic head, or an osteotomy, to alter the angle between the femur and the pelvis.

Osteoarthritis is a disease with social implications. It becomes increasingly common as the number of old people in the country increases. People who are affected are predominantly in the lower income brackets in which labourers and those who do heavy physical work are found. A reducing diet is more

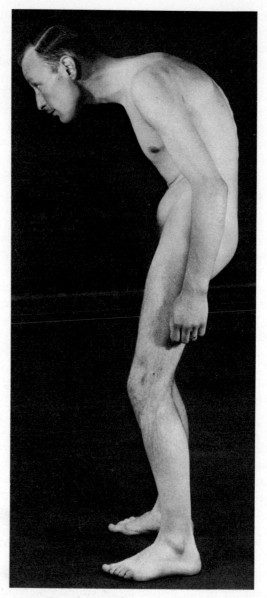

Fig. 106. Ankylosing spondylitis.

expensive than a normal one, since the cheapest foods are carbohydrates like bread and potatoes, which are those to be avoided by heavy people. Fuel costs are high, and it is not easy to keep rooms warm on an old age pension.

Health visitors try to know all the old people in their area, and can offer them advice and help in adapting to their disabilities, and how to obtain the financial benefits to which they may be entitled. e.g. a heating allowance.

ANKYLOSING SPONDYLITIS

This is a progressive spinal arthritis, leading to rigidity of the spine, usually with kyphosis, or forward curvature.

Aetiology. It is a disease of young adults, and affects men far more often than women. The cause is not known, but as in rheumatoid arthritis there are general signs which indicate that ankylosing spondylitis is not simply a joint disease.

Course. The typical patient is a young man, often well built who begins to feel pain in the sacro-iliac joints. He refers to his pain as lumbago. He may have a slight rise of temperature, and the blood sedimentation rate is raised. Unless treatment is effective, the whole spine eventually becomes involved, and stiffens, often with much deformity. In the worst cases, the joints of the ribs with the vertebrae may become fused, and by limiting movement may cause respiratory trouble, the hip joints are affected, and the patient may eventually be crippled.

Treatment. Radiotherapy to the spine is effective in the early stages, and even when the disease is more advanced may halt it. It causes a slight risk of initiating leukaemia, but this risk may be thought worth taking for the results achieved. If the condition involves the rib joints respiration will be affected, and physiotherapy must be used to enable him to make the most of his decreased chest movements.

The usual drugs are used for pain, e.g. aspirin, paracetamol or phenylbutazone. Corticosteroids give some relief, but are prescribed with caution in view of the prolonged course of ankylosing spondylitis.

GOUT

Gout is a condition in which repeated attacks of acute arthritis occur, usually in the big toe joint at first, later on many other joints. It is due to an inborn difficulty in the metabolism of purines, which are related to the proteins.

Aetiology. Gout is hereditary, and almost invariably affects men of more than 40 years old. The purines mentioned above are found especially in the nuclei of the animal cells that make up meat. Internal organs like liver, kidney and sweetbreads have large nuclei, and so contain large amounts of purines. When these are taken in the diet they are broken down and uric acid is produced. This is excreted in the urine as urates. Men who are liable to attacks of gout may precipitate one by heavy eating and consumption of alcohol.

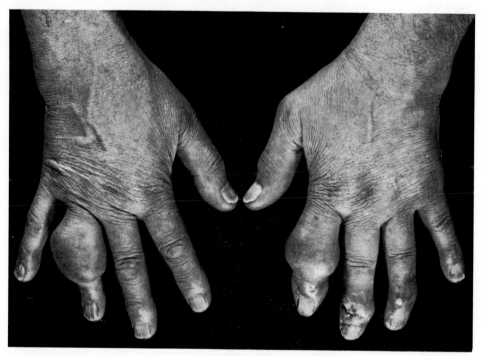

Fig. 107. Gout.

Course. An acute attack may be heralded by indigestion and sometimes frequency of micturition. The big toe joint is almost always the one attacked, and rapidly becomes red, swollen and acutely tender. Patients say the pain is the severest they can imagine; any pressure or jarring of the joint is feared, and they are apprehensive and often acutely irritable. If the blood uric acid is estimated now, it will be found raised above the normal 2 to 6 mg per 100 ml (0·1–0·4 mmol/l).

The acute attack will subside, and the joint returns to normal. Further attacks will occur unless treatment is effective, and urates will be deposited in the joint which eventually becomes arthritic. Other joints may be attacked, and urates may be deposited in cartilage anywhere, especially in the ears, where these chalky masses, or **tophi** may ulcerate through the skin.

In long-standing gout, urinary symptoms may appear. Urate stones may form in the kidneys, and renal failure may lead to uraemia.

Treatment. During the acute attack, the patient should be kept in bed with a cradle over the affected foot. Hot or cold compresses may be comforting, but if the joint is very tender, the foot may merely be wrapped in gamgee tissue. Care should be taken while giving nursing attention or making the bed not to jar the limb. The diet should be lacto-vegetarian, to keep the purine intake low, and fluids must be drunk freely.

Drugs to relieve pain are given in adequate dosage, and a course of colchicine, 0·5 mg two-hourly, is given until the pain subsides. Colchicine is toxic, and may cause diarrhoea and vomiting. If this occurs before the pain has gone, the dose may be decreased, or kaolin and morphine mixture may be given to control the diarrhoea. The drug is stopped as soon as the joint pain has gone.

Treatment between attacks is directed towards facilitating the excretion of uric acid, and so averting attacks of arthritis and stone formation in the kidneys.

As in all patients with arthritis, the weight must be kept down to normal, and the fluid intake should be good. A low purine diet is one that avoids liver, kidney, sweetbreads, brains and fish roe, and includes only moderate amounts of alcohol. Any foods which are found to precipitate an attack should be omitted. In view of the efficiency of drugs in controlling the blood uric acid, severe dietetic restrictions are not indicated. The classical diet used to be one low in purine.

Probenecid (Benemid) lowers the blood uric acid level by promoting excretion in the urine. The dose is 0·5 g three times a day. If joints have become deformed, physiotherapy may be helpful, and if tophi ulcerate through the skin, they should be removed surgically.

Gout is not now a common disease. It appears to have been not unusual in the eighteenth and nineteenth centuries, when gout stools for resting the affected foot were a well-known article of furniture.

"RHEUMATISM"

"Rheumatism" is a word much used by the general public for a variety of painful states in muscles and soft tissues. Doctors often used the term "fibrositis" in days when it was believed that there was an inflammation of fibrous tissue, but no inflammatory changes can be demonstrated in painful areas, and the word is not a real description.

Patients complain of pain, often of acute onset, in soft tissues, usually in the neck and shoulders, back or buttocks. Pain in the lower back is described as "lumbago", and some of these patients will have a more serious condition, due to prolapse of an intervertebral disc (page 406), and these are not included here. Small acutely tender areas can often be found, and neighbouring muscles are in spasm. Since no cause is known, consideration of the circumstances in which "rheumatism" most often occurs may help to adopt means of avoiding and treating it.

"Rheumatism" is commonest in cool, moist climates such as that of Britain, and is often precipitated by exposure to cold, especially in the form of draughts. It occurs most often in those engaged in heavy work, or enjoying strenuous hobbies. Poor posture can cause pain, which in turn may make the posture worse and so establish a vicious circle. Excess weight stretches ligaments and gives rise to pain.

Course. Episodes of muscular pain are very common and most adults experience them at some time. They clear with simple measures like those described in the next paragraph, and only recur at infrequent intervals. In other cases, the condition becomes chronic, and pain and stiffness of varying degree are felt for long periods.

Treatment. Analgesics, warmth and rest are ordered in the acute stage, and if the condition is widespread or severe, rest in bed may be necessary. Electric pads, hot water bottles or hot baths may be used, depending on the site of the pain. Massage will relieve the spasm in muscle, and faulty posture should be corrected by advice and exercise. If tender spots are present, injection of 1 per cent procaine may effect rapid improvement. Obese patients should be advised on how to lose weight.

Those subject to painful attacks should avoid draughts, and getting chilled after exercise. Patients with chronic pain may benefit from spa treatment, in which an intensive course of physiotherapy involving heat, massage and hydrotherapy combines both exercises and rest.

PAGET'S DISEASE OF BONE

This condition was first described by James Paget, a nineteenth-century surgeon. Areas of dense new bone formation occur in the skull, pelvis and large bones, alternating with patches of thinner bone.

Aetiology. It is an uncommon disease of elderly people of both sexes, and the cause is unknown.

Course. The patient may complain of headache, and notice enlargement of the head if the skull is affected. There may be pain in the bones, and forward bowing of the femur and tibia may occur, causing decrease in stature. Fractures happen frequently in the abnormal bones, but will heal with the usual management. Osteogenic sarcoma, a malignant growth of bone, is a less common complication.

Treatment. Calcitonin, a thyroid hormone inhibits bone destruction and aids in remodelling of the abnormal bone and is the current method of treatment. It also seems to help the pain, but other analgesics are usually necessary.

Chapter 13

Diseases of the Skin

The skin is one of the most extensive organs in the body, and since it forms a barrier between the rest of the tissues and the exterior, its great area is subject to many influences both from within and without. In the blood there come to it products of digestion, hormones, bacterial toxins, or drugs that have been taken. From the exterior, the skin is subject to extremes of temperature; sunlight; friction and pressure from clothes made of leather, synthetics and natural fibres coloured with dyes; industrial and household chemicals; cosmetics; plants and animals. The diseases, injuries and reactions of the skin are just as numerous.

The outer layer of the skin, the **epidermis,** is made of stratified epithelium, the upper layers of which are worn away by friction and replaced from the lower layers. The upper ones become progressively thinner and flatter, until the uppermost or horny layer consists only of dead cells. The epidermis has in its upper layers, no nerve endings, no blood vessels at all, and its lower surface is indented so that it interlocks with the dermis or true skin beneath, and cannot be separated from it except by force. The dermis is a layer of loose connective tissue containing the nerves, blood vessels, muscle and glands which perform the functions of the skin.

The skin has many functions, among them the following:

1. It is **protective,** keeping bacteria out of the deeper tissues, and sealing in the tissue fluids. One has only to consider the dangerous loss of plasma and the risk of infection that occurs when burns destroy large areas of epidermis, to realize the importance of this function.

2. It is **excretory,** ridding the body of excess water, sodium chloride and a little urea, through the sweat glands.

3. It **regulates body temperature,** being the principal organ by which heat is lost. Evaporation of water from the sweat glands cools the skin, and by exposing or covering areas of skin one can allow convection currents to cool it, or prevent this happening. When the surrounding air is warm, the blood vessels in the skin dilate, so that heat can be lost by radiation. When it is cold, vasoconstriction occurs, to prevent heat loss.

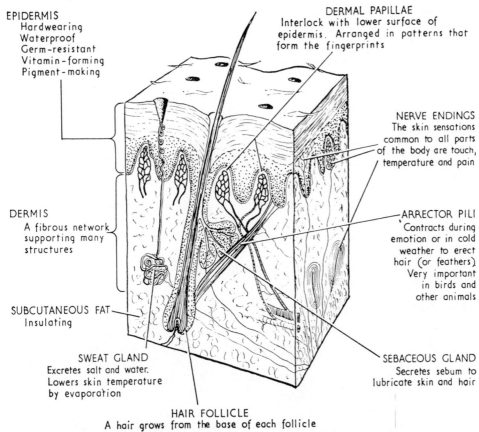

EPIDERMIS
  Hardwearing
  Waterproof
  Germ-resistant
  Vitamin-forming
  Pigment-making

DERMAL PAPILLAE
Interlock with lower surface of
epidermis. Arranged in patterns that
form the fingerprints

NERVE ENDINGS
The skin sensations
common to all parts
of the body are touch,
temperature and pain

DERMIS
  A fibrous network
  supporting many
  structures

ARRECTOR PILI
  Contracts during
  emotion or in cold
  weather to erect
  hair (or feathers)
  Very important
  in birds and
  other animals

SUBCUTANEOUS FAT
Insulating

SWEAT GLAND
Excretes salt and water.
Lowers skin temperature
by evaporation

SEBACEOUS GLAND
Secretes sebum to
lubricate skin and hair

HAIR FOLLICLE
A hair grows from the base of each follicle

Fig. 108. The structure and functions of the skin.

4. It is **secretory,** producing from the sebaceous glands the oily secretion that waterproofs the skin and provides a dressing for the hair.

5. It **makes vitamin D,** when the sterol (7-dehydrocholesterol) it contains is irradiated by the ultra-violet component of sunlight.

6. It is a **sense organ.** The special senses of sight, hearing, taste and smell are localized in small special structures, but touch, pain, heat and cold can be felt all over the body through the nerve endings in the skin.

SKIN LESIONS

The following terms are used in describing the abnormalities of the skin in disease:

Erythema is reddening, as in sunburn.

A macule is an alteration in the colour of the skin in a limited area. They may be areas of erythema; of pigmentation (e.g. freckles) or depigmentation; or may be caused by bleeding into the skin (i.e. purpura). Macules are seen but cannot be felt.

Papules are elevations of the skin, which can be felt.

Vesicles are small blisters; large blisters are called bullae.

Pustules are lesions containing pus. The rash of chickenpox consists of vesicles which become pustules in a day or two.

Weals are raised erythematous lesions due to oedema of the skin; the effects of nettle stings are weals.

Fissures are cracks in the skin, exposing the dermis.

Ulcers are formed by the destruction of the epidermis and part or all of the dermis.

A surface from which serum is exuding is said to be weeping; as the serum dries it forms crusts.

Scales are collections of epidermal cells adhering together to form large or small masses.

PRINCIPLES OF TREATMENT

There are a few skin diseases which are infectious, which can be rapidly and permanently cured. There are more, however, which run a long course, and some which can only be controlled, not completely cured. These can be very damaging to the patient's morale, since he feels other people may find his condition repulsive, may lose sleep through itching, and may have to spend much time each day in applying ointment, which soils the clothes and the bed-linen.

Itching is often a dominant symptom in skin diseases. It leads to scratching, which causes dilatation of the skin vessels, and the increased warmth leads to more irritation. If scratching injures the skin, weeping results and infection may follow. Itching is usually worse when the patient is warm in bed, so that sleep is lost. This cycle must be broken. Enough sedative must be prescribed to ensure sound sleep, and administration of antihistamines by mouth and topical application of crotamiton (Eurax) will also help prevent itching. Applications to an inflamed skin should be lotions, creams or pastes, rather than heavy ointments. If a dressing has to be used, it should be of gauze, and wool should never be applied. Bandages should be openwove or net. Night-clothes should be of cotton rather than wool, and heavy blankets should not be put on the bed. When applications are made to the skin, vigorous cleaning which may injure it must be avoided.

Diet is not of specific importance in most cases of skin disease. Alcohol, which dilates the skin vessels, should be avoided, and large quantities of sugar and chocolate are thought to be harmful to those with acne vulgaris. Patients with allergic conditions must not of course take those foods to which they are known to be sensitive, and should usually avoid those foods which are notorious allergens, such as shellfish.

SOME COMMON SKIN CONDITIONS

ACNE VULGARIS

Acne vulgaris is a common affection of the face, chest and back of young people in their teens and twenties. Acne is often associated with excessive production of the male hormones or androgens, but the immediate cause appears to be the thickening of the mouths of the hair follicles, leading to the retention of sebum. The swollen, inflamed papule thus produced is the comedo, the characteristic lesion of acne. The plugging of the orifice of the follicle is

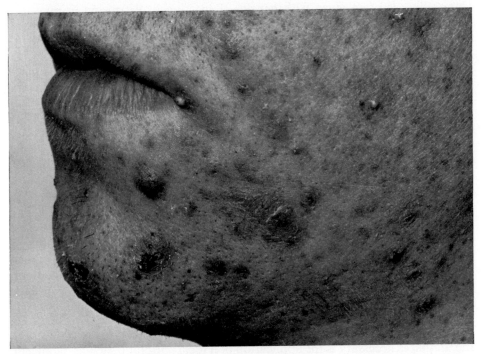

Fig. 109. Acne vulgaris.

probably a response to the production of chemically abnormal sebum acting as an irritant. The distended gland may rupture, and its contents are irritating to the tissues.

Acne is not dangerous to health, and tends to disappear spontaneously before the age of thirty. It causes great misery and social embarrassment to boys and girls at a very important time of their lives, however, and severe attacks may leave permanent scars on the face and shoulders.

The contents of blackheads may be expressed, and the areas affected should be well washed with soap and water twice a day. The usual application is one containing sulphur (e.g. Sulphurated Potash and Zinc Lotion B.N.F.), which causes mild peeling which tends to keep the mouths of the sebaceous glands open. Girls may be treated by small doses of an oestrogen, or female hormone.

General treatment is important. Plenty of fresh air and sunlight, and a low carbohydrate diet are beneficial. A course of ultra-violet light is often prescribed. The patient may be treated twice a week with a dose not strong enough to cause reddening, and each night the face is washed with soap for five minutes. Tetracycline is often given with benefit. If scarring is disfiguring, it may in a few cases, be improved by dermabrasion. A small area of skin is frozen, and the scar tissue removed with a revolving burr or wire brush attached to an apparatus like a dentist's drill. Healing takes place in a week or ten days.

IMPETIGO CONTAGIOSA

Impetigo is an infection of the epidermis, caused by staphylococci or streptococci. It usually affects children, especially those who are undernourished or run-down. The lesions appear most often on the face, especially on the cheeks and chin, but impetigo may be implanted on scratch marks or moist surfaces (such as weeping eczema). If impetigo is present on the scalp, the hair is almost certainly infested with head lice, for which careful search must be made if these are not at once apparent.

The first lesion is a pink macule a centimetre or two across, on which a blister appears. This turns to a pustule, which ruptures and dries to form a yellow crust on an inflamed base. Other lesions appear, especially if the patient is a young child who handles the infected lesions. The condition is contagious, and other children may be infected by manual contact with the patient, or from infected towels.

Treatment. Unless the attack is very severe, there is no fever or general upset, and all that is necessary is the application of a local antibiotic such as neomycin. Tetracycline cream is effective but is not used because the organism may become

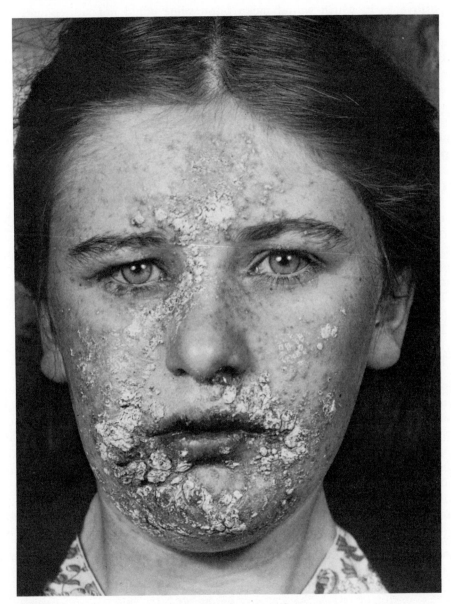

Fig. 110. Impetigo contagiosa.

insensitive to it, which would mean tetracycline could not subsequently be given by mouth for a general infection, such as pneumonia, caused by this organism.

Precautions must be taken against spread of infection to other children, and the patient's pillowslip, sheets and towels should be boiled when the impetigo is cured. As the infection is superficial, scarring does not occur.

RINGWORM

Ringworm is the lay term for tinea, or fungus infection of the skin. Several types of microscopic fungus are involved, and these dissolve the horny layer of the skin to provide nourishment, and also cause acute inflammation. The variety which gives rise to the common name is *tinea* circinata, an infection of the hairless skin, in which the fungus grows outwards from the infected centre, and healing takes place in the centre of the patch. The growing edge is red and scaly, often with vesicles and pustules. It usually affects the neck or forehead, and farmers handling infected calves may contract it on the hands and arms. Griseofulvin should be given by mouth, and the lesions treated with undecylenic acid or Whitfield's ointment.

Tinea is best classified according to the parts affected, and the commonest varieties are:

Tinea pedis (ringworm of the feet).
Tinea cruris (ringworm of the groin).
Tinea capitis (ringworm of the scalp).

Tinea pedis is commonly known as athlete's foot, and is a frequent infection of young adults. It is contracted from the floors of swimming baths and wet bath mats, and causes maceration of the skin in the clefts between the toes, particularly the small ones. The sodden skin peels to expose painful cracks. Whitfield's ointment, which contains benzoic and salicylic acid, is an old and effective remedy, and there are many others. The feet must be washed and dried daily, and the socks or stockings changed daily.

Re-infection or relapse are common, and it is advisable to use an anti-fungus powder e.g. undecylenic acid) after apparent cure. Contact with wet floors and communal mats in bathrooms of hotels or residences should be avoided.

Tinea cruris causes painful, itching red areas in the groins, and is more common in men than women. It is most prevalent in hot weather and hot climates, and is usually transferred by towels to the groins from infected feet, which must be treated. Whitfield's ointment will cure a mild infection, but it may be necessary to prescribe griseofulvin.

Tinea capitis is an infection of the scalp, more common in boys than girls, and never persisting beyond puberty. It causes oval scaly patches from which the hair falls out. The fungus can be identified by examination of infected hairs under the microscope, or by looking at the head with a special lamp (Wood's light), when affected patches will fluoresce and appear bright green.

Treatment is by griseofulvin and attention to local cleanliness. The hair is cut short and Whitfield's ointment is applied to the affected areas. Infection of other children in the family through pillow-cases or hats should be avoided by hygienic precautions.

CANDIDIASIS (THRUSH)

Candida (Monilia) albicans is a yeast-like organism which is commonly present on the skin, but only causes infection if resistance is low or the skin is injured or macerated. It is a common vaginal infection in pregnancy, frequently infects the nail folds of housewives, appears in the mouths of bottle-fed babies, and often causes vulvitis in women with glycosuria. It is also a well-known complication of treatment by the wide-spectrum antibiotics like tetracycline, causing thrush of the anus and vagina.

The antibiotic used is nystatin, which is prescribed as a dusting powder, an ointment, vaginal pessaries or oral tablets. Nystatin is not absorbed from the digestive tract, so is only given by mouth for candidiasis of the bowel. Underlying conditions must be corrected if cure is to be effected. For instance, glycosuria must be controlled, and housewives with nail infection must keep the hands protected while washing up.

PEDICULOSIS

Pediculi or lice are parasites that infest the hairy parts of the body, and live on the blood of the host. There are two varieties of the human louse, one living on the head (pediculus capitis) and one on the body hair (pediculus corporis).

The female head louse lays her eggs or nits on the hair close to the scalp, usually behind the ears or under the occiput. The eggs hatch in about nine days, and the larvae become mature in about another nine days. The eggs are usually more easily seen than the lice unless they are very numerous. The bites cause intense irritation, and the scratches caused may become infected, causing impetigo. Children and woman are more often infested with the head louse than are men, and it is a condition mainly associated with crowded living conditions and poor personal hygiene.

There are many methods of treatment, two effective ones being Dicophane

Application, B.P.C. or Gamma Benzene Hexachloride Application, B.N.F. About 15 ml suffices to treat the scalp. It is applied by a pipette, parting the hair from one side of the head to the other so that the whole scalp is treated. All lice should be killed, but the hair should not be washed for a fortnight, so that larvae emerging from the nits may be killed also. The empty nits should be removed from the hair with a fine, metal comb.

Body lice live chiefly on the clothing and the eggs are usually laid in the seams. The lice feed in the skin, especially in the flexures, and the bites cause scratching that leads to excoriation of the skin. The clothing must be disinfected, and in hospitals this is usually done in a formalin chamber. Thorough dusting with D.D.T. powder is also effective.

The crab louse (*Phthirus pubis*) is not closely related to the pediculi, though its life cycle is similar. The louse lives especially in the pubic hair, where it lays its eggs, and can be found on the skin clinging to the hair. The most usual source of infestation is intercourse with an affected person. Treatment is with D.D.T. powder, or Lorexane cream.

SCABIES

Scabies is caused by infestation with a mite (*Sarcoptes scabiei*). The female burrows in the skin to lay her eggs, and this causes intense irritation. The burrows are about a centimetre long, and contain 30 to 40 eggs, which hatch in about a week. The mites mate on the skin surface, and the pregnant females begin the cycle again. The lesions are usually found in soft skin, in the axillary folds, under the breasts, in the inner sides of the elbows and forearms, and between the fingers. The genitalia, thighs and lower borders of the buttocks are frequently affected.

The burrows appear as straight or wavy lines in the skin, and if one is examined with a lens or watchglass, a small vesicle is seen at one end. If this is opened with a needle the mite can be extracted and the diagnosis confirmed. Although itching is the usual symptom, often scratching has produced dermatitis and pustules. In infants, skin in any part of the body may be attacked.

Infection is by close personal contact, and frequently all members of a family require treatment. The patient takes a hot bath, scrubbing all infected parts with a soft brush and plenty of soap. After this the whole body except the head (which is never infected) is painted with a brush dipped in benzyl benzoate. This is allowed to dry, and a second coat is applied the next day. On the third day the patient has a hot bath, and changes his clothes and bed linen. Since thorough application is necessary for a cure, treatment should be undertaken at a cleansing station if it appears that it cannot be adequately performed at home. All other members of the family must be treated at the same time, or re-infection will occur.

For itching that continues after adequate treatment with benzyl benzoate, Crotamiton (Eurax) is prescribed. This allays the itching, and also has some action against the mite responsible, should any still be present. Further application of benzyl benzoate must not be made, or dermatitis will result.

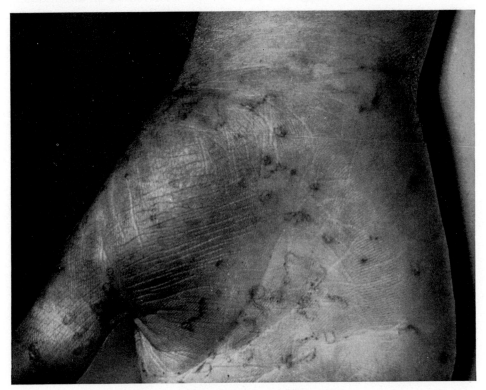

Fig. 111. Scabies showing multiple burrows.

URTICARIA

The lesions of urticaria or nettle rash resemble those caused by the stinging nettle; they are raised red areas, blanched in the centre, and known as wheals. They are due to oedema in the dermis, and are usually intensely irritating. Widespread eruptions are usually due to sensitivity to drugs, such as penicillin, or foods (e.g. shellfish or strawberries). Urticarial attacks may recur frequently in susceptible individuals, and appear to be precipitated by emotional upset. Massive oedema in the subcutaneous tissues (angioneurotic oedema) sometimes occurs in the mouth or throat and if not treated quickly and effectively may cause asphyxia.

In widespread or acute cases, 0·5 ml of adrenaline is given by hypodermic injection, and there is a possibility that tracheostomy may be needed for angioneurotic oedema obstructing the airway. In less severe cases, an antihistamine is given by mouth (e.g. promethazine hydrochloride or mepyramine maleate), and if the sensitizing agent can be identified, it must be avoided. People who are taking antihistamines regularly must be told that they cause drowsiness that may be dangerous to car drivers.

DERMATITIS

Dermatitis means inflammation of the skin. A few cases are due to self-inflicted injuries (*dermatitis artefacta*) and are symptoms of the emotional troubles of hysterical people. A large number of cases are due to agents that reach the skin from the outside, and the condition produced is *contact dermatitis*. Some things, such as excessive heat, light, or caustic chemicals, will injure any skin. There are in addition a large and increasing number of cases of dermatitis which are due to sensitization to substances reaching the skin from outside, or from the bloodstream. The condition produced is *allergic dermatitis*.

The skin reacts in such circumstances with dilatation of the blood vessels, causing heat and redness. If the reaction is a mild one, scaling occurs, and this condition may persist or slowly resolve. A more acute reaction causes vesicles to appear in the skin; these break to leave a weeping surface. Crusting follows, and either scaling and healing, or the outbreak of further crops of vesicles and a repetition of the cycle. *Eczema* is the term often used for this type of reaction.

Allergic contact dermatitis. The substances capable of causing sensitization are very numerous; the most common ones can be classified as follows:

1. Drugs, e.g. penicillin, streptomycin and chlorpromazine. Doctors and nurses giving these should protect their hands, preferably with gloves. When preparing injections, small quantities may be sprayed into the air and reach the face.
2. Cosmetics, e.g. lipsticks and hair dyes.
3. Plants. Primula obconica and chrysanthemums are the most common.
4. Metals. Nickel used in suspenders and to fasten brassiere straps is a very common sensitizer.

5. Industrial chemicals.
6. Dusty substances—flour, cement.

Detergents and soaps which are often thought to cause allergy, appear to act mainly by removing fat from the skin, and exposing it to the action of alkalis.

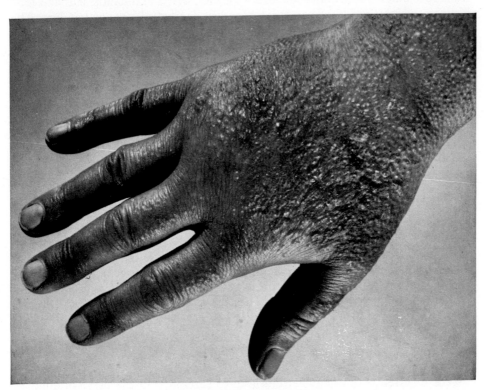

Fig. 112. Contact dermatitis.

Identification of the cause may be easy; (for instance the eruption may occur under the suspenders); but sometimes a careful history of the patient's working habits and hobbies may be necessary, or a patch test may be used to demonstrate sensitivity.

Avoidance of exposure to the offending substance is the first line of treatment. Hydrocortisone ointment usually causes rapid improvement in acute cases; scaly lesions can be treated with Lassar's paste. If the outbreak is very extensive, the patient should be kept in bed, with sedation to prevent scratching. Only mild applications should be used on the skin, and these should be gently applied.

Infantile eczema. This condition is usually easy to diagnose. The eruption occurs on the face and forehead, the shoulders, elbows, wrists and hands, legs and feet, all places which the infant can scratch or rub against pillows or bedding. The cause may be more difficult to determine, but the general treatment in all cases is similar. Scratching must be prevented as far as possible, and bland applications such as hydrocortisone ointment are used. Sedatives such as phenobarbitone, and antihistamines like promethazine hydrochloride may be helpful.

Three groups of children may be distinguished.

a) Those sensitive to a substance in the food, often the lactalbumin in cow's milk. A proprietary food (such as Allergilac) which is free from lactalbumin should replace cow's milk. This cause is not a common one.

b) In some children, the eczema is a manifestation of an allergic disposition that remains throughout life. They may later suffer from asthma and hay fever as well as eczema (Besnier's prurigo). The treatment is directed to the child's emotional state and environment as well as to the skin. Relief of tension and anxiety in the family is important, as well as sedation and treatment of the eczema.

c) Seborrhoeic eczema occurs chiefly in well-fed infants with greasy skins. In spite of the rash and the scratching, the baby may appear in remarkably good health, while the mother seems worn out. Thrush (candidiasis) and staphylococcal infection may be superimposed on the eczema, but will respond to the appropriate antibiotic. Weight reduction on a well-balanced diet should be prescribed. A period in hospital for the baby may allow the mother a period of rest, but the baby must be nursed in a cubicle with precautions to prevent superinfection.

Some children with phenylketonuria have eczema, and the urine of children with eczema should always be tested with Phenistix, since the mental deterioration caused by this condition can be prevented by a diet low in the amino acid phenylalanine which the child cannot metabolize.

Steroid ointments such as hydrocortisone or newer preparations like betamethasone valerate are useful, especially in the flexures, but systemic corticosteroids are not used, because of their side effects and also because their withdrawal is followed by worsening of the eruption.

Energetic and persistent treatment will usually clear the greater part of the eruption, but its return in months or years must be expected. This is a daunting prospect, but patients may truthfully be encouraged by pointing out that new

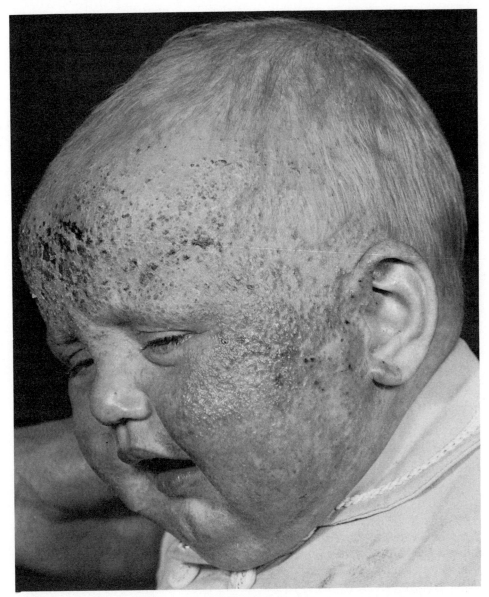

Fig. 113. Infantile Eczema.

remedies are likely to be available, and that long remissions are possible. A holiday in a warm sunny climate is usually helpful, and the use of a sun lamp at home may improve the skin lesions. Fortunately the great majority of patients recover completely by the third decade of life.

EXFOLIATIVE DERMATITIS

Exfoliative means "shedding the leaves", and this form of dermatitis involves desquamation of the whole body. It is rare and may be caused by poisoning by one of the heavy metals (e.g. gold, used for chronic rheumatoid arthritis); drug sensitivity (e.g. barbiturates, penicillin); and extension of some previous skin condition (e.g. eczema, psoriasis).

The epidermis is shed in scales or large flakes, so that the whole body is reddened and tender. Heat loss through the thinned skin is great, and the dermis is vulnerable to infection because of the loss of epidermis.

These two points determine the main aspects of nursing care. The patient should be in a warm room with adequate humidity, and clean linen should be supplied daily or more often if necessary. No one with a septic lesion, however small, should care for the patient. A fluid intake/output chart is kept, and the diet must contain enough protein to make up for that lost in the shed skin. Only bland creams or pastes are prescribed for the skin. If the cause is gold poisoning, a course of dimercaptol (BAL) is given by intramuscular injection, to inactivate the gold.

SEBORRHOEIC ECZEMA

The name of this condition suggests that the cause of this quite common skin complaint is excess production of sebum. This is not entirely true; some metabolic error seems to be present, but most sufferers do have greasy skins. They also have an increased liability to skin sepsis, and this sets up eczema, which may also be triggered off by general infections, or apparently by emotional upsets.

Seborrhoeic eczema most often affects the areas best supplied with sebaceous glands—the scalp, face, chest, back, axillae and groins. All patients have severe dandruff of the scalp, and between attacks this may be the only complaint. Periodically, acute exacerbations causing weeping eczema of the scalp, which spreads to the face, ears and neck and perhaps to the upper part of the trunk. The skin is red and oedematous, and the serous exudate dries in crusts. Cracks occur readily behind the ears. Inflammation of the lid margins (blepharitis) is common, and if left untreated will cause distortion of the lashes, with the risk of injuring the cornea.

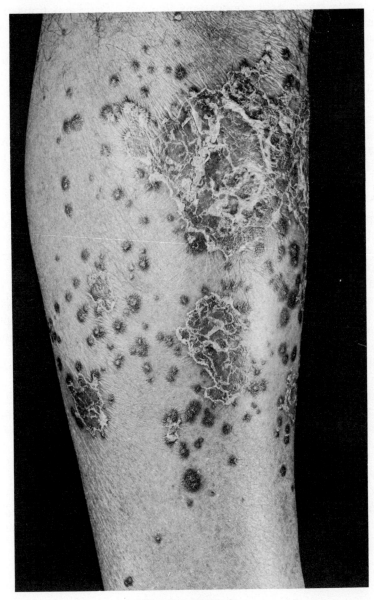

Fig. 114. Psoriasis.

In the acute stage, mild applications like oily calamine lotions or hydrocortisone cream are used. In the chronic condition, the dandruff must be regularly treated by a proprietary shampoo, or one containing cetrimide 1 per cent. For chronic greasy lesions on the trunk, salicyclic acid and sulphur cream is often prescribed. Not all physicians believe that diet is important, unless the patient is overweight, but some advise excluding fried and greasy foods, chocolate, excess sugar and alcohol.

Treatment in this condition is not only of the skin condition; it involves consideration of the whole person and his emotional circumstances and problems. Keeping the scalp condition under control involves much effort on the patient's part, and encouragement is needed.

PSORIASIS

This common skin disease provides the dermatologist with a sizeable part of his work. Not only are there large numbers of sufferers in the temperate zones, but it is exceedingly chronic, and those who have it are subject to recurrences throughout life.

The cause is not known, and probably several factors are involved. Heredity plays some part, and since it is not common in tropical climates, it is believed that lack of sunlight is also involved. It can be precipitated by streptococcal infections, especially in children, and is apparently influenced by hormones, since it often begins at puberty, or the menopause.

The characteristic lesion is a well-defined red area, topped with silvery scales. Sometimes the scales are only obvious if the lesion is scraped; sometimes the scales are thick and piled up.

The site and severity of the lesions are variable. In acute cases almost the entire body is covered, but characteristically there are plaques on the elbows, knees, sacrum, and in the scalp. Patients with chronic psoriasis should have a warm bath at night, and scrub the patches with a soft brush. Afterwards they may apply an ammoniated mercury ointment with tar. Dithranol in Lassar's paste, beginning with $\frac{1}{4}$ per cent and increasing in strength, is another useful remedy. Ultraviolet light treatment may also help to prevent recurrences and lengthen the period of remission. Few patients remain permanently free from psoriasis, but most can keep it under control.

Chapter 14

Diseases of the Nervous System

Anatomy and physiology. Twelve pairs of nerves arise from the brain (cranial nerves), and thirty-one pairs from the spinal cord (spinal nerves). By means of these nerves, information reaches the brain from the exterior about touch, pain, heat, cold, light, sound, taste and smell. From within the body, sensations from joints, tendons and muscles tell of the position of the body. Incoming fibres carrying information of this kind form *sensory* or *afferent* nerves. *Motor* or *efferent* nerves originating in the brain and cord, supply the skeletal muscle of the body. Of the cranial nerves, some are sensory, some motor and some mixed; all the spinal nerves are mixed.

THE AUTONOMIC SYSTEM

The glands of the digestive and respiratory systems, the plain muscle of the intestine, heart and arterioles are not directly under the control of the will. They are supplied by the nerves of the autonomic system which is formed of (two) opposing halves, the *sympathetic* and the *parasympathetic*.

Sympathetic fibres are derived from nerve cells in ganglia on either side of the spinal cord, and they are distributed with the spinal nerves and some of the cranial nerves. When active they constrict the arterioles, thus raising the blood pressure, quicken the heart rate, dilate the pupil, raise the blood sugar and suppress secretion of the salivary and other digestive glands. These actions are the same as those produced by adrenaline from the suprarenal glands, secreted in response to fear or excitement.

Parasympathetic fibres accompany some of the cranial and sacral nerves, the largest part of this system being the 10th cranial nerve, the vagus. When stimulated the parasympathetic relaxes the arterioles, slows the heart rate, constricts the pupil, lowers the blood sugar, and causes secretion from the bronchial and digestive glands.

Most internal organs are supplied with both sympathetic and parasympathetic fibres, and their activities are due to a balance of the two sides.

THE CRANIAL NERVES

1. *Olfactory nerves.* The first cranial nerves convey the sense of smell. From the mucous membrane in the top of the nose its fibres pass through the ethmoid

bone to the olfactory bulb and thence to the olfactory centre in the temporal lobe.

The sense of smell is often temporarily lost when a cold in the head causes swelling and mucous secretion by the nose. It may be permanently lost on one or both sides if a fracture through the anterior part of the base of the skull tears the nerve. Since many flavours are appreciated not by taste but by smell, patients often complain of loss of taste as well.

2. *Optic nerves.* The fibres of the nerve of sight converge at the back of the eyeball and leave in a single bundle. The place at which it leaves is the optic disc, which because there are no nerve cells in it is a blind spot. The two nerves pass through the sphenoid bone, and meet in front of the pituitary gland in the optic chiasma, where the inner fibres from each eye cross to the opposite side. The optic tracts continue backwards and eventually reach the visual centre in the occipital lobes. Sight may be affected not only by the eye conditions which are the province of the ophthalmic surgeon, but by those which affect the optic nerves, such as raised intracranial pressure, tumours of the pituitary gland, diabetes or hypertension.

The optic disc can be seen through the pupil with an ophthalmoscope, and is the only part of the nervous system that can be seen and inspected. The most important pathological conditions that can be seen are:

a) *Papilloedema,* or swelling of the optic disc. It is commonly seen when the pressure within the skull is raised by injury or infection, and in hypertension. Sight is not greatly affected until the condition is far advanced.

b) *Optic neuritis.* The most common cause is multiple sclerosis (p. 402); and sight is diminished even in the early stages of optic neuritis.

c) *Optic atrophy.* This condition results in loss of sight. The causes may be traumatic (e.g. damage to the nerve); nutritional (e.g. prolonged vitamin B deficiency; repeated haemorrhage or severe anaemia); toxic (e.g. syphilis, methyl alcohol poisoning); general disease (e.g. multiple sclerosis).

3, 4 and 6. The oculo-motor, trochlear and abducent nerves serve the muscles that move the eyes. Injury to one of these nerves results in a squint, the direction of which depends on which nerve is affected. Such a paralytic squint causes double vision, or *diplopia.* The autonomic fibres that control the pupil accompany the 3rd nerve. Rise of pressure inside the cranium may compress the 3rd nerve and produce dilatation of the pupil, an important neurological sign, particularly after head injury.

Most squints are not paralytic, but due to weakness of an eye muscle.

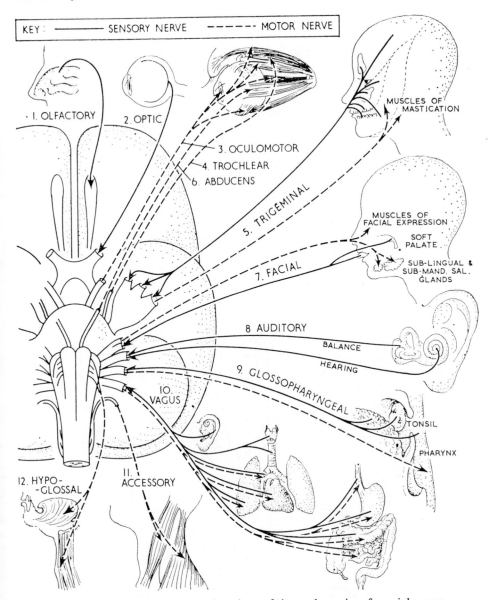

KEY: —— SENSORY NERVE ----- MOTOR NERVE

· I. OLFACTORY

2. OPTIC

3. OCULOMOTOR
4. TROCHLEAR
6. ABDUCENS

5. TRIGEMINAL

7. FACIAL

8 AUDITORY

9. GLOSSOPHARYNGEAL

10. VAGUS

12. HYPO- -GLOSSAL

11. ACCESSORY

MUSCLES OF MASTICATION

MUSCLES OF FACIAL EXPRESSION

SOFT PALATE

SUB-LINGUAL & SUB-MAND. SAL. GLANDS

BALANCE

HEARING

TONSIL

PHARYNX

Fig. 115. The distribution and functions of the twelve pairs of cranial nerves.

Double vision does not occur, and correction can be obtained by orthoptic exercises or an eye operation.

5. The trigeminal nerve is the sensory nerve of the face, and has three major divisions. The upper one (ophthalmic) supplies the forehead; the eye, including the cornea, and part of the nose. The middle (maxillary) supplies the cheek, upper lip and the side of the nose. The lower (mandibular) is sensory to the side of the head, ear, cheek and chin. There is also a small motor part to this nerve, which supplies the muscles of mastication. The most important affection of this nerve is trigeminal neuralgia.

Trigeminal neuralgia is a condition of unknown cause, in which attacks of very severe pain occur in the area served by the nerve. It usually begins in middle age, and is more common in women than in men.

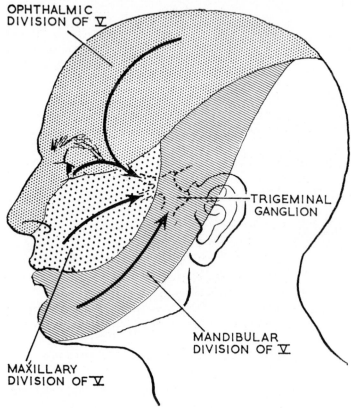

Fig. 116. The areas supplied by the three divisions of the 5th (trigeminal) nerve.

The pain is usually one sided, and is more common in the two lower than in the upper section of the nerve. It is paroxysmal, stabs of pain recurring for a few seconds or minutes. Attacks of pain return for a week or two, then usually disappear for some time. As time passes, the relapses may last longer, and the periods of remission shorter. The pain may be triggered by touching the face, washing, eating, or a cold wind. In a few cases, the intensity of the pain and fear of its recurrence may keep the patient indoors in constant apprehension and even with thoughts of suicide.

Analgesics will be used at first, but in view of the possibility of frequent recurrence, the addictive drugs must not be given. Tegretol sometimes gives good results. Cure can only be affected by abolishing sensation in the affected part of the nerve. If pain is confined to the mandibular section, this can be injected with alcohol, and although sensation eventually returns, the pain may not. If all roots are affected, it is usually necessary to divide the nerve by an intracranial operation. In this case, the cornea will be anaesthetized and glasses with side pieces must be worn to protect the eye from dust that might lead to corneal ulceration. The numbness that follows section of the nerve is unpleasant, but patients who have had severe neuralgia usually find it of small account compared with the pain.

Herpes zoster. The zoster virus attacks the nervous system, and invades the cells of sensory nerves. The first symptom is pain in the area supplied by the nerve, then red patches on which vesicles appear. These crust, and the crusts separate to leave slightly depressed scars. The most serious form is *ophthalmic herpes*, in which the upper section of the trigeminal nerve is affected, because the cornea is involved, and this may lead to blindness from scarring.

Idoxuridine in dimethylsulphonide may rapidly relieve the pain and cure the rash of herpes zoster. If treated very early by intravenous cytosine arabinoside it may be possible to abort the attack. The vesicles on the skin can be kept dry by painting them with collodion. Pain should be relieved by analgesics, but addictive drugs should not be given since sometimes intractable neuralgia develops in the affected nerve, especially in elderly patients. The pain from such neuralgia may lead to depression with suicidal thoughts. Tegretol, an anti-convulsant, is often prescribed for facial neuralgia, sometimes with good results.

The nerves most commonly affected by the zoster virus are the intercostals, and the eruption is known as shingles. The condition is usually unilateral, but both sides can be infected, and the common belief that the patient will die if the eruption meets in the middle is unfounded. As for herpes ophthalmicus, the rash should be painted with collodion, or sprayed with nobecutane, and analgesics should be given for the pain. Loose clothing should be worn until the vesicles have healed.

7. *Facial nerve.* This nerve supplies all the muscles of the face, except the masticatory ones. It leaves the skull with the eighth nerve (auditory) and runs through the parotid gland before it breaks up into its branches. It is accompanied by a sensory branch that supplies taste sensation to the anterior part of the tongue.

Injury to the facial nerve causes paralysis of the same side of the face, which becomes smooth and expressionless. If the patient tries to smile, the movement of the unaffected side is unopposed by the paralysed one.

The facial nerve may be involved in infection in the mastoid region, or in new growths of the parotid gland, or injured by fracture of the base of the skull. The commonest cause of facial paralysis is, however, Bell's Palsy.

The cause of this condition is unknown, but the facial nerve apparently is compressed within its bony canal. It is mainly a disease of adults, usually running a benign course. The paralysis comes on abruptly, and no other symptoms may be present. Patients often ascribe it to cold draughts, but there is no sound evidence that this is so. In mild cases only the lower part of the face is affected; if the upper part is also paralysed, the eye cannot be closed, and tears run down the cheek.

In most cases the paralysis clears completely, though it may take some months. In a few, however, movement does not return. It seems likely that if corticosteroids are given early, this permanent damage can be avoided, perhaps by reducing inflammation around the nerve in its bony canal, and some physicians would prescribe it for all cases except the mildest. The patient should be reassured about the outcome, and if the eye cannot be closed, paroleine drops and an eyeshade may be given to avoid the possibility of injury to the eye. If movement does not return within a few weeks, a malleable wire splint is used to support the mouth on the paralysed side and so prevent stretching of its muscles. One end of the splint is hooked into the angle of the mouth, the other passes behind the ear to keep it in place. If the wire is covered with flesh-coloured plastic it is not too conspicuous in use. Should the paralysis still be complete after twelve months, no cure can be expected, and plastic operations to sling up the affected muscles may be considered. It must, however, be stressed that a favourable outcome is usual.

8. *The Acoustic nerve* is the nerve of hearing, and has a section concerned with balance. Damage to the auditory portion of the nerve causes deafness, or in milder instances tinnitus (ringing in the ears). Damage to the second part of the nerve causes giddiness (vertigo) and loss of balance. Injury to the eighth

nerve is a possible complication of treatment with streptomycin, and nurses should report at once any complaints of deafness, ringing in the ears or giddiness in patients having streptomycin, especially towards the end of their course, or if kidney function is impaired. These three symptoms may accompany many kinds of ear disease. If no organic cause can be found, the condition is called *Ménière's disease*. It is a disease commoner in woman than in men, and usually occurs in middle age or later. There may be long periods of remission, but the condition is progressive, and hearing may eventually be lost. Sedatives are the mainstay of treatment, and a low salt diet with diuretics is often tried and may be continued if the effects are good.

9. *Glossopharyngeal*. This nerve supplies the sensation of taste to the posterior part of the tongue, and is motor to the muscles of the pharynx. Secretory fibres to the parotid gland are distributed with the glossopharyngeal nerve.

10. *Vagus*. The vagus nerve has a very wide distribution in the chest and abdomen, supplies the larynx, bronchi, heart, small intestine, and half the large intestine. The branch that supplies the larynx is occasionally damaged in operations on the thyroid gland, and results in paralysis of the vocal cord on the affected side.

Fainting attacks in young people are often *vasovagal* in origin; unstable vagal action slows the heart beat and allows pooling of the blood in the abdomen. There is pallor, sweating and loss of consciousness. Rest with the head low quickly relieves the attack by allowing blood to return to the brain.

Atropine and hyoscine are widely used before operations because they paralyse the vagus nerve, and this action not only reduces mucous secretion from the airway, but by preventing undue slowing of the heart by the vagus, helps to reduce the risk of cardiac arrest.

11. *Spinal accessory nerve* and 12. *Hypoglossal nerve* are motor to the muscles of the shoulder and tongue respectively.

SPEECH

The ability to speak is complex, but cannot take place unless the speech area in the cerebrum is intact. This centre lies in the temporal lobe and nearby parts of the frontal lobe, on the left side in right-handed people, and vice versa. Difficulty in finding the word wanted is called *dysphasia*, and complete inability to select words is *aphasia*. This is always due to a lesion in the speech centre. The patient may, however, know the words he wants, but finds difficulty in producing them, because the nerves or muscles involved mechanically in speech are not functioning. Difficulty in articulation is *dysarthria*.

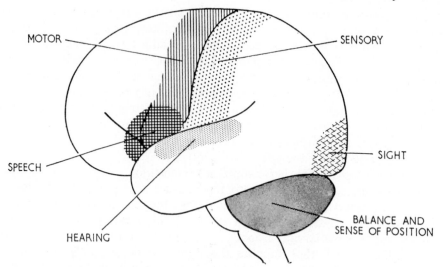

MOTOR

SENSORY

SPEECH

SIGHT

HEARING

BALANCE AND
SENSE OF POSITION

Fig. 117. The main external features of the brain. The central sulcus, or Fissure of Rolando, divides the motor from the sensory cortex.

Patients who are unable to speak may be quite capable of understanding what is said to them, and should be talked to. Some who cannot find the word they want can sometimes describe it, and some produce bizarre terms. Nurses should remember that patients requests mostly fall within a fairly limited range—a bedpan, or urinal, or drink—and they will often be able to interpret the meaning correctly.

THE MOTOR TRACT

Voluntary movement is initiated in a band of nerve cells in the frontal lobes running from the temporal lobe to the vertex in front of the Fissure of Rolando Comparatively large areas are concerned with movements of the face and hand and smaller ones for structures like the abdomen.

The fibres from these motor cells converge and narrow to a compact right and left tract running down through the brain stem to the medulla, where the two cross to the opposite side, so that movement of the right side of the body is controlled from the left hemisphere, and vice versa. These fibres form the *pyramidal tracts*. The brain cell and its fibres form the *upper motor neurone*. The motor impulse is taken on to its eventual destination by a second neurone; for the muscles of the limbs and trunk this begins with a nerve cell in the anterior

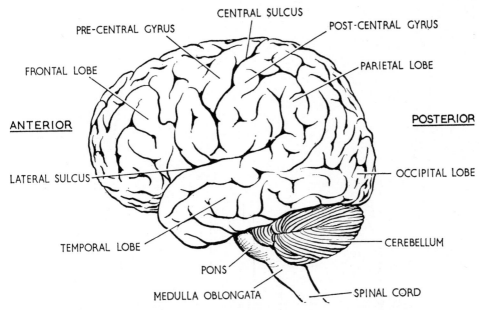

Fig. 118. Location of function in the brain. Below and at the right is the cerebellum, responsible for balance and muscle tone. All the other centres shown lie in the cerebrum.

horn of the spinal cord, from which the fibre travels to the muscle that it activates. This second neurone is the *lower motor neurone.*

Both fibres must be intact if voluntary movement is to take place. Even small movements, however, involve many muscles, some contracting while their opponents relax, and the cell of the lower motor neurone receives stimuli not only from the upper motor neurone, but by fibres from other cerebral centres and from the cerebellum. The fibres form the *extra pyramidal* tracts.

Damage to either the upper or the lower motor neurone will cause paralysis of the muscle supplied, but the clinical picture in the two cases is different. If the upper motor neurone is affected, the lower motor neurone still receives impulses from the extra pyramidal tract. Tone in the paralysed muscle is increased so that there is danger of contracture developing, and the muscle does not waste. Because of the increased muscle tone, the paralysis is termed *spastic.*

If the lower motor neurone is injured, the muscle is cut off from all stimuli; tone is absent, and muscle wasting is marked. This kind of paralysis is flaccid. The differences can be tabulated thus:

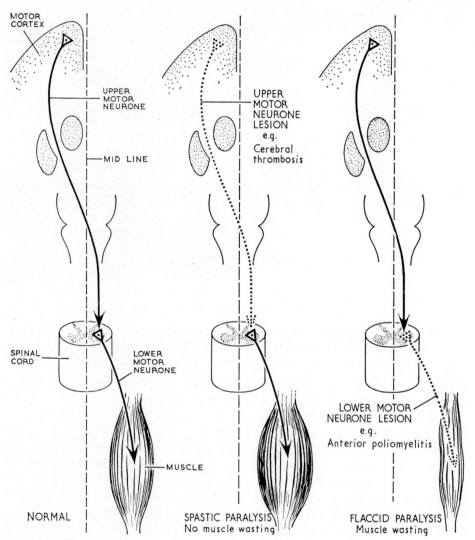

Fig. 119. Paralysis results from loss of function in either the upper or the lower motor neurone. The signs depend on which is affected.

	Upper motor neurone injury (e.g. by a stroke)	Lower motor neurone injury (e.g. in anterior poliomyelitis)
Paralysis	Spastic	Flaccid
Tone	Increased	Diminished
Wasting	Absent	Present

When the motor impulse reaches the junction between the nerve ending and its muscle, a chemical *acetylcholine*, is released, which sets off the muscle contraction. Acetylcholine is destroyed by a tissue enzyme, so that the cycle can begin again. This chemical reaction at the neuromuscular junction is important in several therapeutic procedures and diseases. The curare group of drugs that the anaesthetist uses to induce muscle relaxation exert their action here. The nerve palsies of lead poisoning originate here, and it is failure of the normal mechanism that produces the muscle fatigue of myasthenia gravis.

Finally, there are diseases of the muscles that may cause difficulty in movement, or weakness.

To summarize, disorders of the motor system can arise at one of four levels, and cause differing signs and symptoms.

a) In the upper motor neurone, e.g. cerebrovascular accidents.

b) In the lower motor neurone, e.g. anterior poliomyelitis.

c) At the neuromuscular junction, e.g. myasthenia gravis.

d) In the muscles, e.g. the muscular dystrophies.

MYASTHENIA GRAVIS

This is a disease in which there is abnormal fatigue of striped muscle on exercise. It is a disease of young adults, and the onset is usually gradual. The muscles affected are mostly those supplied by the cranial nerves, that is those of the head and neck, so that speech, swallowing and movements of the eyes are usually the first and sometimes the only ones affected, though spread to the muscles of the limbs and trunk.

Early in the day there may be no symptoms, and these become progressively worse during the day. The lids droop (*ptosis*), and the patient tilts the head back in order to see. Speech becomes slow, slurred and nasal. Swallowing becomes progressively more difficult, so that by the end of the day often only fluids can be taken.

" Gravis " means " serious ", and this disease can be dangerous to life, progressing rapidly to involve most of the muscles, so that pneumonia and respiratory failure may occur. In others, there may be long periods of remission, or the disease may produce only slight symptoms for many years.

Treatment. Physostigmine and its synthetic ally neostigmine destroy cholinesterase, and so prolong the action of acetylcholine. Its effect on a patient with acute myasthenia is dramatic. It can be given by intravenous or intramuscular injection in emergency, but is usually given by mouth in 15 mg tablets. The dose should be the smallest that is effective, since tolerance to it is gradually established. Infections (e.g. colds, influenza) usually make the weakness worse, so that the patient should be protected from them as far as possible. Acute crises of weakness occur from time to time, and the patient should be admitted to hospital, since respiratory failure may occur suddenly and require treatment on a respirator. Thymectomy has often been tried in the treatment of myasthenia, because many of these patients have thymus glands larger than usual, and it gives marked relief in some cases.

MUSCULAR DYSTROPHIES

Under this heading are grouped a set of conditions with a predisposition to run in families, all of which cause degeneration of striped muscle, and its gradual wasting away, or replacement by fat. Severe weakness and disability may be caused eventually, and these people do not usually live long. Gradually increasing muscle weakness limits the patient's activities, and so reduces his social contacts unless his relatives, doctor and nurses actively seek ways of preventing this. Weakness of the respiratory muscles leads to poor chest movements and inability to cough, so that eventually diminished lung function leads to pneumonia, which may prove fatal. The patient must be protected from respiratory infection, and the help of a physiotherapist in the home is invaluable. The home nurse will be a regular visitor in connection with toilet needs, and will be alert to notice the first signs of chest infection, so that treatment can be started early.

PSEUDOHYPERTROPHIC MUSCULAR DYSTROPHY

This condition is described as an example of the congenital muscle diseases. The sufferers are almost always boys, and the first symptoms appear in early childhood. The child walks badly, standing on a wide base, with the normal lumbar curve exaggerated. If he falls, he has difficulty in standing again; typically he gets on his knees, and pushes himself up by pressing his hands first on his knees, then on his thighs, a manoeuvre called " climbing up the legs ". The weakness surprises the parents, since the child looks strong, because the muscles appear large and well-developed. They are in fact being replaced by fat. Gradually this fat disappears, and the true extent of the muscle wasting can be seen. Eventually the boy usually dies of pneumonia, as described above.

No cure is known, so effort is directed towards supplying the parents with means of care, e.g. wheel chairs or bed rests. The home nurse and the health visitor may help to solve some of the domestic problems. Parents are often helped by joining the Muscular Dystrophy Association, which provides money for research and so allows parents to feel that they are doing something about these sad conditions. Other parents are often able to give support and answer questions.

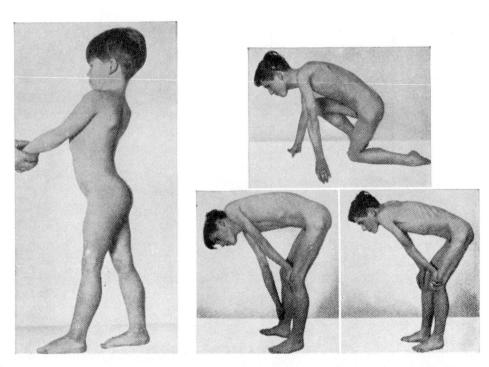

Fig. 120. Progressive muscular dystrophy.

A. Note the marked lordosis, winged scapulae and pseudohypertrophy of the calf muscles.

B. In rising from the prone position the patient "climbs up his own legs".

(Reproduced from Textbook of Paediatrics, Fanconi and Wallgren,
William Heinemann Medical Books Ltd.)

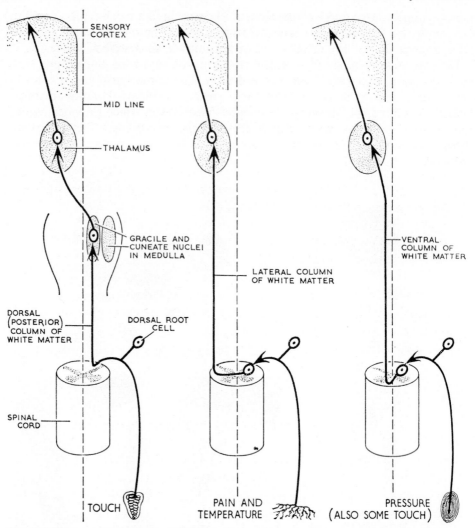

Fig. 121. The sensory pathways. Fibres carrying sensations of pain, temperature and pressure cross on entering the cord. Most touch fibres cross to the opposite side in the medulla.

THE SENSORY SYSTEM

Two main kinds of information are sent to the brain:

    a) sensations from outside the body which are received by the skin. These are of pain, heat, cold and touch;

b) sensations from within the body, from joints, tendons and muscles, which tell of the position of the limbs and trunk. Sensory fibres entering the spinal cord cross to the opposite side, either in the cord or in the medulla. The sensory cortex, in which feeling is recorded lies posterior to the fissure of Rolando, immediately behind the motor area.

The sensory pathway may be interrupted in the peripheral nerve, in the spinal cord, or in the brain. Loss of sensation is not only a deprivation, but a danger because of the risk of injury to the skin, especially from burns, when the patient does not realize he is touching something hot. If the power of movement is lost as well as sensation, the skin is especially vulnerable, and nurses caring for paralyzed patients are aware of the need for regular turning to relieve the pressure on the anaesthetic skin.

Reflexes. A reflex is an automatic response to a sensory stimulus. In its simplest form it is a withdrawal reaction, as when the bare foot encounters something sharp. The spinal cord, the brain and the autonomic system may

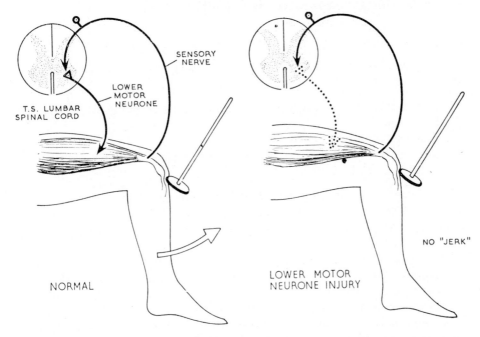

Fig. 122. The knee jerk is a simple example of a reflex. If part of the reflex arc is not functioning (e.g. the lower motor neurone injury) the reflex is lost.

take part in reflex reactions, and several reflexes are tested by the physician in examination of the neurological patient. These are common examples.

a) *Pupillary reflex.* If a light is directed on to the pupil, it should contract. Nurses caring for a patient who has had a head injury or a craniotomy examine the pupils regularly to see if they are active and equal. Increasing dilatation of the pupil indicates that the 3rd cranial nerve is being subject to pressure within the skull.

b) *The knee jerk.* If the patellar tendon is tapped the quadriceps extensor muscle contracts, and the knee straightens momentarily. If the lower motor neurone is injured, the knee jerk is absent. If the upper motor neurone is injured, although the patient cannot move his leg, the knee jerk is present because the spinal pathway is still intact, and is usually brisker than normal.

c) *Plantar reflex.* If the sole of the foot is firmly stroked the big toe flexes. In disease of the nervous system, it may go up (dorsiflex) instead; this abnormal response is called the Babinski response.

THE MENINGES AND THE CEREBROSPINAL FLUID

The brain and the cord are covered with a triple layer of protective membranes, the *meninges*. These are from without inwards:

1. The dura mater, a tough layer in which some of the great vessels of the brain run.
2. The arachnoid.
3. The pia mater, a thin membrane clinging closely to the surface of the brain and cord.

These membranes are extensive, and meningitis (p. 74) is therefore a severe illness. The space beneath the arachnoid is filled with the *cerebrospinal fluid* which is of the greatest importance in the physiology and the pathology of the nervous system.

In each cerebral hemisphere is a cavity, the *lateral ventricle* in which cerebrospinal fluid (C.S.F.) is formed. From the two lateral ventricles it drains backwards and downwards to the centrally placed third ventricle and thence by the narrow *cerebral aqueduct* to the fourth ventricle, out through the roof of this ventricle into the subarachnoid space. The C.S.F. is constantly circulating and is returned to the blood from the arachnoid into the veins in the skull.

If there is an obstruction to the passage of the C.S.F. through the ventricles,

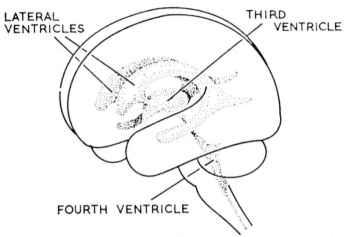

LATERAL VENTRICLES

THIRD VENTRICLE

FOURTH VENTRICLE

Fig. 123. The position of the four ventricles of the brain.

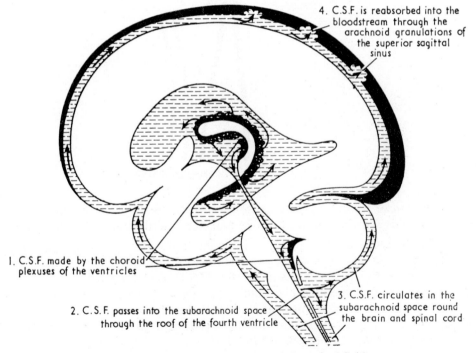

4. C.S.F. is reabsorbed into the bloodstream through the arachnoid granulations of the superior sagittal sinus

1. C.S.F. made by the choroid plexuses of the ventricles

2. C.S.F. passes into the subarachnoid space through the roof of the fourth ventricle

3. C.S.F. circulates in the subarachnoid space round the brain and spinal cord

Fig. 124. The circulation of the cerebrospinal fluid.

or if its reabsorption from the subarachnoid space is delayed, hydrocephalus (p. 412) will result.

Examination of the ventricular system and its contained fluid yields important information. C.S.F. can be withdrawn by inserting a needle and stilette into the subarachnoid space between the lumbar vertebrae, or (a slightly more dangerous procedure) below the foramen magnum. Accidental

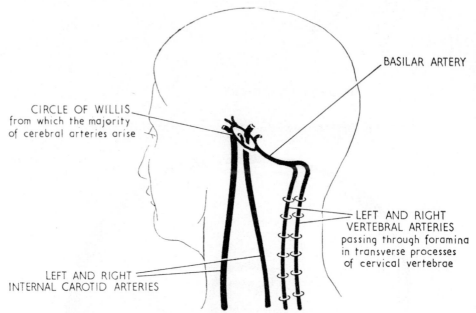

Fig. 125. The arteries that supply the brain.

introduction of infection would cause meningitis, so sterile technique must be rigorous. The information that can be gained by lumbar puncture includes:

a) The pressure of the C.S.F., which is normally 100–150 mm of water.
b) Whether a spinal block is present. Pressure on the jugular veins should cause a rise in the pressure of the C.S.F. (Queckenstedt's test) if the circulation of the fluid is normal.
c) Whether bacteria are present, and what they are.
d) Whether the chemical constituents are normal. Levels of protein, sugar, and chlorides may be changed.
e) A positive Wassermann reaction may be present indicating late syphilis.

The shape, size and position of the ventricles may be altered by disease, especially by intracranial tumours. The ventricles can be visualized in two ways by means of an X-ray. A burrhole can be made into the skull, and a needle through which air is passed; introduced into a lateral ventricle this will make the ventricles visible on X-ray. This procedure is *ventriculography*. Another method is to introduce air by lumbar puncture with the patient in a sitting position; so that air rises to fill the ventricles. This is *air encephalography*.

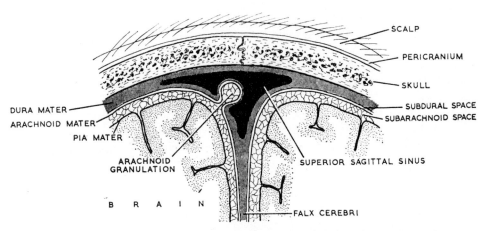

Fig. 126. Blood returns from the brain in spaces between the layers of dura. These are called sinuses; the superior sagittal sinus shown here runs between the two halves of the cerebrum.

CEREBROVASCULAR DISEASE

If the blood supply to the brain is interrupted for more than four minutes at normal temperatures, life cannot continue. The brain is supplied by four major arteries; two vertebral arteries pass up through the transverse processes of the cervical vertebrae, and in front of them are the two internal carotid arteries. These four connect with each other under the base of the brain, and from the circle thus formed, arteries are given off to the whole of the brain. The venous blood is finally collected into spaces in the dura, the venous sinuses. It passes downwards to the lateral sinus, lying close to the mastoid process, and thence into the internal jugular vein on its way back to the heart.

INTRACRANIAL BLEEDING

Haemorrhage within the skull may be:

A. Meningeal;
   1. extradural
   2. subdural
   3. subarachnoid

B. Intracerebral.

MENINGEAL HAEMORRHAGE

A blow on the top of the skull may rupture the middle meningeal artery, so that bleeding occurs between the skull and the dura, and an *extradural haematoma* collects. The typical story is that the patient, who may have lost consciousness after the blow, makes a recovery, but subsequently becomes drowsy, and lapses into coma, with dilatation of the pupil on one side, and paralysis of one side of the body. Treatment is surgical. The important point as far as the nurse is concerned is to recognize the signs of rising intracranial pressure—drowsiness, slow pulse, pupil dilatation—since if treatment is not undertaken the patient will die.

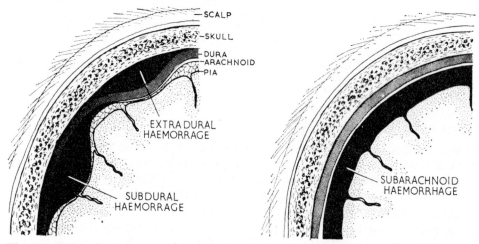

Fig. 127. Types of intracranial haemorrhage. These include bleeding between the skull and the meninges (extradural); between the dura and the arachnoid (subdural); and into the cerebrospinal fluid.

Subdural haemorrhage is usually from veins and capillaries, and is much slower in its onset, which may take days or even weeks. The injury may have been forgotten so that a patient may arrive in a medical ward with signs suggestive of a growth in the cranium. After bleeding has ceased, the haematoma may continue to grow in size by absorbing fluid (osmosis). Headache, drowsiness, paralysis and fits may be features. Ventriculography may reveal the nature of the condition, and *angiography*, by the injection of a radio-opaque dye into the internal carotid artery, may be helpful. The treatment is surgical.

Subarachnoid haemorrhage. Bleeding into the subarachnoid space may be caused by injury, but is more commonly due to an *aneurysm* of an artery at the base of the brain, or to an arterio-venous aneurym, which is a mass of connecting arteries and veins.

The onset is often extremely sudden, with very severe headache, vomiting, and loss of consciousness. If still conscious, the patient is restless, irritable, has *photophobia* (dislike of light) and has neck stiffness. Lumbar puncture reveals that the C.S.F. contains blood.

The prognosis in this condition has been much improved by surgical intervention. If the facilities are available, carotid angiography is undertaken, and the neurosurgeon may be able to clip the neck of an aneurysm, if this is present, or may decide to tie the internal carotid artery on the affected side.

If these facilities are not available, or the patient is old, medical treatment consists of nursing the patient in a quiet place, undisturbed by direct light, and giving analgesics for the headache. Chlorpromazine may help to relieve the vomiting. The fluid intake must be adequate but not excessive.

Only about a third of the people who have a subarachnoid haemorrhage will recover without surgical treatment, and of these another third are likely to suffer a second attack.

CEREBROVASCULAR ACCIDENTS

There are three ways in which the event known to the lay public as a stroke may be caused. A vessel in the brain may be blocked by a clot, or by an embolus, or it may rupture and allow haemorrhage into the brain.

Cerebral thrombosis. Clotting in a brain artery is usually associated with atheroma in elderly patients, and the neurological signs depend on which artery is affected. The patient often feels unwell for minutes or even hours beforehand as the clot develops. In most cases, if the artery is of any size, the pyramidal tract is affected, and paralysis of one side (*hemiplegia*) appears. Vomiting is common, and consciousness is often lost. The face is flushed, the pulse slow and full, the respiration labouring and stertorous. The paralysis on the affected side appears flaccid at first, but as the initial shock passes off, tone returns. Speech is lost if the clot is in the dominant hemisphere. Often the patient lies with the head turned to one side, with the eyes looking in the same direction. Urinary retention or incontinence may occur.

The area in the brain from which blood has been cut off (infarct) is oedematous, and this compresses neighbouring vessels. If the patient survives, some recovery of function takes place as oedema subsides and a collateral circulation opens up, so in many cases the symptoms improve over a few days or weeks. The face usually recovers first, then leg movements, and finally the arm. Fine movements of the hand are the last to return, and often they never do. If paralysis remains, the muscles become spastic and unless treated effectively the elbow and wrist and fingers will become flexed. Speech may return, or may be considerably affected.

Treatment. This falls into three parts:
1. The measures necessary to preserve life in the initial phases.
2. The rehabilitation required when recovery begins.
3. Teaching the patient and his relatives how life at home may be possible if there is loss of function. If disability is severe, return home may not be possible.

The patient is put to bed, and a free airway maintained by a correct position and if necessary suction. Saliva tends to accumulate in a paralysed cheek and must be removed. Charts of the temperature, pulse, respiration and blood pressure are kept, the pupils and the colour observed, cyanosis being treated by oxygen. If coma persists, intravenous or nasal feeding will be begun.

Regular turning from side to side will help to prevent pneumonia and relieve pressure on the skin. The eyes are bathed and paroleine drops instilled; the mouth is cleaned; soiled linen is changed, and the skin protected from incontinence by silicone cream. The limbs must be put through a full range of passive movements daily, the feet are supported to prevent footdrop, and the fingers of the paralysed hand supported with a light plastic splint.

When consciousness returns oral feeding may be begun, with precautions against choking. A spoon, or feeder or a drinking straw can be used, whichever seems best suited to the needs. Patients who cannot speak must be offered a urinal or bedpan regularly, to avoid incontinence. It is quite easy to assume that patients who are unable to speak are also incapable of understanding. To speak to an adult in babytalk, to speak loudly as if he were simple, or (worse still) not to talk to him at all indicate lack of imagination. Take the patient's good hand when you speak to him, so that by pressure he can show understanding, and ask questions which can be answered by a nod or shake of the head.

Physiotherapy is begun as soon as possible. Patients are first taught to turn themselves in bed, then how to sit up. As soon as sitting balance is restored, standing and walking with the help of a tripod stick is taught. Even severely handicapped patients may be taught how to get up from a chair and get to the lavatory unaided, and this is a big step towards independence and the possibility of return to home.

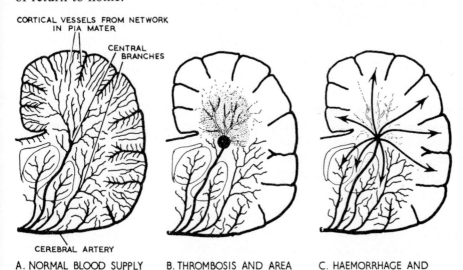

A. NORMAL BLOOD SUPPLY   B. THROMBOSIS AND AREA   C. HAEMORRHAGE AND
                            OF INFARCT   POSSIBLE SPREAD OF DAMAGE

Fig. 128. Cerebrovascular accidents.

A. Shows the normal cerebral vessels.
B. A thrombus cuts off the blood supply to a limited area of the brain.
C. Haemorrhage from a ruptured vessel tracks in all directions in the brain tissues and causes extensive damage.

Frustration and attacks of depression are common and easy to understand and must be met with sympathetic reassurance. Occupational therapy may help to strengthen muscles and regain movement, and those who have lost the use of the right hand must be encouraged to write with the left. Speech therapy may be necessary for some.

The possibility of return home for a handicapped patient depends on his circumstances and the competence of relatives to undertake his care. The welfare worker and health visitor may confer on this, and give advice about the position of the bed, and small adjustments that may be helpful. A non-slip mat in the bath, a handrail in the lavatory, a pulley over the bed are examples.

As the number of elderly people increases, so will the number of those who suffer cerebral thrombosis. Preservation of function and independence and restoration to home life where practicable are therefore of much social importance.

Cerebral embolism usually occurs in patients with heart disease, especially those with atrial fibrillation which may permit the formation of blood clot in the atria. The onset of the stroke is sudden, but the symptoms are similar to those of cerebral thrombosis, and indeed these two conditions cannot always be distinguished from each other. The treatment is the same in both, but in cerebral embolism the condition which gave rise to the embolus must also be treated.

Cerebral haemorrhage occurs when a vessel ruptures, and blood escapes into the brain tissue. Since this is soft, the bleeding tends to continue, and the swelling ruptures neighbouring vessels. Such haemorrhage tends to spread, and is usually fatal in a few hours or days. If the patient recovers he is managed in the same way as other patients with cerebro-vascular accidents.

Venous sinus thrombosis. Clotting in a venous sinus of the brain usually occurs as the result of infection spreading from a neighbouring structure. For instance, mastoid infections used not uncommonly to cause lateral sinus thrombosis, before antibiotic therapy made ear infections less dangerous. The symptoms are fever, swinging hectically, with shivering and sweating, headache and vomiting.

Thrombosis in the cavernous sinus is rare and may result from boils on the upper lip, and causes pain and swelling around the eye. Treatment of either is by the appropriate antibiotic.

Temporal arteritis. In this disease of elderly people there is inflammation of medium sized arteries, especially the temporal and occipital arteries. The cause is unknown.

There may be a long period at the onset when there are no specific symptoms to point to the diagnosis. The temperature rises a little in the evening, and there may be vague aches and pains and loss of weight. This may go on for some weeks, and then severe headache begins, usually over the temples. The scalp may become so tender that the hair cannot be touched. The temporal arteries become thickened and tender.

In nearly half the people who have temporal arteritis the retinal artery is also affected and so the sight is affected, and may eventually be lost. Treatment with a corticosteroid, such as prednisolone, must be given as early as possible in the course of the disease, if eye complications are to be avoided.

INFECTIONS OF THE CENTRAL NERVOUS SYSTEM

Cocci, bacilli, viruses and spirochaetes may infect the nervous system and its covering membranes as they do other systems of the body. Inflammation of the cord is **myelitis;** anterior poliomyelitis is described on page 393. Inflammation of the brain is **encephalitis;** and of the meninges **meningitis.**

The layer of the meninges most often affected in meningitis is the arachnoid, and since the cerebrospinal fluid lies beneath it, there is every chance for infection to become widespread. Infections may reach the meninges from the blood stream, through penetrating wounds, and from structures like the middle ear or the upper respiratory tract.

The organisms that most often cause meningitis are:

a) Pyogenic cocci. Meningococcal meningitis has been described on page 74. Pneumococci and staphylococci may be responsible.

b) The tubercle bacillus.

c) Viruses.

Meningitis used to be a much-feared condition with a high mortality, but effective treatment is available against the dangerous organisms, while the virus infections are rarely fatal. In countries where diagnosis can be made early and effective treatment begun, the outlook has improved greatly.

Signs and symptoms. Whatever the cause, there are certain signs common to all forms of meningitis. There is a day or two of general signs of infection, e.g. **malaise,** with sore throat, joint pains and a little **fever. Headache** develops early, and rapidly becomes severe, spreading down the neck and back. **Vomiting** and **photophobia** are usual. **Drowsiness** and **irritability** follow the patient tending to lie on his side with the back to the light, resenting interference. If an attempt is made to flex the head towards the chest, the neck is found to be stiff, and this **neck rigidity** is a very important diagnostic sign. In children the neck spasm may be so severe as to cause **head retraction,** and sometimes all the muscles of the back are in spasm, causing arching backwards of the body, or **opisthotonos. Kernig's sign** appears; if the hip is flexed, and an attempt then made to straighten the knee, it will be impossible or very painful to the patient. Unless treatment is effective **paralyses** of eye muscles appears and coma supervenes.

The diagnosis may be made on the clinical signs, but **lumbar puncture** must be performed as soon as meningitis is suspected in order to find the organism responsible, and the antibiotics to which it is sensitive.

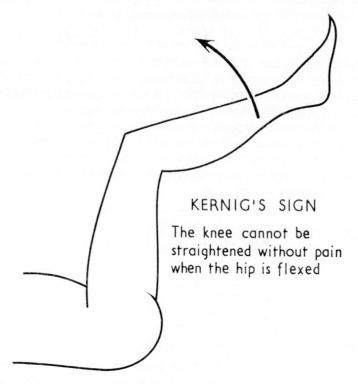

KERNIG'S SIGN

The knee cannot be
straightened without pain
when the hip is flexed

Fig. 129. Kernig's sign.

Pyogenic meningitis. Pneumococcal meningitis may complicate pneumonia, and septic infections from the middle ear or the mastoid process. If such a septic focus is presented, it must be treated.

The patient is nursed in a quiet room without bright light shining on his face. He is usually more comfortable on his side because of the neck stiffness, and the head of the bed may be raised to reduce intracranial pressure. Bedsides are necessary for a restless or drowsy patient. Specific treatment should be started as soon as possible. Sulphadiazine reaches the cerebrospinal fluid in good concentration, and is often prescribed in combination with an antibiotic, like penicillin or tetracycline. The fluid intake must be recorded and an adequate level assured. A restless patient will need sedation.

Tuberculous meningitis. This condition was at one time always fatal, but since the introduction of effective anti-tuberculous drugs the majority of patients who are diagnosed early can be saved. Since this form of meningitis is secondary to tuberculosis elsewhere in the body, a fall in the incidence of tuberculosis means that there will be fewer cases of meningitis.

The onset is slower than in pyogenic meningitis, but the pattern described above gradually develops. The prognosis is better the earlier treatment is begun. Streptomycin is given by intramuscular injection, and isonicotinic acid hydrazide (I.N.A.H.) by mouth. Treatment must be continuous for at least three months, and watch must be kept for such symptoms as giddiness and deafness that indicate that streptomycin is affecting the inner ear. Streptomycin used to be given into the C.S.F. by daily lumbar puncture, and although this may be necessary for adults, children (who form the majority of patients) can usually be cured by intramuscular injection.

Viral meningitis. Virus infections are not yet amenable to antibiotic treatment, but the majority of patients recover without specific drugs. The course resembles that of meningitis due to other causes.

"Meningism" is a term used when a patient has signs suggestive of meningeal irritation, but the cerebrospinal fluid is sterile.

ENCEPHALITIS

Encephalitis is inflammation of the brain, and the main symptoms resemble those of meningitis, with fever, headache, vomiting, drowsiness and often fits, which increase in severity as the inflammation spreads. There is little neck rigidity, Kernig's sign is negative, and the cerebrospinal fluid is normal in pressure, and usually sterile, since encephalitis is usually caused by a virus.

Since viruses are not susceptible to antibiotics, there is no specific treatment. The patient is nursed with attention to fluid balance, sedation for restlessness, and physiotherapy to prevent pneumonia. Corticosteroids may be ordered to reduce the swelling of the brain. This is especially useful in the encephalitis that very occasionally follows vaccination against smallpox, or virus infections such as measles and mumps.

An epidemic form, encephalitis lethargica or sleeping sickness, occurs from time to time, though it has been uncommon for some years. The last epidemic in Europe was in the early 1920's. The symptoms were as described above, and in addition patients suffered disturbance of the normal sleep rhythm, being drowsy by day and wakeful at night. Most patients recovered, but some showed (often years later) the symptoms resembling those of Parkinson's disease

(p. 400). The causal virus has never been discovered. "Slow" viruses exist, with an incubation period varying from months to years, causing disease in animals and (more rarely) in man.

CEREBRAL ABSCESS

Septic infection may spread to the brain directly from an infected mastoid, or by embolus from the lungs if a lung abscess or bronchiectasis is present. An abscess may form in the cerebrum, most commonly in the frontal or temporal lobes. The outlook is most favourable if the organism can be identified, and the appropriate antibiotic given, and also if the abscess is single. Its position may be found by X-ray, a burrhole made, and the abscess contents aspirated. As healing occurs, the septic focus diminishes in size and becomes surrounded by a thick layer of fibrin, and eventually it may be possible to excise it.

SYPHILITIC INFLAMMATION OF THE NERVOUS SYSTEM

If syphilis is inadequately or ineffectively treated, some years later the central nervous system may become involved in chronic inflammation. Such cases were quite common at the time when the treatment of syphilis was long and difficult, but the introduction of penicillin reduced the incidence dramatically, and diseases of the kind described in this section are not now common. The number of people with acute infectious syphilis is still rising, but if these are treated in the early stages, neurosyphilis can be prevented. The central nervous system can be involved in three ways.

1. *Meningo-vascular syphilis.* The small arteries of the brain and meninges are inflamed, and clots in them give rise to sudden paralysis of a limb, or of symptoms which depend on the organs supplied. They may include the structures supplied by one of the cranial nerves, especially the oculomotor nerves. Neck rigidity, mental confusion, and difficulty in speech are other symptoms sometimes seen, depending on the situation and the extent of the inflammation. The Wassermann reaction of the blood is positive, and often that of the cerebrospinal fluid as well.

2. *General paralysis of the insane.* The nerve cells of the brain are attacked in this condition and the name indicates that both the motor system and the higher cortical centres are involved. The mental signs usually appear first. The patient may become morose, apathetic, suspicious and neglectful of his personal appearance, or may suffer from delusions of grandeur, full of alarming schemes

for making money or improving his business, or imagining himself to be some-one famous or powerful. Fits are common, and gradually paralysis appears. Since this is due to injury of the upper motor neurone, it is spastic in type. In untreated cases, the patient sinks into complete helplessness and mental vacuity due to atrophy of the brain cells.

3. *Tabes dorsalis.* The structures affected are the sensory roots of the spinal nerves, and there is degeneration of the tracts that take information to the brain about the position of joints. Lack of this information means that the patient has to rely on sight for knowledge of the position of his body, and so finds it difficult to get about at night, and tends to be unsteady when the eyes are closed, for example, when washing the face. The patient walks with the feet wide apart, putting them down with a stamp.

Involvement of the sensory roots causes sudden stabbing pains in the limbs and along the course of the intercostal nerves. These are so severe that they are called **lightning pains.** Loss of sensation in the bladder causes retention of urine, with overflow incontinence. Joints, especially the knees, may be affected by destructive but painless inflammation. Trophic ulcers may occur on the feet, especially under the big toe. The pupil of the eye may still constrict when focusing on near objects (i.e. it reacts to accommodation) but does not respond to light. This is termed the **Argyll Robertson** pupil, and is highly characteristic of meningo-syphilis.

Treatment. Since the conditions described are degenerative, treatment can only arrest the condition, and cannot reverse changes that have already occurred. The earlier treatment is begun, therefore, the better the results will be. A course of penicillin is begun, a total of 20,000,000 units being given over 10 to 12 days. The Wassermann reaction is checked, and the course repeated after 3 months unless all signs of active disease have disappeared.

ANTERIOR POLIOMYELITIS

Anterior poliomyelitis is caused by a virus which affects nervous tissue and has a special affinity for the anterior horn (motor) cells of the spinal cord, and those of the medulla. It used to be known as infantile paralysis, because the victims were once almost invariably young children. Nowadays many older people are attacked, and this is thought to be because immunity can be pro-duced by subclinical infection, and with rising standards of hygiene fewer people become immune in this way in infancy.

Poliomyelitis is most common in the summer months, and occurs both in epidemic and sporadic form. Until the introduction of immunization, there were many outbreaks of the disease in countries with a high standard of hygiene, but now it is to be hoped that this disease will rapidly become unusual in countries with an immunization programme.

The virus enters the body by the mouth, and invades the intestinal mucous membrane, and thence reaches the bloodstream. Active immunity may be acquired at this stage, so that the disease progresses no further, but in the absence of such immunity the nervous system is invaded, and the motor cells of the cord and medulla attacked, as mentioned above.

Poliomyelitis then may run only a mild course, without obvious involvement of the nervous system, or may progress to become a major illness.

1. **Minor form.** The patient has a cold, with headache, mild fever, sore throat and malaise. These symptoms are of course not specific, so it is unusual for the illness to be diagnosed at this stage, unless an epidemic is in progress and doctors are alert to the possibility. Sometimes the condition is recognized by hind sight, when another member of the family develops a severe illness.

2. **Major form.** The symptoms are more severe, with fever up to 103° or 104°F (39·4° to 40°C). The muscles of the back and limbs are painful, vomiting and anorexia are common, and there gradually follow the signs of meningitis, such as photophobia and neck rigidity. The patient is apprehensive and miserable, resenting any touch or movement. Lumbar puncture produces cerebrospinal fluid which is clear and contains many lymphocytes.

Although the patient is severely ill, the majority do not progress beyond this stage, and recovery ensues. The treatment is that of any feverish patient, but if the illness is diagnosed the family must be kept in quarantine under supervision, and must be taught how to avoid infecting others by faecal contamination.

In the most serious cases, between the second and tenth day of the illness paralysis becomes apparent. Sometimes this may affect so few muscles that the disability is not noticed till the patient resumes activity, while in others it may involve all four limbs, the respiratory and swallowing muscles. Since the lower motor neurone is affected, the paralysis is flaccid, tendon reflexes are lost, and rapid extreme muscle wasting occurs. Retention of urine is common, especially if the trunk muscles are involved.

The paralysis reaches its height in a day or two, and in a week some recovery often begins to take place, and this may eventually be complete. In three months the extent of the residual paralysis is usually clear, though with physiotherapy improvement of function may go on for months.

Treatment of the major illness. General measures to maintain fluid intake, prevent pneumonia and pressure sores, relieve pain and retention of urine are taken, and the patient is nursed with precautions to prevent spread of infection to others. The most important aspects of treatment are the care of the paralysed muscles and watch for complications.

When a muscle is paralysed, the pull of its antagonists is unopposed and will cause severe deformity, and the paralysed parts must be supported in a position to prevent this. A fracture board is used beneath the mattress, and the measures taken depend on which muscles are affected. The feet must be supported to prevent foot drop, a small pillow or roll beneath the knees maintains a little flexion, and the arms should be slightly abducted if the deltoid is paralysed. A small pad is kept in the palm of the hand to keep the thumb abducted and the fingers slightly flexed. Light splints may be required, easily detachable so that limbs may be put through a full range of passive movement daily. Painful muscle spasm may be eased by hot fomentations.

Once the disease has become inactive, intensive physiotherapy is given to restore those muscles which are incompletely paralysed. Exercises in slings or in a pool are especially valuable. After six months no further recovery of nerve cells will occur, but improvement of function may go on for years as the patient learns to make the best use of partially affected muscles. Later still, orthopaedic operations such as arthrodesis may stabilize weak joints, and tendon transplants may increase useful movement.

The two most feared complications are bulbar paralysis and respiratory failure.

a) **Bulbar paralysis.** On the second or third day it may be noticed that there is difficulty in swallowing, nasal speech, increasing secretion in the pharynx, rapid pulse and drowsiness. Although this complication is a grave one, if the patient survives, there should be a complete recovery. The head must be lowered to allow postural drainage of secretions, and pharyngeal suction is usually required. Feeding must be by nasal catheter, with aseptic technique, using every precaution to ensure that fluid does not enter the airway. Should respiratory failure also occur, the outlook is considerably worse.

b) **Respiratory paralysis.** Although this may occur quite suddenly, there are usually warning signs such as dyspnoea, restlessness, cyanosis, and decreasing chest movement. Treatment should be undertaken early, or the lungs will become increasingly consolidated with secretion.

Tracheostomy is performed, a cuffed tube is inserted, and the patient connected to a positive-pressure ventilator. The old tank respirator is now rarely used, as it made nursing exceedingly difficult, and if bulbar paralysis was present, drew secretions into the lungs and soon led to death.

Prevention of poliomyelitis. Two vaccines are available for producing active immunity. The older is the Salk vaccine, which is a killed culture of all three viruses that cause poliomyelitis. It is given in three doses by intramuscular injection.

The Salk vaccine consists of live but weak virus, which is given by mouth on a lump of sugar. This vaccine has now been widely used in Britain.

During an epidemic, certain measures can be taken, in addition to mass vaccination, to lower the incidence of paralytic cases. It is known for instance that bulbar paralysis may follow tonsillectomy, so operating sessions in the throat department should be suspended. Intramuscular injections for children should be avoided, since these may precipitate paralysis in the muscles used. Over-strenuous activity is unwise, and public swimming pools, should be closed. Doctors are alert to recognize the minor form of the disease, and to isolate suspected sufferers.

EPILEPSY

Brain cells show electrical activity, and it is the record of this activity which constitutes the **electroencephalogram.** This is an important aid in the diagnosis of intracranial conditions, since the normal pattern is changed by disease, such as new growths inside the skull. In epilepsy, there is abnormal electrical activity in some part of the cortex, which from time to time triggers off attacks in which consciousness may be lost and fits occur. Though one usually thinks of fits as being motor in form, these attacks sometimes consist of unusual sensations, feelings, thoughts, and behaviour. Apart from those who actually have "fits", there are many people who show a typically epileptic pattern of encephalogram but never have an obvious attack. There is a family tendency to such a pattern.

Epilepsy in its major form has been described in literature since classical times, but several different manifestations are now grouped under this term. They may be considered under these headings:

1. **Idiopathic epilepsy.** There is no ascertainable physical disease in the brain to cause the fits, which may be of two kinds.
   a) Major epilepsy, in which convulsions with loss of consciousness occur. This is what the lay public understands by epilepsy.
   b) Minor epilepsy, in which brief attacks of confusion and dizziness occur, without the patient falling or having a convulsion. Since a patient with minor epilepsy may sometimes have a major fit, there seems no very sound reason for dividing these patients. There is no doubt, however, that

patients who only have minor fits have a better social prognosis than those who have major ones.

2. **Petit mal.** Children may suffer brief attacks in which they become for a moment vacant in expression, may drop what they are holding, even occasionally tumble over. The attacks are momentary, though they may be very numerous sometimes, and the child resumes activity at once. These attacks of petit mal may occur in children who also have major fits, but not uncommonly they are the only manifestations, and if this is so, the child frequently grows out of these attacks, which never recur.

3. **Focal epilepsy.** The attacks only affect one part of the body. They are always due to local disease of the brain, such as a new growth, or scarring, or adhesions between the meninges and the brain. Focal attacks which begin always in the same site, and spread in a regular way to involve first one side of the body and then the other are called **Jacksonian** fits.

Major epilepsy or grand mal. The characteristic fit often begins with a warning sensation of **aura.** This feeling is always the same; the patient may see a light, feel constriction in the chest or experience a smell. The aura is short-lasting, and is followed by loss of consciousness; the patient falls, and there is a rigid contraction of the whole body. The arms are flexed, the legs extended, the back arched, the head extended and the jaws clenched. Breathing ceases, so that intense cyanosis develops. This is called the **tonic** phase of the fit. In a few moments, jerky movements of face and limbs begin, the jaws open and close, often biting the tongue. This is the **clonic** part of the fit. The movements may become violent, and the bladder is often emptied involuntarily. The movements gradually die away, and the patient lies deeply unconscious, with flushed face and absent pupillary reflexes. The coma may last for a few minutes, or for hours, and the patient wakes in bewilderment, and then if permitted falls asleep. During the confused stage he may perform acts which he cannot subsequently remember, and which may harm himself or others (**post-epileptic automatism**). Occasionally patients pass from one fit into another, a condition called **status epilepticus.**

Once a fit has begun, nothing can stop it, and help is directed towards safe-guarding the patient during the attack. If he is in danger from fire, or traffic, or from injury by nearby objects, he must be protected. It is commonly advised that something be placed between the teeth to prevent the tongue being bitten, but this is not usually practical when the fit occurs in a public place; fragile objects are bitten through, and metal ones may break the teeth. Collar and tie may be loosened, and care must be taken that the airway is not obstructed, e.g. as it may be by lying face down in a pillow. The patient should not be left alone until he has recovered consciousness.

Treatment aims at abolishing fits by the regular and continuous administration of anti-convulsant drugs. A barbiturate such as phenobarbitone is usually given, and a drug of the hydantoin group, such as phenytoin sodium (Epanutin). The dosage and the drugs that will abolish fits are found, and this régime must be rigorously and continuously followed. The dose should not be reduced until the patient has had no fit for a minimum of two years, and then reduction must be very gradually undertaken, since sudden withdrawal may precipitate status epilepticus.

A patient in status epilepticus must be under continuous observation to prevent injury or obstruction of the airway. The temperature is taken hourly, since high fever may result from the excessive muscular activity. This must be prevented or treated by tepid sponging, or use of an electric fan. Paraldehyde 10 ml and/or phenytoin sodium is usually given by intramuscular injection.

Petit mal. Ethosuxamide is usually effective in controlling the attacks in children. The tendency to spontaneous cure as the child grows up has already been noticed.

All fits, especially focal epileptic attacks demand careful investigation (e.g. by carotid angiogram and encephalography) to determine the cause. Tumours, abscesses, scars or arterio-venous aneurysms may be capable of surgical cure. Even though fits are focal in origin, surgery is not always effective.

Social aspects of epilepsy. Epilepsy often begins in young adults, and sometimes becomes inactive as time goes on. In most cases, attacks can be prevented if an adequate drug régime is meticulously followed, but the possibility of a fit occurring still remains. In a few, the fits cannot be controlled by drugs without producing toxic effects, and life in an institution must be accepted.

Young people are often overwhelmed when told of their diagnosis, and need counsel and support in many ways. Suitable work and hobbies must be found. Work that involves exposure to undue risk from machinery, or fire, or falling from a height must be avoided. Most games and sports are suitable, though swimming alone, or horse riding, or sailing single-handed would be unwise. Employers should always be told of the condition, and a tolerant and helpful attitude by fellow employees may be produced by teaching the simple precautions to be taken during a fit.

Alcohol is bad for the epileptic and should be avoided. The epileptic is legally barred from driving and this is a great hardship, but the safety of others as well as the patient is of paramount importance. If there have been no fits for two years, and if drugs have been withdrawn with no ill effects, the condition may be supposed to have been arrested, and application may be made for consideration.

The question of marriage is always raised, and provided the partner knows the diagnosis and is prepared to live with it, a happy life and a stable environment is of great benefit to the epileptic. The chance of children being affected is little greater than chance, unless both partners are epileptic, when the risks are increased.

MIGRAINE

In migraine there are severe recurrent paroxysms of headache, due to alteration in the blood flow of the vessels of the brain. The attack begins with an aura, usually of a visual kind. The patient may see flashes of light, sometimes of vertical lines called fortification spectra, or may find the visual field is decreased. Numbness or tingling of the face may be experienced. Within minutes headache develops, often severe enough to cause vomiting, and lasting for several hours, unless treatment interrupts it. The headache is incapacitating, the patient feeling unable to do anything but lie down in the dark until it is over. The aura is thought to be due to constriction of the vessels inside the skull, and the ensuing headache to dilatation of the external arteries of the head and face.

No cause is known, but there is a tendency for migraine to run in families. Patients are usually young adults, tense and conscientious in nature, who get headaches after periods of hard work or anxiety, or before the menstrual period. In some patients attacks may be precipitated by constituents of chocolate. Migraine tends to become less severe, and sometimes to disappear as the patient gets older.

Treatment. Many patients fear the onset of the next headache and if they are tense and anxious sedation by diazepam or one of the many other tranquillizers will benefit them and may reduce the number of attacks.

The most effective treatment of a severe attack is ergotamine tartrate, given as early as possible, and preferably by injection. Those who are capable of learning to give themselves hypodermic injections should be taught to do so. Patients should be told that, though painful, migraine is not dangerous and that attacks will diminish in frequency.

THE BASAL GANGLIA

Most of the nerve cells of the cerebrum are on the outside, forming the cerebral cortex, but there are in addition masses of nerve cells deep in the white matter or nerve fibres. These are known collectively as the **basal ganglia,** and they may be thought of as the remains of a primitive motor pathway, which has lost in importance as the cerebral cortex increased in size and complexity.

If the basal ganglia are affected by a group of diseases, muscular movement and tone are upset, tremor and rigidity being the usual results. There are several rare diseases which affect the basal ganglia, and one common one, Parkinson's disease, or **paralysis agitans.**

PARKINSON'S DISEASE

Paralysis agitans is a disease of elderly people, the leading symptoms being tremor, or muscular rigidity, or both. When the clinical picture is fully developed it is characteristic. The face is expressionless, and speech is indistinct and monotonous. The posture is stooping, with knees and elbows flexed, and when at rest there is coarse tremor, especially noticeable in the thumb and fingers ("pill-rolling" movement). This tremor may improve when movement is undertaken; it is difficult to believe, for instance, that a patient with a marked tremor can pick up his cup of tea, but as he does so the tremor stops. Walking is done in small shuffling steps, often with the arms hanging. Sweating and increased salivation may occur, indicating that the autonomic system is involved. The mental powers are often unaffected, though the slowness of speech may mislead strangers.

The final transmission from a nerve fibre to its target cell is by a chemical. Acetylcholine has been mentioned in connection with myasthemia gravis, and noradrenaline is well known for its sympathetic effects. In paralysis agitans, areas of the cerebellum and midbrain become depleted of a chemical transmitter, dopamine, allowing unopposed action by acetylcholine. Treatment therefore aims either at replacing the dopamine, or by blocking the action of acetylcholine. *Levodopa* is converted into dopamine in the brain and is most effective in reducing rigidity. The dose is gradually increased until maximum benefit is obtained. Effects such as nausea and sleeplessness may limit its use, and patients with longstanding disease may not be able to tolerate a dose adequate to relieve their symptoms. *Orphenadrine* may be used if levodopa is not well tolerated.

Anticholinergic drugs are useful in treating tremor and salivation. *Benzhexol* is effective, and may be used with levodopa. A variety of other drugs may be tried alone or in combination. These will improve the symptoms, but do not halt the progress of the degeneration.

Surgical treatment gives good results in selected cases. Patients should not be too advanced in age, or suffering from vascular disease, and the best results are achieved in unilateral Parkinsonism. The operation consists of the destruction of one of the basal ganglia, the globus pallidus, on one or both sides. The effects of operation are not always permanent, and in all cases social care is important. The patient is helped to maintain good grooming, nutrition should be satisfactory, and the patient should be encouraged to maintain social interests and contacts as long as possible.

DEGENERATIVE DISEASE OF THE NERVOUS SYSTEM

Motor neurone disease affects the anterior horn cells and the fibres of the pyramidal tract. The symptoms depend on the level at which the disease occurs.

It most commonly begins between the ages of 40 and 60. Weakness and wasting usually begins in the hands and shoulders and spreads to the muscles of the trunk and legs. If the brainstem is affected, difficulty in speech and swallowing occurs, and there is a danger of inhalation pneumonia. If the pyramidal tract is affected first, there will be muscle spasticity, but wasting and weakness eventually supervene.

There is no curative treatment for this degenerative condition. Care is directed to promoting comfort, maintaining morale and nutrition, and preventing pneumonia. Patients eventually realize that they are receiving no treatment, and have to face the fact that they will progress to complete helplessness. An effort must be made to supply aids (such as house modifications, a wheelchair, invalid car or electric typewriter) quickly, or before relief arrives the patient may have deteriorated past the point where he can make use of it. Relatives have a very trying time, and need sympathetic support.

Syringomyelia is a degenerative disease in which a cavity appears in the spinal cord. The extent of the symptoms depends on how far down the cord the cavity extends. It involves the fibres that record pain and temperature, so that the patient finds he burns or injures his hands without noticing it at the time, although his sensitivity to touch is not impaired. Wasting may become marked as time progresses.

Treatment. Deep X-ray to the affected region of the cord has sometimes appeared to delay extension of the cavity. Progress of the disease is often slow, and there may be many years of life of moderate comfort. The patient must be taught self-protection from stoves and hot dishes, and to avoid the use of hot water bottles.

Cerebral (cortical) atrophy, or degeneration of the brain, occurs as a result of cerebro-vascular disease or injury, or perhaps of causes still unknown. Memory and intellect progressively deteriorate, until the patient can no longer order his affairs, or even recognize his relatives.

The treatment of the degenerative nervous conditions is sad for the physician, who does not know the cause and cannot effect a cure. For the nurse, the opportunity to promote comfort and provide assistance is always present.

DEMYELINATING DISEASE

Most nerve fibres are covered with a sheath of myelin, which insulates them from their neighbours and is essential to their proper function. In some diseases, the myelin sheath of certain fibres disintegrates, and the function of these fibres is lost. Scar tissue is formed around them, which may prevent nerve fibres regenerating, and also involve healthy ones as it contracts in the way all scars do. There are several demyelinating diseases, but only one, multiple disseminated) sclerosis, is common.

Multiple sclerosis. Sclerosis means hardening, and the term refers to the patches of scar tissue that occur in the nervous system. The reason for their appearance is still unknown, and since they can appear anywhere the signs and the progress of the disease are variable.

Multiple sclerosis usually begins in young adults, and is an uncommon disease outside the temperate zones. Symptoms appear as the result of demyelination, then settle down again, only to recur later. Eventually the scarring process leads to permanent loss of function in the parts affected. It is therefore a disease in which there are alternate remissions and relapses.

The symptoms depend on the part of the nervous system affected. Changes in one optic nerve causes loss of sight in one eye; affection of the oculo-motor nerves produce double vision (diplopia), a common complaint. Cerebellar sclerosis causes ataxia, and affection of the pyramidal tract causes spastic weakness, and bladder symptoms such as urgency of micturition. The downhill progress may be rapid, but may take many years, and sometimes the condition becomes stationary, and no further deterioration follows. Typically, however, the patient finally becomes bedridden, with paraplegia and urinary incontinence.

Management. No cure is yet known, though corticosteroids sometimes have a temporary beneficial effect. The problem of the physician is to enable the patient to support life under the conditions which the disease imposes.

Since the early symptoms are transient, they may often be thought of as neurotic, or the doctor may prefer to avoid disclosing the diagnosis until it can no longer be kept secret. In either case the patient may feel bitter, thinking either that the doctor did not realize what was wrong, or practised deception. Everyone must be considered individually, but it is probably better to disclose the diagnosis as soon as possible, since it is a great shock if the patient learns it accidentally. In the early stages, it is always possible to give a hopeful view, stressing the likelihood of remissions, and the possibility that these may be prolonged, and that many years of active life may lie ahead. As with all chronic diseases of unknown cause, there is always the possibility that a cure will be discovered from which the patient can benefit.

In the late stages, when the patient is bedridden, prevention of flexion contractures, bed sores and urinary infection are the primary considerations.

The Multiple Sclerosis Society may give helpful support not only to patients, but to their relatives.

CONGENITAL SPASTIC DISEASE

Congenital spastic paralysis (or palsy) is caused by failure of cerebral cells to develop, or damage to them at birth. The causes of such injury include prematurity; prolonged labour due to uterine inertia, asphyxia of the newborn. Like the damage to brain cells that occurs if cardiac arrest lasts more than a few minutes, this condition is caused by interruption of the oxygen supply to the cortex. In another group of cases, rubella (German measles) causes this and other congenital abnormalities.

If the basal ganglia are affected, there are spontaneous involuntary movements, sometimes rhythmical, sometimes jerky or irregular. Intelligence will be normal if the cerebrum is not involved. If the cerebellum is affected, muscle tone is reduced. Involvement of the pyramidal tract results in paralysis, and since the upper motor neurone is the one damaged, the paralysis is spastic in type. Sometimes only the lower limbs are affected (diplegia), or all four limbs may be spastic.

The symptoms may be noticed soon after birth, the tone of the baby's muscles being increased, or they may become gradually apparent during the first year of life. The changes are always symmetrical, both sides of the body being more or less equally affected. Sometimes only the legs are affected (spastic diplegia), sometimes all four limbs are involved. Involuntary movements often take place.

If the child can walk, it will be only with difficulty. The thighs and knees are pressed together, the calf muscles are contracted so that the heels do not reach the ground; the method of walking thus produced is called the scissors gait. There may be curvature of the spine, and the neck may be either flexed or extended.

Treatment. If mental power is not severely affected, physiotherapy should be begun at an early age, to prevent contractures and increase the power of voluntary movement by passive and active means. Once the child possesses some power in its muscles, tenotomy to release contractures may help to restore more natural movement. Provided intelligence is normal, persistent and lengthy treatment on these lines may permit the spastic to earn his own living.

One of the sad facts about spastic disease is that many of the sufferers are first children, since birth hazards tend to be greater in the first born. Parents often fear to add another child to the family in case it is similarly afflicted, or may be so preoccupied with the care of the spastic child that they feel they cannot give time to another. Sometimes they feel guilt which reassurance cannot assuage. Joining a society of parents with such children may help them by allowing to share their problems, and to benefit from the experiences of others. Such societies may also help to mould public opinion towards acceptance of these handicapped children into the community, by inducing tolerance to their muscular disability.

THE SPINAL CORD AND ITS NERVES

Thirty-one pairs of nerves are given off from the spinal cord, each being formed by the union of a sensory (posterior) and motor (anterior) root, and also containing fibres from the autonomic system. In the thoracic region, these nerves pass singly from the cord and run in the grooves below the ribs to be distributed to the trunk and abdominal wall. In the cervical and lumbar areas, the nerves join together to form networks called **plexuses,** from which the individual nerves arise. From the first four cervical nerves is formed the **cervical plexus,** the most important branch of which is the **phrenic** nerve, which passes down through the chest to supply the diaphragm. The **brachial** plexus, from which the nerves to the arm are given off, is derived from the last four cervical nerves and the first thoracic. The **lumbosacral** plexus, supplies nerves to the legs. Individual nerves may be injured, or many of them may be affected together by general disease or deficiency.

Brachial plexus. This plexus lies behind the clavicle in the neck and passes into the axilla, is derived from the 5th, 6th, 7th and 8th cervical roots, and the 1st thoracic. It is occasionally injured during delivery, if difficulty is experienced in extracting the shoulders, and traction is made with the neck drawn to one side. After birth the baby's arm is noted to be limp, lying at the side with the elbow extended and the back of the hand turned forward. Recovery is usual, and in the meantime the arm must be supported with the shoulder abducted and the elbow flexed to a right angle. This is simply done by putting a bandage round the wrist and fastening it to the top of the cradle so that the hand is level with the chin.

Injury to the brachial plexus may occur if the shoulder is dislocated, or is over-abducted and extended for some time, as is possible during a surgical operation if the arm is being used for intravenous therapy, or a breast amputation is being performed. Care over the patient's position will avoid this accident.

It is not uncommon for a small extra rib to arise from the last cervical vertebra, and although in most cases it gives no trouble, such a rib or fibrous bands associated with it may press on the brachial plexus and give rise to symptoms. These usually do not occur until adult life, when the dropping of the shoulder girdle brings the accessory rib into contact with the brachial plexus.

The condition occurs most often in women, and in the right arm. They feel numbness, tingling and pain in the hand and fingers, usually in the area served by one of the brachial nerves. The skin may be hot or cold, and wasting of muscles may occur.

Complaints of this kind indicate the need for a general examination, to exclude conditions such as pernicious anaemia with involvement of the nervous system, and local examination is also made to exclude the possibility of, for instance, the carpal tunnel syndrome (p. 406). Mild pain may be relieved by support in a sling, avoiding carrying heavy shopping baskets, and physio-therapy to improve the muscle tone. Sometimes surgical removal of the rib is necessary, especially if there is muscle wasting.

Nerves of the upper limb. Three large nerves arise from the brachial plexus, the radial, the median and the ulnar. The **radial nerve** passes around the back of the humerus on its way to the thumb side of the forearm and hand. It is often contused when the humerus is fractured, or if the back of the arm is allowed to rest on the edge of an operating table, or on anything hard, while the patient is unconscious. The most noticeable sign is wristdrop, since the radial nerve supplies the extensor muscles of the wrist and fingers. Although the radial nerve is a mixed one, the effects of injury fall mostly on its motor section.

The **ulnar nerve** is most susceptible to injury where it runs past the inner epicondyle of the humerus into the forearm. Everyone knows how a knock here, on the "funny bone" will cause tingling in the little finger side of the hand. Paralysis causes a claw-hand, with the joints between fingers and hand extended, and the last joints of the fingers flexed.

The **median nerve.** Injuries involving only this nerve are uncommon. Just as the effects of injury to the radial nerve are mostly motor, so those of the median nerve are mainly sensory, and such injuries cause much pain. The best known condition involving the median nerve is the **carpal tunnel syndrome.** The flexor tendons of the muscles of the hand, and the median nerve pass into the hand under a band of fibrous tissue in the wrist, and the nerve may be compressed here. Sufferers are usually middle-aged women, often overweight, who use the affected hand vigorously in work or play. The hand tingles, but especially at night, so that much sleep is lost, and pain or numbness is felt in the three middle fingers. Avoiding over-use of the hand, a light plastic splint to rest the hand in the neutral position, analgesics and perhaps the injection of hydrocortisone into the carpal tunnel may give relief. Sometimes it is necessary to open the carpal tunnel to relieve the pressure on the nerve, though this may weaken the grip of the hand by also loosening the flexor tendons.

THE NERVES TO THE LOWER LIMB

The nerves to the leg which arise from the lumbosacral plexus are:

1) The **femoral** nerve supplies the quadriceps muscle on the front of the thigh and may be involved in fractures of the pelvis or other injuries. The most important feature is the loss of power to extend the knee, which flexes when any weight is put on it, so that a knee cage is necessary if walking is to be undertaken.

2) The **sciatic** nerve, which leaves the back of the pelvis at the great sciatic notch. It supplies the muscles of the back of the thigh and all those of the leg below the knee. Affection of this nerve by a prolapsed intervertebral disc is considered below. The sciatic nerve divides the medial and lateral popliteal branches; the latter is exposed to injury as it winds around the neck of the fibula on the outer side of the leg below the knee. Here it may be compressed by a badly applied splint or a tight bandage. The sciatic nerve itself may be injured by badly placed intramuscular injections into the buttock, and nurses who undertake this common procedure should never relax the precautions that ensure that these injections are given into the upper outer quadrant of the buttock. Injury to the sciatic nerve causes drop foot, with cessation of movement below the knee. Walking is only possible by flexing the knee high enough to raise the paralysed foot clear of the ground.

3) The **obturator** nerve emerges from the obturator foramen to supply the adductor muscles on the inner side of the thigh. It is rarely injured alone.

SCIATICA

This term was formerly much used to mean an inflammation of the sciatic nerve, but now it is believed that most patients with pain in the sciatic nerve have suffered a herniation of an intervertebral disc. The bodies of the vertebrae are joined together by pads of fibrocartilage, the interior of which is semifluid. Muscular efforts or unusual movements may cause rupture of the vertebral ligaments, with escape of some of the substance of a disc into the vertebral canal, usually in the lumbar region, and this presses on a nerve root. Another cause uncommon, but important, is malignant pelvic disease.

Acute pain is felt in the back, and intense muscle spasm renders it rigid. The normal lumbar curve is flattened, so that the buttocks are less prominent than usual. Pain is usually felt in the leg in the distribution of the sciatic nerve,

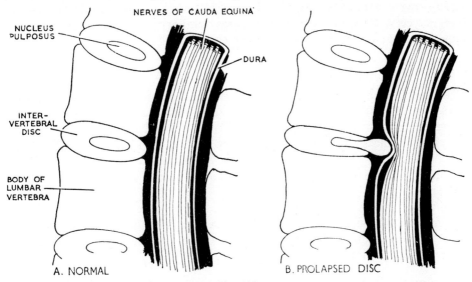

NERVES OF CAUDA EQUINA

NUCLEUS PULPOSUS

DURA

INTER-VERTEBRAL DISC

BODY OF LUMBAR VERTEBRA

A. NORMAL

B. PROLAPSED DISC

Fig. 130.

A. The bodies of the vertebrae are joined by pads of fibrocartilage, the intervertebral discs.

B. The disc may rupture, especially in the lumbar area, and the soft nucleus pulposus may prolapse and imitate nerves of the cauda equina.

though this may arise later than the back pain, and persist longer. The pain is made worse by any muscular strain such as coughing or sneezing.

People in acute pain must be put to bed, lying flat on a firm mattress, and given sedation sufficient to allow them to relax. As soon as the acute pain is relieved physiotherapy must be begun to strengthen the muscles of the back and to restore the usual lumbar curve. Active extension exercises must be practised regularly, and for increasing periods, and may need to be continued for years to maintain good muscle tone and posture and so avoid a relapse.

If the condition does not respond rapidly to treatment, or the acute pain continues, pelvic traction may be used to immobilize the lumbar spine and permit healing. A plaster jacket or an orthopaedic corset may be necessary to allow the patient to get about without pain.

Operation to remove the prolapsed part of the herniated disc is sometimes undertaken, if prolonged bed rest and traction fails to remove the pain, or if sciatica is recurrent.

Prolapse of an intervertebral disc may also occur in the cervical region, causing severe pain in the arm, and in middle-aged people degenerative bony changes (**cervical spondylosis**) may cause similar symptoms. Treatment is support of the neck with a fitting plastic collar.

PERIPHERAL NEUROPATHY

This used to be called peripheral neuritis. Neuritis means inflammation of a nerve, but inflammation in the common sense does not occur, and the more general term neuropathy is now used. The peripheral nerves are susceptible to toxic substances and to lack of necessary nutrients, and loss of function may ensue under such circumstances. Sensory symptoms include pain, numbness and tingling, while motor effects are muscle wasting and weakness, and absence of reflexes.

Deficiency states in which polyneuritis occurs are subacute combined degeneration of the cord with pernicious anaemia (page 158) and beri-beri due to vitamin B deficiency (page 34). Toxic causes include alcoholic poisoning, lead poisoning and diabetes.

Alcoholic neuropathy. Alcohol in excess is an acute poison to the central nervous system, inhibiting the higher cortical centres, and causing ataxia, double vision, difficulty in speech and eventually coma. Chronic alcoholism affects the liver and the brain, and also has a profound effect on the patient's nutrition, since he may have little interest in, or even money for, food. His diet may therefore be short of vitamin B and his inflamed stomach may inhibit its absorption. Polyneuritis is quite common in heavy drinkers, presumably as a result of this deficiency. A noticeable feature of the neuritis is that superficial sensation in the arms and legs is diminished, but deep sensation is heightened, so that pressure on the muscles of the calves or forearms is intensely painful. Treatment is by administration of vitamin B complex, and the avoidance of alcohol.

Lead poisoning is an industrial disease of people who work with it, and may also be acquired by taking contaminated food or drink. Those who live near motorway junctions with heavy traffic are exposed to an atmosphere contaminated with lead in petrol fumes. Children may also acquire it by chewing cot rails or toys with lead paint on them. The lead is deposited in bones, affects blood formation, causes muscle palsies and may be stored in the brain, especially in children.

The muscles affected are mainly those which receive most use, and in manual workers these are the extensors of the wrist and fingers, so that wrist drop is the commonest nervous symptom. As in all kinds of poisoning by heavy metals, there is abdominal colic, and albuminuria indicates that the kidneys are affected.

There are many ways in which the incidence of lead poisoning can be reduced by improving industrial processes, and prohibiting the use of lead paint on children's toys. If wrist drop is present, the wrist should be supported in a sling or splint. In severe cases, excretion of the lead can be encouraged by the use of dimercaprol.

Diabetic neuropathy is thought to be due to disease of the small vessels that supply the nerves, and is a complication of poorly controlled diabetes. The symptoms are mainly sensory, with burning pain and numbness in the hands and feet. Effective control of the blood sugar should arrest the condition but may not cure it.

Acute infective polyneuritis is a not very common condition that begins with a feverish episode. The chief effects are motor, and the paralysis may be widespread, usually including a bilateral facial paralysis. As in alcoholic neuritis, the muscles are often very tender.

During the acute stage, the patient is kept at complete rest, and must be fed. Corticosteroids appear to hasten the recovery, which is usually complete.

PARAPLEGIA

Paralysis and loss of sensation which is equal on both sides of the body is termed **paraplegia**. Such a lesion is always in the spinal cord, and the extent of the damage depends on the level in the cord at which the damage is sustained. If it is high in the cervical cord, death may occur from respiratory paralysis. If it is above the level of the brachial plexus, all four limbs may be affected (**quadriplegia**). If the lesion is in the lumbar region, sphincter control is lost and so is sensation and movement of the legs. If the trouble is below the level of the second lumbar vertebra, where the cord ends, the nerves of the cauda equina are compressed, and there is incontinence, and anaesthesia of the perineum and the inner side of the thighs. The onset of paraplegia may be acute or gradual.

ACUTE PARAPLEGIA

Complete interruption of the cord may occur in fracture-dislocations of the spine, or in vertebral collapse due to a secondary carcinoma. The result is the sudden onset of a flaccid paralysis, with retention of urine and faeces. At this stage the patient is in danger of developing trophic ulcers on the buttocks, heels and great trochanters, and urinary infection in the atonic bladder. If retention with overflow develops, the risk of ulceration of the moist skin will be increased. The flaccid limbs must be maintained in a good position, dorsi-flexion of the feet being the most important point. The bladder must be catheterized at eight-hourly intervals with careful aseptic technique, and sulphadimidine is given as a precaution against urinary infection. The patient must be turned two-hourly to relieve pressure on susceptible areas, and enough attendants should be available to lift him, as dragging may injure the skin. A ripple mattress is a help in keeping the skin over the pressure areas intact.

It must also be remembered that the patient's upper half is just as important as the paralysed part. Paraplegia due to a fracture-dislocation is often a sudden catastrophe occurring in a young patient, and he must be helped to realize that there are activities and chances of enjoyment still open to him. He is encouraged to use his arms, on the strength of which much of his ability to help himself will depend, to eat plenty of protein and to drink well in order to reduce the possibility of urinary infection.

Within two or three weeks of the injury, the state of spinal shock passes off, and reflex activity begins again in the paralyzed part. Because the pyramidal tracts are damaged, the tone in the flexor muscles increases, so that hips and knees flex, and any stimulus, such as nursing attention or the weight of the bedclothes causes intense spasm, though voluntary movement is not possible. At the same time, bladder tone increases, and automatic micturition begins to take place at intervals. The risk of bed sores, though always present in para-plegics, becomes slightly less acute. Attempts are now made to induce automatic reflex activity of the bladder by suprapubic pressure at regular intervals, or by injection of carbachol. If incontinence occurs, a urinal may be worn. The colon must not be allowed to become distended with faeces, but aperients should be used with caution. Patients who can manage it should be taught how to evacuate the rectum manually. Flexion deformities of hips and knees must be prevented by physiotherapy and muscle relaxants may be required if spasm is troublesome.

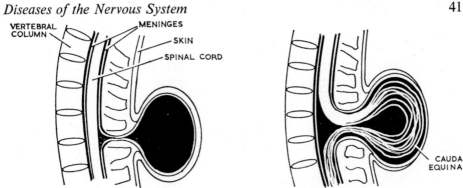

Fig. 131.

A. Meningocele. The external swelling contains meninges and cerebrospinal fluid.

B. Meningo-myelocele. The swelling contains nervous tissue, and there is always some loss of function.

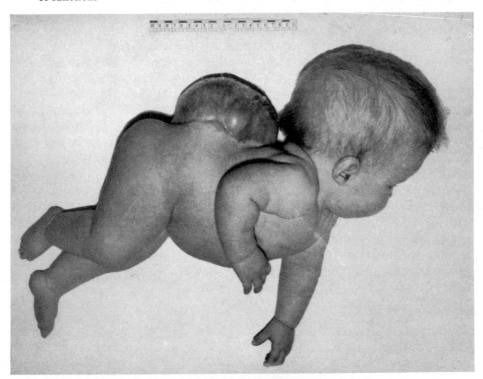

Fig. 132. Meningo-myelocele.

CHRONIC PARAPLEGIA

Paraplegia may come on gradually if spinal compression is due to a new growth of the cord or the meninges. A proportion of these are innocent, and following their removal the paraplegia may be relieved. **Myelography** is often a help in diagnosis; a radio-opaque dye is introduced into the spinal canal through a lumbar puncture. Paraplegia may also occur in connection with general diseases such as subacute combined degeneration of the cord, multiple sclerosis, or lymphadenoma. The treatment then is that of the primary condition, as well as the management of the paraplegia.

SPINA BIFIDA

The neural arch of each vertebra is a ring of bone springing from the body and surrounding the spinal cord. It is formed by the two laminae and the spinous process, and occasionally complete development fails to take place, and there is a congenital gap in the neural arch. This condition is called **spina bifida.** If the gap is small, it may cause no trouble, and will only be detected on X-ray **(spina bifida occulta).** If it is larger, the meninges may bulge through it, causing a soft swelling, usually in the cervical or lumbar region, called a **meningocele.** If nervous tissue prolapses into the swelling, it constitutes a **meningo-myelocele.**

With both the latter conditions, there is a risk of skin ulceration allowing infection to enter and produce meningitis. A meningo-myelocele is usually associated with deformities of the limbs, such as clubfoot, and often causes paraplegia with incontinence. There is little hope of life with a large lesion unless the sac can be excised and the gap closed. Even if this is successful, a proportion of these children later develop hydrocephalus.

In the 1960s much work was done to establish the value of intensive surgical treatment by closing the meningo-myelocele, orthopaedic operations for those with the possibility of walking, and establishment of an ileal bladder to control incontinence. It became clear that life of a kind was often preserved at the expense of comfort and happiness both for the patient and the parents, and that while each case must be considered on its merits, efforts to preserve a severely deformed infant by artificial means were misplaced.

HYDROCEPHALUS

The presence of too much cerebrospinal fluid under pressure constitutes hydrocephalus or water on the brain. The sutures are separated, so that the head is enlarged. This condition may be present before birth, and may obstruct delivery by the natural channel. In other cases it begins to develop soon after birth.

There are two varieties; in obstructive hydrocephalus the exit from the lateral ventricles is blocked, and they become progressively distended, thinning the layer of brain above them and pushing the cranial bones apart. In communicating hydrocephalus the flow through the ventricles is normal, but there is a blockage in the subarachnoid space which prevents reabsorption of the cerebrospinal fluid into the blood.

In some cases the hydrocephalus becomes stationary, but usually it is progressive, the head becoming too large for the child to lift and the eyes turned downwards. Some children are mentally retarded, but in others the intelligence is little affected. The decision as to whether to operate is always a difficult one, but if it is to be undertaken, the earlier it is done the better. Many operations have been devised, the most popular today being the insertion of a Spitz-Holter valve. One end of a tube is inserted into a lateral ventricle, through the skull and the other end leads into the jugular vein. There is a valve in the tube, and this can be pressed through the skin to pump the fluid from the ventricle into the vein, and thus keep the tube patent. Although there are some good results, it seems likely that even better procedures will be devised.

Chapter 15

Psychiatry

By Linford Rees
M.D., B.Sc., F.R.C.P., P.R.C.Psych., D.P.M.
Professor of Psychiatry, St. Bartholomew's Hospital, London
President of the Royal College of Psychiatrists

DEFINITIONS

Psychiatry is the branch of medicine which deals with illnesses which predominantly affect a person's mental state and behaviour. A Psychiatrist is a medically qualified doctor who has spent 5 years to 7 years in postgraduate training in psychiatry. **Psychology** is the science of mental life and behaviour. A Psychologist is a person who has passed a degree in psychology and his work in the clinical sphere consists of carrying out measurements of intellectual capacity, intellectual deterioration, personality, vocational aptitude, etc. Psychology is to psychiatry as physiology is to medicine.

THE SCOPE OF PSYCHIATRY

Nearly half of all hospital beds in England and Wales are for mentally ill or mentally subnormal patients. This only provides an indication of psychiatric illnesses requiring in-patient treatment. A better measure of the prevalence of mental illness is given by surveys which estimate that between 15 per cent and 25 per cent of all patients seen by the general practitioner suffer from psychiatric illness or have some important psychiatric or psychological aspect contributing to the illness or disability.

One woman in six and one in nine men are treated for a psychiatric disorder in hospital during some period of their lives. In England alone in one year 24 million working days are lost because of psychiatric illness.

AETIOLOGY AND CLASSIFICATION

The causation of psychiatric illnesses is usually multiple with genetic, constitutional, environmental, physical and psychological factors playing a role in different illnesses. Some causes may be regarded as essential, that is, without them the disease would not develop. Genetic factors are probably essential for the development of schizophrenia and certain types of affective illness. Even in these disorders other factors are often necessary to make this genetic pre-disposition actually manifested in disease. These are sufficient causes which determine the appearance of the illness at a particular time in a person's life and are as important as the essential causes.

Classification: Psychiatric disorders may be classified as follows:

1. **Organic Mental States** a) Acute and subacute.
   b) Chronic, including dementia.
2. **Affective disorders.** Here the predominant change is in the patient's mood. Affective disorders include:
   a) Anxiety states.
   b) Depressive states.
   c) Hypomanic and Manic states.
3. Schizophrenia.
4. Hysterical disorders.
5. Obsessional disorders.
6. Personality disorders.
7. Mental handicap.
8. Psychosomatic disorders.

ACUTE ORGANIC MENTAL STATES

An acute organic mental state in its most marked form is called **delirium.** In less severe form are subdelirious states and acute confusional states. These conditions are due to infections such as pneumonia or typhoid fever or to toxic or metabolic disturbances, to cerebro-vascular accidents or head injuries. (1) The fundamental feature of delirium is clouding of consciousness which causes the patient to have difficulty in grasping and comprehending his surroundings. He is puzzled, perplexed and bewildered. (2) He is disorientated of time, place, and with regard to persons, e.g. he may not be able to give the correct day, week, month or year; he may not realize where he is and he may mis-identify the people around him, taking them for people he knew previously. (3) Disturbances of perception occur; the patient may misinterpret stimuli, that is, he experiences **illusions;** or he may experience **hallucinations,** that is, he may have a perception with sensory vividness in the absence of an external stimulus. Visual hallucinations are particularly common in delirium. Hallucinations occur in a setting of clouded consciousness in delirium in contrast to schizophrenia where the hallucinations are usually auditory and occur in a setting of clear consciousness. (4) As the patient has difficulty in understanding and grasping what is happening around him, he tends to be suspicious and may even develop delusions of persecution. (5) Patients tend to be restless and tend to get more confused at night.

SUB-DELIRIOUS STATE

Here the clouding of consciousness is less marked and less persistent. The patient is more interested and anxious to get into contact with the environment than with delirium, and awareness fluctuates a great deal. The patient during more lucid moments realizes he is ill and is perplexed and anxious about his symptoms, particularly illusions and hallucinations.

The chronic organic mental states may be due to a whole series of pathological conditions such as (1) the condition may be a degenerative disorder which is primary, e.g. senile and presenile dementia, Huntington's chorea. (2) Cardiovascular disease, including arteriosclerosis and hypertension. (3) Inflammatory; syphilis, encephalitis, etc. (4) Cerebral tumour. (5) Metabolic, endocrine and nutritional disorders. (6) Intoxications, poisoning or anoxia. (7) Trauma. All these processes may lead to a loss of mental capacity which is termed dementia.

Dementia is a loss of mental capacity which shows itself mainly in a failure of memory at first for recent events and subsequently for remote events as the condition progresses. There is also an impairment of comprehension and judgment, emotional instability and deterioration in behaviour. The failure of memory in dementia is due to a failure of retention due to organic damage to the cerebrum.

One of the most common forms of dementia is due to old age—senile dementia. The term senescence is applied to the normal process of growing old and is characterized by a gradual falling off in mental and physical capacity and a tendency to become more restricted in interest and more rigid in outlook. Senile dementia is a pathological state in which the changes of senescence have developed to such a degree that they interfere with a person's wellbeing, adjustment and behaviour. Senile dementia is characterized by a progressive deterioration of memory and thinking, emotional instability, loss of interest and initiative, and lack of responsiveness in emotional reactions. The patient tends to become increasingly self-centred, irritable, difficult and intolerant of any change. The patient is usually worse at night and often creates problems by turning on taps and forgetting about them. They will turn on water taps and forget about them and flood the house, or endanger the occupants by turning on the gas taps and forgetting to light them. Any sudden change in their environment such as moving house or having a new domestic servant tends to be very upsetting and may cause the patient to become highly suspicious or even to develop severe ideas of persecution.

The treatment of acute and chronic mental syndromes is primarily directed towards the underlying cause, e.g. toxic, metabolic, or infective, cerebral-syphilis, tumour, high blood-pressure, etc.

Nursing Management. During his more lucid moments the delirious and sub-delirious patient can be helped by a calm and soothing approach which helps to reduce his fears and agitation. If the patient's behaviour is disturbed he may need sedation. Barbiturates often make the patient worse, and should be avoided. Phenothiazine drugs, such as chlorpromazine, given in adequate doses are more helpful.

The patient should be kept in a part of the ward where he will not be distressed and confused by the various ward and patient activities. He should be nursed by as few people as possible. At the appropriate time he will need to be given simple information regarding his whereabouts, the time of day, how long he has been in hospital. Any sources of worry or emotional disturbance should be excluded as far as possible. The same principles of nursing care apply to patients with dementia who need a simple environment with a regular routine and avoidance of sudden change, familiar faces, simple tasks, and careful attention to nutrition and physical health.

AFFECTIVE DISORDERS
DEPRESSIVE STATES
Depression can be a symptom or a disease. A depressive illness is one in which the primary and dominant change is a change in mood which is fixed and relatively persistent. The mood change in depression may vary in severity in different patients, ranging from mild despondency to the most severe and abject despair which probably represents the most intense form of suffering experienced by man. The depressed patient looks unwell, pale, dejected in appearance. His muscle tone is poor, his hair is lustreless, eyes look dull, tongue is furred, breath offensive. The following are characteristic features:

The patient notices that everyday tasks become very difficult, e.g. making conversation is a burden and meeting people previously liked now becomes something he wishes to avoid. He loses interest in things that he previously enjoyed. His thoughts tend to be painful and, much as he may dislike it, he tends to be self-centred, continually talking about his symptoms. He tends to depreciate himself and to have feelings of unworthiness and, sometimes, guilt feelings. Many patients are slowed in their intellectual functions (**retardation**), but others are restless in a repetitive manner (**agitation**). The patient has the characteristic difficulty in concentration and coping with everyday things or getting through even simple tasks. Appetite is impaired and there can be marked weight loss within a short period of time. Sleep disturbances are invariable. When anxiety is present there may be difficulty in going off to sleep. In many patients there is a tendency to wake up early feeling worse in the morning and to improve later in the day.

Many patients will not complain of depression as such; instead they will say that they feel ill or may report a variety of bodily complaints such as indigestion, pains in various parts of the body, loss of energy, constipation and loss of appetite.

VARIETIES OF DEPRESSIVE ILLNESS

In general it may be said that there are two main varieties of depressive illness. (1) **Reactive depression** which is the response to environmental stress, loss, catastrophe, or other traumatic experience. Reactive depressions usually show a great deal of anxiety and tend to be worse later in the day. (2) Some depressions can come on out of the blue, even when everything in the patient's life is going on all right. These are termed **endogenous depressions** and they are usually more severe, with greater weight loss and characteristically early waking with a diurnal variation in which they are worse in the morning and better later in the day.

In severe depression, particularly if there is marked self-depreciation, there may be a risk of suicide and it is important to remember that the old saying, that a person who talks about it never will commit suicide, is incorrect. Any person who is very depressed and self-depreciatory and expresses suicidal thoughts must be taken seriously.

There is an increased risk of suicide if the patient is socially isolated, e.g. living on his own without ready access to friends or relatives.

Treatment. In mild reactive depressions discussion and help by means of social and symptomatic measures may be all that is necessary. In more severe depressive illnesses, active treatment either in the form of antidepressant drugs or, in very severe cases, by convulsive therapy is needed.

Nursing Care. Depressed patients tend to neglect themselves and may not take adequate nourishment or clothe themselves satisfactorily or look after their personal hygiene. They should be treated sympathetically and should not be forced to do things which they find too difficult. The advice to pull themselves together is totally inappropriate as they would be the first people to do this if it were a matter of exercising willpower.

HYPOMANIA AND MANIA

These are affective disorders in which the mood change is one of elation and excitement. In these disorders we see symptoms and behaviour which are the antithesis of those seen in depression. The patient looks well, his eyes are bright, he is active and energetic and interested in everything. He shows great pressure of activity, both in speech and in behaviour. He talks incessantly, makes jokes and puns, tends to be interfering and managing. He feels confident and that nothing is too much for him to cope with and that no task is insuperable. He is distractable, any passing stimulus may take his attention away from the activity in hand. His talk tends to be detailed and circumstantial but usually reaches the goal, in contrast to schizophrenia. He is enthusiastic and his enthusiasm is infectious. However, if thwarted he will become angry and irritable.

Usually he does not realize that he is ill and will not seek medical advice. Hypomanic and manic patients usually come to the notice of the police, social authorities or doctors because of their behaviour, for example, they may spend more money than they possess, or because of their sex drives or because of overactive disturbed behaviour.

They need very little sleep and spend their day in incessant activity.

Treatment. Treatment of hypomania and mania is by means of drugs such as chlorpromazine and Haloperidol. Lithium can be given which is also effective but probably less so. Some patients will respond to a course of electro-convulsive therapy.

ANXIETY STATES

Anxiety is a normal emotion which helps us to keep alert, on our toes, and maintaining our activities at a reasonable standard. Severe anxiety reactions may occur as a result of a frightening experience such as being nearly run over by a motorcar when crossing the road which in normal health usually passes off after a little time. An Anxiety State is an Affective Disorder in which the primary and predominant change in mood is one of anxiety of such a degree and persistence that it affects wellbeing, adjustment and efficiency. Anxiety states may be mild or severe, acute or chronic, continuous or episodic.

The understanding of the various manifestations of anxiety states is helped if we consider the biological significance of anxiety and fear. In the animal kingdom an animal presented with a threat, e.g. from another animal, reacts by mobilizing its resources for action either for fighting or running away. Various bodily changes which occur are similar to those which occur in anxiety states in man. Blood is redirected from the skin and digestive tract, where it is not needed during the emergency, to the muscles where it is needed for emergency action. Thus the blood vessels to the skin and alimentary canal become constricted, whereas the blood vessels to the muscles become dilated. The heart beats more quickly to carry oxygen to the muscles more rapidly, voluntary muscles become very tense so that the animal can spring off for action immediately. In man, the increased muscular tension causes such symptoms as tremors, tension headaches, pains in the shoulders, arms, neck, back, etc.

The sympathetic nervous system is predominantly involved in mobilizing resources for action. The parasympathetic, particularly the sacral parasympathetic, may also come into action as it subserves the total effectiveness of the organism by evacuating the bladder and bowel and thus getting rid of unnecessary weight.

The patient with an anxiety state is in a constant state of apprehension. He tends to speak in a high-pitched, rapid voice. He meets trouble half-way and constantly needs reassurance. Some patients will have an irrational, morbid fear of a thing or situation. This is termed a phobia. If such a fear plays a prominent part in the illness it is termed a phobic anxiety state.

Aetiology. The causes of anxiety states may be regarded as arising from the individual and his environment. Certain people have very anxious personalities, are anxiety-prone, and some entire families are characterized by anxiety, apprehension and over-protective attitudes. Environmental stresses variously interact with the individual's predisposition to anxiety state. During the last war it was clearly demonstrated that soldiers differed only in the amount of stress they could stand before developing an anxiety state. Some broke down with minimal stress, e.g. that caused by regimentation or separation from home, whereas others needed prolonged and severe stress before breaking down. Severe or prolonged stress over a period in anyone can result in acute anxiety state. Fatigue, excessive responsibility, certain physiological changes, particularly in women at the premenstrual phase, are conducive to the arousal of anxiety; interpersonal problems and inner conflicts may also be contributory factors.

Treatment. The physician must take a full history, carry out a thorough physical examination, discussing, explaining and reassuring the patient. Supportive treatment with guidance and helping the patient to cope with everyday problems is needed. Symptomatic treatment consists of the use of anti-anxiety drugs to relieve symptoms and to encourage the resumption of normal activities. In some patients psychotherapy of varying intensity may be needed, depending on the needs of the patient. For phobias, particularly those which are mono-symptomatic or limited in number, desensitization by behaviour therapy is one of the most promising methods of treatment. Under sedation sufficient to keep him calm and relaxed, the subject of fear is introduced to the patients attention. If he becomes fearful, sedation is increased till he can relax again. The object is gradually to enable the patient to confront the anxiety-making situation without fear.

HYSTERIA

Hysteria must not be confused with malingering. Malingering is when a patient states he has a symptom when he knows he hasn't.

Hysterical symptoms, although not based on organic disease, are nevertheless real and in varying degrees incapacitating to the patient.

Hysteria is a condition in which the patient develops symptoms resembling those of organic disease without such disease being present or, if present, sufficient to account for the symptoms, for some real or imaginary gain without the patient being fully aware of the motive and nature of his symptoms. People often use the term hysteria to denote histrionic and emotional behaviour, but in clinical practice it is necessary for the term to be reserved for those psychogenic illnesses having a motive of gain.

The mechanism underlying hysteria is "dissociation" whereby a part of the stream of consciousness becomes detached and submerged from the main stream of consciousness. This state of dissociation occurs in predisposed persons when faced with difficult situations, problems, or stresses and for the purpose of achieving something; whether this is a real gain in the eyes of other people is not relevant. The development of the hysterical symptom resolves a conflict and the patient is characteristically calm and unconcerned about his symptoms—the typical *belle indifférence*. The degree of calmness and indifference which is associated with hysteria is dependent on the extent to which the anxiety arising from the confronting problem or conflict is resolved by the development of the hysterical symptom.

The dissociated stream of consciousness is apart and its contents cannot be communicated to the main stream of consciousness. This is why the patient is unaware of the nature and the motivation underlying his symptoms.

As an example of the development of an hysterical symptom one may take the case of the soldier in the front line of battle. The soldier is in conflict due to his instinctive need for self-preservation pulling one way and the duty of a soldier governed by his sense of discipline pulling the other. If he is a person predisposed to develop hysteria this conflict will be resolved by the appearance of an hysterical paralysis of the legs which makes him incapable of carrying on his duties as a soldier and resolves his conflict and associated anxiety feelings. Hysterical symptoms can mimic any organic disease. The important thing to remember is that hysterical symptoms, in so far as they are controlled by a part of consciousness, although dissociated, involve functions which are under voluntary control. The form of the hysterical symptom corresponds with what the patient regards as being typical of the disease rather than necessarily conforming to similar conditions of organic origin. For example, hysterical anaesthesia tends to end at joint levels such as the glove and stocking anaesthesia, hysterical paralysis of the legs is associated with a bizarre gait and examination shows contraction of opposing muscle groups. Hysterical loss of memory is usually related to some distressing event.

Hysterical fits are distinguished from major epileptic fits by the fact that they do not conform to the sequence of events of major epilepsy and show evidence of retention of volition; for example, the patient will bite, scream, kick or react in a purposeful manner to stimuli. None of these could occur if consciousness were completely lost as it is during epileptic fits.

Hysteria developing for the first time in middle age or later should suggest the possibility of an overlying organic disease.

Nursing Management. Undoubtedly the most important rule is to ignore the symptoms as far as possible and to direct one's attention to the patient himself. The patient should be dealt with firmly but with understanding and encouragement. There is never any need to treat hysterics harshly or unkindly.

Hysterical symptoms may be removed by suggestion under hypnosis or by intravenous barbiturates, but it is important to explore the causes of the symptom, that is, the underlying conflict, and to help the patient to deal with this, otherwise the patient may develop another hysterical symptom in place of the one removed by treatment. It is desirable that nothing should be done to reinforce any invalid attitudes on the part of the patient and the sooner the patient can be made ambulant and engage in normal activities the more will his recovery be helped.

OBSESSIONAL ILLNESS

Obsessional symptoms may occur as a part of a psychiatric illness such as a depressive state, or sometimes in schizophrenia. It may constitute the entire illness which is then termed an obsessive compulsive illness.

Obsessional symptoms are usually thoughts, fears or impulses to action, which repeatedly intrude themselves into the patient's consciousness. They characteristically have a feeling of compulsion which the patient tries to resist but cannot get rid of even though he realizes that the obsession is irrational. The most important characteristic is the tendency to resist.

Obsessional symptoms may take the form of recurrent thoughts which the patient is unable to get rid of, sometimes repetitive phrases or tunes. They may take the form of ruminations, the patient being persistently troubled by such thoughts as "What is the meaning of life? Why are we living?" etc. Obsessional doubts refer to actions which the patient has carried out, for example, the patient may need to check repeatedly that he has carried out an action such as switching off the lights, turning off the gas taps, etc. Obsessional acts are referred to as compulsions which includes such symptoms as compulsive washing, a compulsion to touch things. The obsessional illness causes a great deal of distress and anxiety to the patient.

Nursing Management. It is important to remember that nearly half of the cases of obsessional illness will clear up spontaneously. It is important to help the patient to accept and understand his symptoms rather than for him to spend a great deal of effort and willpower in trying to get rid of them which, in any event, is impossible. If the patient can learn to accept and cope with his symptoms this will relieve a great deal of the anxiety. In some patients the anxiety and distress is of such a degree that drugs such as Diazepam, Chlordiazepoxide have to be given. In some patients psychotherapy may be necessary but this is notoriously difficult in obsessional states and hallucinogenic drugs like lysergic acid are used to facilitate psychotherapy. Intractable cases which have not responded to any form of treatment and which are associated with severe distress need a prefrontal leucotomy for relief or recovery.

Obsessional symptoms occurring during a depressive illness usually clear up with treatment of the underlying depression.

SCHIZOPHRENIA

The term schizophrenia is derived from Greek and means splitting of the mind. The splitting of mental functions in schizophrenia is quite dissimilar from the dissociation found in hysteria. It is rather a fragmentation or disintegration of mental functions causing a disconnection in thinking, feeling and behaviour. In the normal healthy person thoughts, feelings and actions are in agreement with each other. In schizophrenia there tends to be an incongruity between emotions and thinking, and between emotions and behaviour.

The main features of schizophrenia are as follows:

1. Withdrawal, Introversion, Autism.
2. Splitting of (a) thinking processes, (b) emotional reactions, (c) behaviour.

3. The development of delusions, particularly of persecution.
4. The occurrence of hallucinations in a setting of clear consciousness.

These various components of schizophrenia symptomatology vary according to the subtype of schizophrenic illness.

Introversion, withdrawal or autism is characterized by increasing detachment of interest from the environment. The patient prefers to be alone and tends to spend a great deal of time thinking. He lacks energy, initiative, drive, willpower, He shows a decrease in or lack of natural affection. Replies to questions tend to be brief and uninformative.

An extreme example of introversion is stupor in which the patient shows diminished response to stimuli and little spontaneous activity despite the fact that consciousness is clear.

Thought Disorder is one of the characteristic features of schizophrenia. In the early stages the patient's conversation is noted to be vague, woolly and un-informative. The patient notices that his thoughts will suddenly stop or that thoughts appear to be inserted into his mind. In severe cases speech may be incomprehensible due to incoherence. The patient interprets these phenomena as belief that people are controlling his thoughts, influencing his thoughts, hypnotizing him.

Emotional reactions. In schizophrenia there tends to be a general emotional flattening, but sometimes emotions are clearly incongruous with a situation or with a person's behaviour. They may suddenly burst out laughing in an in-appropriate and fatuous manner without provocation. They may look very depressed and yet feel very happy, they may describe severe delusions of per-secution, yet be unconcerned or even quite happy whilst relating them.

Disconnection of behaviour may show itself in isolated tics or mannerisms, or in stereotyped repetitive activity. In some types of schizophrenia the patient may show automatic obedience, will obey any commands or repeat everything that is said to him, or mirror the actions of the person he is with. In some patients uncomfortable postures can be imposed; this is known as waxy flexibility. Sometimes the patient may have spontaneous utterances of speech which are meaningless, or spontaneous outbursts of behaviour which may be aggressive and which arise apropos of nothing or his surroundings.

THE PARANOID DISPOSITION AND THE DEVELOPMENT OF DELUSIONS

A delusion is a false belief which is not amenable to persuasion or argument and which is not shared by other members of the group of society in which the person holding it lives. Delusions in schizophrenia are often bizarre and may relate to bodily functions (hypochondriacal delusions), to persecution (paranoid delusions), to feelings of grandeur (grandiose delusions). The most common delusions in schizophrenia are paranoid delusions.

The paranoid tendency is one in which the person tends to attribute to the outside world something which in fact arises within him. In its mildest form this may take the form of ideas of reference in which the patient believes that people are paying attention to him, talking about him, passing remarks about him. In the most complex form the system of delusions of persecution may develop to an elaborate degree based on a central delusion that some organization such as the Masons or Jesuits are plotting against him.

HALLUCINATIONS

The most common hallucinations in schizophrenia are hallucinations of hearing (auditory hallucinations). These occur in a setting of clear consciousness in contrast to the hallucinations found in delirium or sub-delirious states which are commonly visual and occur in a setting of clouded consciousness.

The following varieties of schizophrenia are described, although some patients may show features of one form at one stage of the illness and features of another form at another stage.

SIMPLE SCHIZOPHRENIA

Here the main manifestation is withdrawal of interest with ideas of reference. It is usually of gradual onset and tends to have a poor prognosis.

HEBEPHRENIC SCHIZOPHRENIA

This is characterized by emotional incongruity and thought disorder.

CATATONIC SCHIZOPHRENIA

This tends to have a sudden onset and is characterized by phases of over-activity and sometimes phases of under-activity which are referred to as catatonic stupor. It is in catatonic schizophrenia that one sees the manifestations of disconnection of behaviour and motor symptoms to a marked degree, such as echolalia (repeating what has been said to them), echopraxia (repeating and copying actions of other people), the maintenance of imposed attitudes and postures, waxy flexibility (flexibilitas cerea).

PARANOID SCHIZOPHRENIA

This tends to be of later onset and is characterized by a better preservation of personality than the previous varieties. It is characterized by a marked development of paranoid delusions which may be changeable and fleeting, or may become fixed and develop into a complex as in paraphrenia, which is a term given to one variety of paranoid schizophrenia which is characterized by a more or less systematized series of delusions and by the presence of hallucinations.

Causation. There is very strong evidence to indicate that there is a genetic predisposition to schizophrenia which is demonstrated by the fact that the incidence of schizophrenia increases according to the closeness of blood relationship of the relative. For example, the incidence in the general population is 1 per cent, in brothers and sisters of schizophrenic patients 5–15 per cent, in non-identical twins 5–15 per cent, and in identical twins between 50–70 per cent. Not all persons who carry the genetic predisposition to schizophrenia actually manifest the disease. Sometimes the condition develops insidiously; in other patients it may be precipitated by physical illnesses such as infections; by childbirth, or by dieting with loss of weight. Environmental factors may also bring out the predisposition, e.g. faulty parental attitudes and stresses at any age.

Treatment. Treatment of schizophrenia nowadays is by the use of phenothiazine drugs combined if necessary with electro-convulsive therapy. In the chronic schizophrenic patient, rehabilitation and employment in suitable work play an important role as well as the phenothiazine drugs.

The Role of the Nurse. As the nurse spends more time with the patient than the doctor and other medical workers she has an important part to play in the general therapeutic regime. Although schizophrenic patients are sometimes difficult to contact and establish a relationship, the nurse by showing interest and giving encouragement can develop a relationship which is therapeutically valuable. Schizophrenic patients need a general regime of interest, encouragement and activity in which the occupational therapist, doctors and nurses all contribute.

PSYCHOPATHIC PERSONALITY

The term psychopathic personality is used to denote individuals who for a large part of their lives have shown behaviour characterized by episodes of abnormal behaviour which is usually anti-social. They have a tendency to act on impulse to satisfy the needs of the moment without due regard to the consequences. They are unreliable, lack persistence, change jobs frequently and are unable to establish consistent good interpersonal relationships. They sometimes show mood swings from short periods of depression to elation. They are unable, despite average or above-average intelligence, to learn from experiences, they make the same mistakes repeatedly. They are, in general, emotionally immature, self-centred and impulsive. Their immaturity is not only shown in their emotional reactions but is also seen in the electro-encephalogram which shows features characteristic of a much younger person.

The term psychopathic personality therefore carries a connotation of constitutional inadequacy that shows itself not in psychiatric illness but in abnormalities of behaviour.

Genetic and environmental factors are important; many psychopaths have had an unsettled and insecure early upbringing with lack of consistent maternal and paternal guidance.

Some psychopaths are aggressive; these tend to show episodes of violence, sometimes a blind rage. Many of these show abnormalities in the electro-encephalogram with peaks of high voltage electricity. Such patients may often do quite well with epanutin and amphetamine medication. Emotional reactions and behaviour disturbances have been reported to be helped by a recently introduced drug called Pericyazine (Neulactil), but the value of this drug has yet to be established. Group therapy sometimes helps them, such as that provided in the Henderson Hospital, Belmont, Surrey. Fortunately some patients with psychopathic personalities sometimes improve with age in the late thirties or forties.

They are often unwilling to seek treatment. If they request it, treatment must be aimed at increasing stabilization by means of occupational therapy, group therapy, the use of drugs and vocational placement. Only too often the psychopath blames other people rather than himself and is reluctant to consider that he has a problem or that he needs treatment.

MENTAL HANDICAP

Mental handicap (synonyms-subnormality amentia, mental retardation, mental deficiency.) Mental subnormality is a state of arrested development of the mind existing from birth or from an early age. About 5 per cent of all babies born are retarded to some extent. Some of these do not live long and many suffer from physical malformations. During the school age period between 1 per cent and 4 per cent of children are mentally subnormal. The Mental Health Act defines two types of mental handicap from the legal point of view, namely, Subnormality and Severe Subnormality.

Subnormality refers to an arrest of the development of mind which prevents the person from looking after himself or his affairs or from being able to be taught to do so. The intelligence range in this group is roughly between 50 IQ and 70 IQ. (Intelligence Quotient.)

Severely subnormal patients have an intelligence quotient below 50 and are dependent upon other people for survival, for cleanliness and personal care. They are divided into two grades: the medium grade with an IQ between 25 and 50, and low grade patients with an IQ below 25. Medium grade patients have the characteristics of subnormal patients.

Subnormality accounts for by far the largest proportion of mentally handicapped patients. The upper level of the IQ range merges into the lower range of the normal frequency distribution of intelligence. IQ is not the best guide to the social and medical importance of mental handicap, as psychological, educational and emotional factors determine the behavioural problems associated with mental handicap.

As children, subnormal patients lack alertness, curiosity and spontaneity compared with the normal child. They are inert, passive, easily ruled and credulous. Patients at the upper intelligence ranges of subnormality may show no obvious signs of mental retardation but are often late in passing the milestones of development. They fail to make progress in ordinary schools and often have to be transferred to special classes or special schools. After school they may settle down to a simple routine job provided it is within the limits of their mental capacity and provided they are relatively stable.

MEDIUM GRADE PATIENTS

These have an intelligence quotient ranging from 30 to 50. They are incapable of earning their living and fending for themselves in society, but can be taught to look after themselves, to wash, dress and feed themselves. They are incapable of learning in ordinary schools and can be helped at occupational centres, and later may even be found work in a sheltered workshop.

SEVERELY RETARDED

These are patients with an IQ below 30. This group tends to have a greater incidence of physical abnormalities, expectation of life is limited—some die within the first two years of life. The most common causes of death are intercurrent infections such as pneumonia.

Causation. Genetic and environmental factors contribute and interact in the production of mental subnormality. Many cases of mental subnormality, particularly at the higher IQ range, are in fact the lowest range of the normal distribution of intelligence. Some are due to single genes; for example, phenylketonuria, galactosaemia, are transmitted by a single recessive, whereas tuberose sclerosis is transmitted by a single dominant. Some conditions are due to chromosome abnormalities such as Downs' syndrome (mongolism) which is due to an extra chromosome. Other chromosome abnormalities are Kleinfelter's syndrome and Turner's syndrome.

Mental subnormality may be the result of events during pregnancy such as German measles, toxoplasmosis and kernicterus as a result of Rhesus incompatibility or the effect of teratogenic drugs such as thalidomide. Sometimes the cause is at birth, e.g. brain damage, cerebral haemorrhage or excessive oxygen given to premature babies. Causes operating in early infancy and childhood include lack of thyroid secretion giving rise to cretinism, kernicterus, damage due to encephalitis, head injury or schizophrenia. Many forms of mental subnormality have clearly elucidated biochemical abnormalities, e.g. phenylketonuria and galactosaemia. Controlling these by appropriate dietary means can enable the child to develop normally.

Treatment and Training of the Mentally Subnormal—It has been found that 8 per 1000 of the population are mentally subnormal, but at the most only two of these will need admission to hospital. The majority, both children and adults, can be looked after at home or under special conditions.

The need for hospital admission is mainly determined by behavioural difficulties or other social factors. In recent years there has been an even greater tendency to keep mentally subnormal persons outside hospitals for training as useful members of the community. They can attend occupational centres, training centres, and children of school age can receive special education at special schools or special classes.

In hospital, patients are given training and education suitable to their ability, and adult patients are given instruction in social behaviour and are trained for various types of employment. Industrial workshops are used, and some patients may be used in simple repetitive work remuneratively outside hospital.

In recent years an increasing number of mentally subnormal patients are being successfully cared for in the community in preference to hospital admission.

PSYCHOSOMATIC DISORDERS

The term psychosomatic is used in two distinct senses. One usage applies to an attitude to disease in general in which the physician pays attention to psychological as well as physical factors in any disease. The use of the term psychosomatic to an approach to illness would include all forms of illness.

I will use the term psychosomatic disorder more strictly to denote those illnesses with a physical lesion or manifestation in which both physical and psychological factors play a demonstrable role. The role may be demonstrated by clinical observation or by experimental studies.

Used in this sense psychosomatic disorders usually have a genetical and constitutional predisposition as well as having psychological and physical precipitations of attacks of the disorder.

The following illnesses are usually regarded as being psychosomatic disorders in the sense that good medical practice demands the study of psychological aspects with as equal thoroughness as the physical causes.

1. **Respiratory System.** Vasomotor Rhinitis.
   Hay Fever.
   Asthma.

2. **Alimentary System.** Peptic Ulcer—Gastric
   Duodenal.
   Ulcerative Colitis.
   Irritable and spastic colon.

3. **C.N.S.** Migraine.
   Cerebral Haemorrhage.
   Cerebral Thrombosis.

4. **Locomotive System.** Fibrositis.

5. **Skin.** Chronic urticaria.
   Neurodermatitis.
   Eczema, etc.

6. **Circulatory System.** Hypertension.
   Coronary Diseases.

7. **Endocrines.** Thyrotoxicosis.
   Diabetes Mellitus.
   Menstrual disorders.

Psychosomatic disorders in general tend to be due to multiple factors, for example, attacks of asthma may be precipitated by infections and allergic reactions as well as emotional tension. There is experimental and clinical evidence to suggest that these factors exert additive effects. For instance, a person may react strongly to a given allergen when he is emotionally tense but may not show any clinical manifestations to the same dose when he is relaxed. In coronary disease dietary factors the amount of exercise, the existence of arteriosclerotic changes will all predispose to coronary thrombosis. In some patients the experience of emotional stress may determine the time at which a patient has a coronary thrombosis. There is evidence that emotional tension increases the coagulability of the blood.

In psychosomatic disorders it is important for the physician not only to take into account the possible physical factors which contribute to the causation of the disorder but to assess whether emotional factors are playing a role, and in order to do this he must know the patient with regard to personality make up and social circumstances.

METHODS OF TREATMENT

Psychotherapy Treatment. Psychotherapy is treatment involving communication between the patient and the therapist with the aim of modifying and alleviating illness. It may vary from being supportive, which deals with current problems, to help the patient overcome his symptoms and cope more satisfactorily with these and with life generally, to intensive, prolonged individual psychotherapy on Freudian or Jungian lines. This involves many visits a week and may take some years.

Group Therapy whether psychoanalytically orientated, or educative and explanatory may also be helpful in treating patients. The group is usually about 8 in number and is economical on the doctor's time.

Hypnosis. Hypnosis is a state of artificially induced increased suggestibility in which the patient's awareness becomes restricted to the hypnotist. The hypnotic state can vary in depth; deep hypnosis can be induced in about 5 per cent only of the population. Some people can never be deeply hypnotized. Hypnosis must be used judiciously, not merely to remove symptoms but to elicit the nature of underlying emotional conflicts and problems and to facilitate the recall of forgotten experiences which may be emotionally important, to release distress in past experiences or to modify symptoms and attitudes.

Abreactive techniques. In addition to hypnosis certain techniques may be used to facilitate abreaction, that is, the release of emotion attached to experiences which are buried and which may be producing symptoms. Intravenous Sodium Amytal, intravenous methedrine, hallucinogenic drugs, gaseous anaesthetics such as ether and nitrous oxide have all been used to induce a state of narcosis which facilitates exploration and abreaction.

BEHAVIOUR THERAPY

During recent years new methods have been devised to alleviate behavioural problems and symptoms within a comparatively short period of time by controlling the patient's learned behaviour. Behaviour therapy is a form of psychotherapy which attempts to alter beneficially, human behaviour and emotions by the application of the laws of modern learning theory.

Behaviour therapy is used for the treatment of neurotic symptoms which in this context are defined as a very persistent habit of unadaptive behaviour acquired by learning.

Behaviour therapy uses the following technique of re-learning and unlearning in the treatment symptoms.

(1) Aversion therapy
(2) Negative learning or extinction based on negative practive
(3) Reciprocal inhibition based on relaxation
(4) Implosion therapy. (Flooding)
(5) Operant conditioning.
(6) Modelling.
(7) Shaping.

1. *Aversion Therapy*

Aversion conditioning is achieved by associating stimuli relating to the symptom to be treated with unpleasant effects following the adminstration of apomorphine, emetine or by the administration of a painful electric shock. The latter enables a more precise timing in the occurrence of the effect of the noxious stimulus and the stimuli related to the symptom to be treated.

Aversion therapy is used when the symptom or pattern of behaviour is pleasurable to the person, e.g. alcoholism, transvestism, homosexual inclinations, etc.

2. *Negative Learning or extinction based on negative practice*

This has been used in the treatment of involuntary movements such as tics. If consists in getting the patient to adhere to a rigid schedule of massed practice to voluntarily carrying out the movements of the tic at intervals throughout the day. This sets up a state of inhibition which impairs or prevents the appearance of the tic movements.

3. *Reciprocal inhibition based on relaxation*

Many forms of neurotic behaviour are acquired in an anxiety-generating situation.

Treatment can be used on the suppression of anxiety responses by responses which are physiologically antagonistic to anxiety.

Systematic desensitization, which consists of enquiring first of all into the stimulus situations which provoke anxiety in the patient and to rank these stimuli in order from the most to the least disturbing, i.e. a hierarchy of stimulus situations.

Then the patient is asked to visualize the least disturbing stimulus when he is in a state of relaxation produced by hypnosis or intravenous anaesthetic.

Whenever marked disturbance occurs the therapist withdraws the stimulus and calms the patient.

Each stimulus is visualized for 5–10 seconds and 2–4 items presented in each session, each item usually being presented twice.

As soon as the patient is able to visualize the items without disturbance, the therapist moves on to the next item in the next session.

Eventually the patient is able to visualize all the former noxious stimuli without anxiety and this ability to imagine the noxious stimuli with tranquility is transferred to the real life situation.

4. *Implosion therapy* (*Flooding*)

This method in contrast to systematic desensitization the patient is confronted in imagination or reality with his most feared situation or stimulus at once and encouraged to remain in contact with that situation until the evoked anxiety subsides. Flooding is particularly effective for treating animal phobias.

5. *Operant Conditioning*

Operant behaviour usually affects the environment and generates stimuli which "feed back" to the organism. Any response or behaviour which is rewarding and therefore reinforcing increases the likelihood of further similar responses.

This method has been used with varying degrees of success in the treatment of behaviour disorders in children, in multiple tics, hysterical symptoms, stammering, etc. [*continued on p. 437*

TABLE 1

Approved Name	Trade Name	Usual Daily Dose Range mg.	Principal Indications	Limitations, side effects, toxic and adverse effects
		Low High		
ANTI-ANXIETY Amylobarbitone	Amytal	1–4·5	Anxiety	Addiction if dose is high
Chlordiazepoxide	Librium	15–60	Anxiety, increased muscular tension	Ataxia, drowsiness, constipation, weight gain
Diazepam	Valium	6–30		
Nitrazepam	Mogadon	5–20	Anxiety, Insomnia	
Medazepam Promazine	Sparine Nobrium	75–400	Elderly patients anxiety and agitation	
		Low High		
ANTI-PSYCHOTIC **Major Tranquillizers** *Phenothiazine derivatives* Chlorpromazine	Largactil	75–800	Overactive and disturbed behaviour in various psychotic disorders	Little use for anxiety states. Limited value for inert and apathetic schizophrenia
Prochlorperazine	Stemetil	15–100	Vomiting, Tinnitus, prevention of migraine. Schizophrenia, including inert and apathetic patients	Dystonic reaction in higher doses

Approved Name	Trade Name	Usual Daily Dose Range mg.	Principal Indications	Limitations, side effects, toxic and adverse effects
Perphenazine	Fentazin	6–64	Schizophrenia. Disturbed behaviour in psychiatric and physical disease	Dystonic reaction in higher doses
Trifluoperazine	Stelazine	3–30	All types of schizophrenia. Low doses for anxiety symptoms	Extrapyramidal side effects frequent
Fluphenazine	Moditen	0·5–12·5	Mainly for preventing anxiety and tension	Extrapyramidal side effects frequent
Fluphenazine enanthate	Moditen enanthate	12·5–25 by injection at intervals	Modern treatment of schizophrenia	Extrapyramidal side effects frequent
Fluphenazine decanovate	Modicate	12·5–75 by injection at intervals	Modern treatment of schizophrenia	Extrapyramidal side effects frequent
Pericyazine	Neulactil	7·5–60	Behaviour disorders, schizophrenia, severe anxiety states	Drowsiness, necessitating careful adjustment of dosage
Thioridazine	Melleril	30–600	As tranquillosedative in neuroses and psychoses	Side effects frequent
Butyrophenones Haloperidol	Serenace	2–15	Hypomania, mania, schizophrenia	Marked extrapyramidal effects

Approved Name	Trade Name	Usual Daily Dose Range mg.		Principal Indications	Limitations, side effects, toxic and adverse effects
		Low	High		
ANTI-DEPRESSION *Tricyclic* Imipramine	Tofranil	50–150		Endogenous depression	Anti-cholinergic, hypotension, extra-pyramidal, confusional state, rash
Amitriptyline	Tryptizol	50–250		Depression and anxiety	Anti-cholinergic, hypotension, confusional state, rash
Nortriptyline	Aventyl	30–150		Depression with apathy	Anti-cholinergic, hypotension, confusional state, rash
Trimipramine	Surmontil			Depression, tension	Anti-cholinergic, hypotension, confusional state, rash
Dibenzepin	Noveril	240–480		Depression with apathy	Anti-cholinergic, hypotension, confusional state, rash
Protriptyline	Concordin	15–30		Depression with apathy	Anti-cholinergic, hypotension, confusional state, rash
Chlorimpramine	Anafranil	75–15		Depression	Anti-cholinergic, hypotension, confusional state, rash

Approved Name	Trade Name	Usual Daily Dose Range mg.	Principal Indications	Limitations, side effects, toxic and adverse effects
Monoamine Oxidase Inhibitors Mebanazine	Actomol	15–30		Autonomic reactions, hyperreflexia, peripheral oedema
Phenelzine	Nardil	15–75	Depressive illness of mild or moderate severity	Autonomic reactions, hyperreflexia, hypertension, hepatic pathology
Isocarboxazid	Marplan	10–30		Autonomic reactions, hyperreflexia, hypertension, hepatic pathology, blood dyscrasia, peripheral oedema
Nialamide	Niamid	35–300		
Tranylcypromine	Parnate	10–30		Autonomic reactions, hyperreflexia, hypertension, severe headaches occasionally occur

6. *Modelling*
This is a technique used with flooding or desensitization in which the patient sees the therapist enter the phobia situation and induces the patient to do so.

7. *Shaping*
Shaping is based on operant conditioning principles. The patient is systematically instructed to do what he fears and is rewarded by the therapist with praise

when he succeeds and with no response if he fails. This method is useful in the treatment of phobias and obsessions.

It may be said that behaviour therapy achieves the best results in persons who previously were reasonably well adjusted and who have a limited number of symptoms. In many patients symptoms and unadaptive behavioural responses continue autonomously, even when the original psychodynamic factors cease to be important or active.

PSYCHOPHARMACOLOGY

During the past decade many new drugs have been introduced which have revolutionized psychiatric treatment. They may be conveniently classified according to their main clinical effects into (i) anti-anxiety drugs, (ii) anti-psychotic drugs (major tranquillizers), (iii) anti-depression drugs. (Vide Table on p. 434.)

Anti-anxiety drugs. These include well known and long used drugs such as barbiturates and chloral. The new drugs in this series include diazepam (Valium), chlordiazepoxide (Librium), and nitrazepam (Mogadon). These new drugs differ from barbiturates insofar as they act mainly on subcortical structures, especially those concerned with emotional reactions. They also act on the pathways which are concerned with muscle tension. Their action is two-fold: to relieve anxiety by affecting the higher emotional centres and partly by inducing increased muscular relaxation.

Major tranquillizers. The best known in this group are the phenothiazine derivatives which are used in the treatment of schizophrenia and over-active disturbed behaviour in all psychiatric conditions including mental sub-normality, dementia and hyperkinetic states in children and for relieving tension and distress in physical illnesses. They are also used to help relieve pain and distress in inoperable carcinoma. The drugs in the phenothazine series vary in their action. Briefly, drugs such as chlorpromazine are used when disturbed behaviour, anxiety and tension are prominent in schizophrenia and other severe psychiatric illnesses. The more potent derivatives such as Stelazine, Dartalan, are preferred to chlorpromazine for schizophrenics who are inert, apathetic and disinterested.

Anti-depression Drugs. These include the central nervous system stimulants such as (i) amphetamines, (ii) the monoamine oxidase inhibitors, and (iii) tricyclic antidepressants. Central nervous system stimulants such as amphetamine and similar compounds were the only drugs available for alleviating depression prior to 1957. They were of limited value, their effect was transient followed by a latent state of fatigue and irritability, tolerance and dependence developed and addiction not infrequently occurred.

The two first important drugs for treating depression were Iproniazid, a monoamine oxidase inhibitor, and Tofranil, which is chemically similar to chlorpromazine and is one of the tricyclic group of antidepressants.

Monoamine Oxidase Inhibitors (MAOI). It has been shown that these drugs in experimental animals increased activity, alertness and responsiveness which has parallel with an increase of adrenaline and serotonin in the central nervous system. Serotonin and noradrenaline are broken down by monoamine oxidase which is inhibited by this group of drugs. Some of these drugs produce jaundice and liver damage and others produce an intense, severe headache due to fluctuating high blood-pressure. The MAOI drugs in current use are Marplan, which is probably the safest but takes time to produce its effects; Parnate, which is quick acting but has a high incidence of side effects; Iproniazid, which is very effective but should only be used by a specialist; Nardil, and Actomol also tend to produce a variety of side effects. Patients on these drugs have to be advised not to eat cheese, Marmite, nor to take any proprietary medicines without informing the doctor. Certain beverages such as Marmite and Bovril and certain cheeses contain tyramine, which interacts with the MAOI drugs to produce a very intense and incapacitating headache.

MAOI drugs mainly help the less severe and atypical sorts of depression. In some patients they are the only drugs which are effective.

The tricyclic antidepressants are the drugs of choice for the treatment of mild or moderately severe endogenous depression.

All antidepressants may take two weeks to produce their effects. If no benefit occurs after three or four weeks it is pointless carrying on with that particular drug. If one is changing from an MAOI drug to a tricyclic antidepressant a period of time must elapse in view of the possibility of severe effects due to interaction.

Lithium Therapy

Lithium Carbonate has been used for treating mania and hypomania for many years. The most important and significant use of Lithium Carbonate is for the prevention of recurrent attacks of affective disorders, (depression, anxiety, mania). To achieve the best results, the blood level of Lithium must be kept within prescribed limits. Lithium preventive therapy has to be continued indefinitely. It has transformed the level of thousands of sufferers who were previously incapacitated by recurrent attacks of depression and or, hypomania or mania.

Electroconvulsive therapy. This is induced by passing a current through the front part of the head which induces a major epileptic fit for therapeutic purposes. The treatment is given under the effect of an intravenous anaesthetic and a muscle relaxant such as scoline. It is given once or twice a week. It is the treatment of choice for severe endogenous depressions.

Prefrontal Leucotomy. This is used when other methods have failed and when certain requirements are fulfilled. The operation consists of cutting fibres going from the frontal lobe to the thalamus. It has the effect of relieving anxiety, tension and depression. In selecting patients for the operation, (1) emotional distress must be present; (2) the personality must be reasonably stable and well adjusted, as people with psychopathic traits may be made worse; and, (3) the family and home circumstances must be accepting, helpful and encouraging during the post-operative period which is so important for rehabilitation.

ALCOHOLISM AND DRUG DEPENDENCE

ALCOHOLISM

Alcoholism is a pathological state in which the person becomes dependent on alcohol and suffers an impairment in personality and efficiency as a result. Characteristically, alcoholics tend to start drinking early in the day and have periods of amnesia or blackouts after drinking.

A variety of syndromes may be associated with alcoholism. Delirium tremens is an acute confusional state showing all the features of delirium together with tremors of the limbs. The Korsakoff syndrome is a condition in which the person has a marked memory failure for recent events and shows a tendency to confabulate to fill in the gaps of memory. Prolonged alcoholism may result in dementia or may result in various psychiatric syndromes such as alcoholic paranoid states and alcoholic hallucinosis which are believed to be related to schizophrenia but made manifest by chronic alcohol consumption.

Treatment. The treatment of alcoholism is first of all to get the patient into hospital to be "dried out". During this process of withdrawal from alcohol, drugs such as diazepam are invaluable by relieving the emotional distress of the withdrawal state and also by preventing the development of epileptic fits which might otherwise occur. Another useful drug is heminevrin which similarly has sedative and anti-convulsant properties. After this drying-out process the important treatment begins which consists of psychotherapy in the form of individual or group therapy, and the patient should be advised to join an organization like Alcoholics Anonymous which has a high success rate in preventing relapse to alcoholism. In patients who need an additional support to help them to withstand temptations to resume drinking they may be given drugs such as antabuse or temposil which interact with any alcohol ingested and produce unpleasant symptoms and general malaise. It should be noted that if the patient on these drugs takes a large amount of alcohol it presents a real hazard and may prove fatal. The patient is usually given a test dose of alcohol prior to leaving hospital so that he knows what will happen if he does take alcohol whilst on these drugs.

DRUG DEPENDENCE

The term "drug dependence" is used to include the term "drug addiction", "drug habituation" and all types of drug abuse. Drug dependence is a state which arises from repeated administration of a drug on a periodic or continuous basis. It is characterized by a strong drive, need or compulsion to continue taking the drug and there is always a psychological dependence and in some drugs a state of physical dependence also occurs. Physical dependence results from an altered physiological state of the body which necessitates continued administration of the drug in order to prevent the appearance of a characteristic series of symptoms referred to as the abstinence syndrome or withdrawal state. Drug habituation refers to a strong need or compulsion to continue taking the drug on which he is emotionally dependent but he does not develop the withdrawal state characteristic of physical dependence. The manifestations of drug dependence and the characteristics of the withdrawal state vary with the nature of the drug itself. All the drugs of dependence have powerful actions on the nervous system, and they produce harmful effects on the individual and also are usually harmful to society as a whole. Thus, opiates, including heroin and allied drugs, produce a lack of energy and drive and a decrease in productivity. Alcohol, barbiturates and allied hypnotic and sedative drugs produce manifestations of drunkenness, inco-ordination, faulty judgement and impairment of efficiency. Drugs like amphetamines, cocaine and marijuana in high doses may produce a toxic psychosis which resembles schizophrenia. Similarly, the withdrawal state varies according to the type of drug. Opium alkaloids, heroin and synthetic analgesics produce a state of physical dependence with the withdrawal syndrome being characterized by a nervous irritability and autonomic symptoms mainly affecting the parasympathetic nervous system. Drugs such as alcohol, barbiturates, paraldehyde, chloral, meprobamate and glutethimide produce a withdrawal syndrome characterized by delirium and/or convulsion. Drugs which have a stimulating action on the central nervous system such as cocaine and the amphetamines, produce a withdrawal syndrome characterized by depression, sleepiness and lack of energy.

In the last decade, there has been a very rapid increase in the number of individuals who mis-use drugs. This applies to heroin, amphetamines, marijuana and barbiturates.

Treatment. The treatment of drug dependence consists first of all in establishing good rapport and a therapeutic relationship with the patient. This is the most important single factor in treatment. Many heroin addicts can be successfully treated as out-patients, as the recently established drug dependency clinics have demonstrated. At one time it used to be believed that it was only possible to treat heroin addicts successfully if they had a period of treatment as in-patients. The withdrawal from the drug is usually carried out gradually in the case of heroin and other opiates and with barbiturate drugs. Amphetamines and cocaine can be stopped abruptly because the withdrawal syndrome is not hazardous. The withdrawal from heroin can be helped by giving phenothiazine drugs or giving methadone. The withdrawal of the drug is only a relatively minor part of the treatment and the most important aspects of treatment are the utilization of all measures to help the patient's rehabilitation back into work in society without the need for taking drugs. The follow-up period may involve psychotherapy, group therapy, vocational placement and the use of social agencies in order to help the patient establish himself as a healthy, useful member of society.

It should be noted that the mortality rate of heroin addicts is much greater than the corresponding age group in the general population. The deaths are usually due to taking, unwittingly, an excessive dose of the drug or may result from infection due to faulty hygiene in the administration of the drug.

COMMUNITY CARE

In the United Kingdom the policy of the Health Departments is to promote the care of the mentally ill and the mentally retarded in the community. The establishment of psychiatric units in general hospitals serving a defined catchment area has facilitated community care of psychiatric patients. Local authorities, sometimes helped by voluntary organizations, are expected to provide workshops for training and rehabilitation, occupation centres, day centres, hostels and group homes for a number of patients to live in and run themselves. The use of long acting neuroleptics, such as Modecate and Depixol, is a significant advance in the community care of schizophrenics, and continued therapy with neuroleptics is an important factor in preventing relapse in schizophrenia. There is an increasingly important role for the psychiatric nurse in community care.

Chapter 16

Care of the Old

More people survive into old age now than at any other time, and so the number of old people in the community is constantly rising. The preservation of mental and physical activity in the old is therefore important not only for the happiness of the individual, but also because it will reduce the demands on communal resources for care.

The diseases from which the old suffer are not different from those of younger adults, except that the incidence of degenerative disease (e.g. arteriosclerosis) and of carcinoma is considerably higher. The normal process of aging does, however, render people more liable to accidents and infections, and since the old have often outlived relatives and friends, the social aspects of their condition may be of greater importance than the medical ones. Women tend to live longer than men, so that the oldest group contains more females than males.

People who are self-supporting are sometimes incapacitated permanently as the result of an accident or illness which would be minor to a younger person. The protection of the old from accidents or infections is therefore an important aspect of geriatric care, and nurses are often in a favourable position to provide the advice and help that old people and their relatives need.

The effects of age vary markedly from one individual to another, but every system eventually shows the effects of senescence, and these may be classed as follows:

1. *MUSCULO-SKELETAL*

Loss of calcium from the bones and thinning of the intervertebral discs must cause decrease in height, often accentuated by bowing of the spine. Muscles waste and stiffen, and the old may suffer fractures from very small accidents or stumbles, because they have lost the agility to right themselves after minor losses of balance, and the bones are fragile. Fracture of the neck of the femur is the best known of such injuries, and Colles' fracture of the wrist due to falls on the outstretched hand is also common. If nutrition is good, fractures will heal even in the very old, and the effects of confinement to bed, if required, may be worse than those of the fracture.

Osteoarthritis (p. 340) of some degree usually occurs in weight bearing joints such as those of the spine, hips and knees. Even if not painful, it causes loss of mobility and increases the liability to trip or lose balance.

Loss of calcium from the jaw bones may mean that dentures which once fitted no longer do so. If they are left out, nutrition may suffer, and so may morale. Loss of pride in the appearance and grooming is insidious and destructive, and many factors may contribute to it. Decreasing manual dexterity leads to spilling of food. Laundering clothes is either laborious or expensive. The patient may fear to sit down in the bath if he lives alone, and so may abandon the habit of bathing.

2. *CARDIO-VASCULAR*

Hardening of the arteries leads to a rise in the systolic blood pressure, and hypertension is a common cause of heart failure in the old. Coronary artery disease and cerebrovascular accidents frequently occur.

Restriction of the blood supply to the legs and feet may cause cramp in the calves, and complaints of burning pain in the feet at night. If arterial disease is advanced, senile gangrene of the feet may result.

3. *DIGESTIVE*

Although old people living alone may feel little interest in preparing food for themselves, meals are usually enjoyed if they are cooked and served for them. As muscle tone becomes weaker, sphincter control may be uncertain when the faeces are fluid.

4. *URINARY*

As long as the mental functions are well preserved, bladder control is usually normal unless some complicating condition such as prolapse of the uterus or hypertrophy of the prostate gland is present.

5. *TEMPERATURE-REGULATING*

Subcutaneous fat usually decreases with age, so that the body becomes less well insulated against heat loss. Bodily activity diminishes, and these two factors combine to cause susceptibility to cold which is often one of the greatest afflictions of the old. The skin temperature is often about 97°F (36°C) and an axillary temperature which would be normal in someone younger may indicate the start of an infection.

6. *RESPIRATORY*

Increasing rigidity of the rib cage diminishes the amount of respiratory movement, and renders the elderly susceptible to respiratory infections such as bronchitis and pneumonia.

7. *AUDIO-VISUAL*

Though many old people retain hearing and vision unimpaired, senile cataract is a common cause of decreasing sight, and some deafness frequently occurs.

CARE OF THE OLD AT HOME

The family doctor, the health visitor and district nurse are all able to offer help and advice to old people and their relatives on the maintenance of health. Most of the old live at home, either alone or with relatives, and this is in general preferable to living in an institution.

Very many old people are anxious about money; the cost of living continually rises, while pensions remain fixed, or rise slowly, and the real value of savings falls. The ability to afford good food, adequate heating and clothing decreases. The old must be made aware of the funds that are available to them in case of need from welfare sources.

Obvious dangers in the home should be rectified as far as possible. Loose mats, worn carpets and unguarded fires are obvious examples. Gas fires and stoves that need lighting with a match sometimes allow accidents because the gas is turned on and the lighting forgotten.

Cold is a great enemy, and the value of exercise as well as warm clothing must be remembered. In very cold weather old people should be visited frequently, and if they are not well the temperature should be taken with a low-register thermometer, when figures below normal (hypothermia) may be found. The patient should be re-heated slowly in a warm room, and a broad spectrum antibiotic given to help prevent pneumonia.

The food taken should contain average amounts of protein (meat, fish, eggs or cheese) and fresh vegetables or fruit. Unfortunately these are the more expensive foods, and pensioners may economize on these, which may lead to anaemia and chronic sub-health. "Meals on Wheels" is a service available in many areas through the Women's Royal Voluntary Services, and provides a midday meal ready cooked.

Taking a bath unaided can be dangerous, and some local authorities provide bath attendants to help the district nurse by assisting the elderly with their toilet. Care of the feet is of the greatest importance, and chiropody is often needed. Shoes and socks or stockings should be well fitting, and if tinea is present it should be treated.

The bowels should act regularly. "Diarrhoea" is sometimes a complaint when the rectum is irritated by the presence of impacted faeces, which can be detected by digital examination.

Exposure to the risks of upper respiratory infection should be avoided as far as possible. Colds should be treated, and the risk of mild upper respiratory infection spreading to the chest should be remembered. Advice should, if necessary, be given on the hygiene of food, such as the protection of meat from flies.

Deafness and failing sight are not inevitable accompaniments of age, and should be investigated to see if they can be relieved. Syringing the ears to free them from wax may improve hearing, and age is no bar to a successful cataract operation.

Increasing difficulty with bladder control is often a problem of age. Sometimes it is associated with prolapse of the uterus, enlargement of the prostate gland, or urinary infection, and these may be corrected. The fluid intake should be adequate, or the urine will be concentrated and so more irritating to the bladder, but large quantities of diuretic fluids like tea and coffee should not be taken just before bedtime. A commode by the bed at night may be an advantage, and old people ought always to have a bedside lamp so that if they have to get up at night there is no risk of a fall in the dark.

Incontinence of urine is often the final cause of old people having to leave home and enter an institution, and if relatives are prepared to cope with this problem at home they should be given every help. The difficulties are chiefly those of laundering and drying clothes and linen, and some local authorities will help with this. Plastic sheeting and incontinence pads may also be available, perhaps from voluntary organizations such as the British Red Cross. Faecal incontinence is usually associated with cerebral damage, and if it occurs in old people who appear well-orientated, the possibility of impacted faeces should be borne in mind, and rectal examination made.

Apathy is a great enemy of health and happiness in the aged, and is usually due to lack of occupation and of sensory stimulus. Those who can read, talk to visitors, watch television or listen to the radio can maintain contact and interests. People who have nothing to do feel valueless, and tend to neglect diet and grooming.

Relatives sometimes need advising against over-protectiveness. An old person who is well fed and housed may still be unhappy if expected to spend the day sitting in an armchair. Minor tasks and small responsibilities should always be given as long as the physical state allows, and this will maintain morale and self-esteem.

THE OLD IN HOSPITAL

The old are subject to most of the acute medical and surgical emergencies as the young, and all acute wards have a number of old patients. The most important point in their management is that besides the dangers inherent in their primary condition, the old are especially threatened by the risks of confinement to bed.

These are hypostatic pneumonia and venous thrombosis leading to pulmonary embolism in the early stages; if the patient has to remain in bed for some time, pressure sores, contractures and incontinence may develop unless effective precautions are taken. Disinclination to get up again may also develop.

Breathing exercises and percussion of the chest by the physiotherapist should begin on admission to prevent pneumonia, along with calf massage and passive leg movements to avert thrombosis. As soon as possible, the patient should be helped out of bed to stand with assistance, and to spend some time sitting up well supported in a comfortable chair.

The pressure areas, especially the sacrum and the heels, should be examined and treated regularly. Dark marks on the heels indicate approaching skin necrosis, and measures should be taken at once to relieve all pressure with ankle pads or something similar.

Old people who are alert and well-orientated at home often appear to deteriorate sharply in hospital, because they are confused by their new surroundings and the speed of events. They are often sleepless and restless at night, and if barbiturates are given their confusion is usually worse. If a sedative is needed glutethimide or chloral hydrate is the most suitable.

Social problems associated with the discharge of old people from acute wards are severe. Those who were previously self-supporting may now be incapable of looking after themselves in their former homes. Relatives who have had the aged living with them may feel unable to resume the burden. It may be possible to send the patient home if he can be given a home help and support from the health visitor. Some local authorities have small flats especially for the aged, and there are homes in which the tenants have their own rooms or flats, and some supervision and help. Some may be fit for discharge to an old people's home, but some must go to a geriatric unit or hospital for rehabilitation or as permanent inmates.

GERIATRIC UNITS

On admission to a geriatric ward, a careful assessment of the patient's particular problems is made. The physician looks for the presence of organic disease, and at the nutritional state, the mental condition, and whether the patient has bladder and rectal control. He can then define his aims and make a realistic forecast of the improvement that can be expected.

The acute complications of confinement to bed have been discussed. The chronic results are contractures, decalcification of the skeleton, incontinence and mental apathy. Patients must therefore not be confined to bed if they are capable of activity, though it is equally wrong that those suffering from terminal or disabling disease should be made to sit in chairs.

Incontinence is one of the major problems in a geriatric ward, depressing to the morale of patients, staff and visitors. If the load of work on the nurses is such that patients capable of being got up must lie in bed, a high level of incontinence will result. Regular offering of urinals or bedpans will reduce the level. Up-patients must be escorted to the toilets, which should be adequate in number and accessible, since the old often suffer from urgency of micturition.

Faecal incontinence may be reduced by giving a bedpan in the morning and allowing adequate time for defaecation. Administration of a suppository regularly will empty the rectum, and may ensure relative cleanliness. Impaction of faeces must be avoided by recording the bowel actions and taking measures if this occurs, otherwise spurious "diarrhoea" results and constantly soiling follows.

It is often supposed that geriatric wards have lower staffing requirements than acute wards, but the number of nursing tasks in a chronic ward often exceeds that in general wards. Enough nurses should be available to change as often as necessary the soiled bedding, which should be put in plastic bags and sent to the laundry, not sluiced in the ward. Ward ventilation should be good.

Contractures of joints and wasting of muscles are still an almost inevitable accompaniment of confinement to bed, unless effective counter measures are taken. The active treatment of hemiplegia following cerebral thrombosis (p. 385) has considerably reduced the number of such patients.

The management of a ward of geriatric patients must be considerably more relaxed than in an acute ward. This is home for a great many of the patients, and comfortable chairs, a dining area, television and adequate space to keep clothes and belongings are all essential.

CARE OF THE DYING

When a diagnosis of incurable disease has been made, a decision must be reached by the physician as to how much information should be given to the patient. Hard and fast rules have little place in such a situation. If the physician feels that all patients have a right to know that they are dying, some who have no wish to have this brought to their attention will be burdened by this information. If it is felt that patients should not be told, there are some who will be impatient of evasion, and have a real desire to know their prognosis. The needs of every person must be considered individually.

Near relatives must always be honestly and fully informed of the diagnosis and outlook. In many diseases, no cure may be known, but this does not mean that effective treatment may not become available and a person with an incurable condition that runs a long course may live long enough to benefit from research. It will be recalled that diabetes in young people was once a fatal disease, until insulin was brought into use.

Nurses do not have the necessary detailed knowledge of disease and prognosis to answer accurately the question, "Am I going to die?". They can usually recognize the people who want reassurance, not truthful information. It is equally important to recognize the people who really want to know, and to see that they have an opportunity to talk about it to the physician.

The terminal stages of disease may be sad or unpleasant, but should never be painful. The choice of the correct analgesic and the regime to be followed should ensure this. Even when the doctor feels that no more treatment is available, his visits to the patient will still be appreciated by the patient and his relatives. The nurse of course never reaches a stage when there is nothing more that she can do for the dying patient. Cleanliness, fresh linen, a moistened mouth, a comfortable position, freedom from pain, and an atmosphere of peace and tranquillity can usually be arranged.

Patients rarely say "I can't bear it", it would be a reflection on medical care if they did, but relatives not infrequently do, and need support and sympathy. They often feel they have no useful part to play in the closing scenes, and must never be made to feel superfluous. They should be allowed to participate in every possible way, and helped to feel that their presence is welcome if they wish to be there at all times.

Further reading

An Investigation of Geriatric Nursing Problems in Hospital by Exton-Smith Norton and McLaren. Publisher: The National Corporation for the Care of Old People 1962.

Nursing the Psychiatric Patient by Joan Burr. Baillière Tindall and Cassell 1967. Chapter 14.
The Last Refuge by Peter Townsend. Routledge and Kegan Paul 1962.
Principles of Rehabilitation by W. Russell Grant. E. & S. Livingstone Ltd.

Chapter 17

SI Units

In 1960 the General Conference of Weights and Measures adopted an International System of Units (Système International d'unites), abbreviated in English to SI Units. The aim was to produce a coherent system of measurement that would apply to all scientific disciplines, throughout the world. The advantages to medicine when all countries use the same code are clear. Doctors and nurses in large numbers work in countries other than their own, and universal adoption of the same measuring system will promote easy understanding. Physicists, chemists and engineers will use the same units as doctors. Scientific journals throughout the world will employ comparable measurements. As SI units are now used in school, entrants to hospital in future will already be familiar with them, but those trained in earlier methods will need to work at thinking in SI units. They should carry a conversion card in the pocket, and notice especially those areas in which difficulties may arise, because of reading or writing errors, or with abbreviations.

SI units are based on the metric system, and some of the adopted terms are already familiar to us, and some are not used in our type of work. Below are listed the independent base SI units and their symbols.

Quantity	Base unit	Symbol
Length	metre	m
Mass	kilogram	kg
Volume	Litre	L
Time	second	s
Electric current	ampere	A
Thermodynamic	kelvin	K
Luminous intensity	candela	cd
Amount of substance	mole	mol

From these are derived other units, and there follow the ones important in medicine

Quantity	Base unit	Unit symbol
Energy	joule	J
Force	newton	N
Power	watt	W
Pressure	pascal	Pa
Temperature	degree Celsius	C

The base unit is often inconveniently large or small for the purpose for which it is to be used. There are prefixes that can be used to show multiples and sub-multiples of the base unit. Indices can also be used to express both, but both parties engaged in communicating in indices must be quite sure they understand the mathematics involved. Indices should not be used in the prescription of drugs.

Prefix	Symbol	Indices	Value
tera	T	10^{12}	1 000 000 000 000
giga	G	10^{9}	1 000 000 000
mega	M	10^{6}	1 000 000
kilo	k	10^{3}	1 000
hecto	h	10^{2}	100
deca	da	10^{1}	10
deci	d	10^{-1}	0·1
centi	c	10^{-2}	0·01
milli	m	10^{-3}	0·001
micro	μ	10^{-6}	0·000 001
nano	n	10^{-9}	0·000 000 001
pico	p	10^{-12}	0·000 000 000 001
femto	f	10^{-15}	0·000 000 000 000 001

It will be noticed that the groups of three noughts in the column on the right are separated not by the comma usual in England, but by a space. This is to avoid confusion with continental countries where a comma is used for the decimal point.

Many of these prefixes are already familiar to nurse e.g. centimetre, kilometres, milligram. The most likely source of error is distinguishing between milligram and microgram (mg and μgm). When micrograms are being used in prescribing, the unit should be written out in full. Nurses who are not completely confident in their reading of a prescription must consult the prescriber; a milligram is a thousand times greater than a microgram, and to mistake one or the other would involve a thousand-fold error in drug administration.

Dietetic calculations

Dietitians and workers in nutrition have used some SI units for years, and the metric units of weight and of volume are familiar to us. The new unit of energy, the joule, must now be incorporated into the system, and will give rise initially to need for adjustment. The energy which food can generate has hitherto been expressed in kilocalories (kcals) is now given in joules, or, since this unit is inconveniently small for some requirements, in kilojoules (kJ) or megajoules (MJ). The list below gives some conversion figures.

1 kcal = 4·2 kJ
1000 kcal = 4200 kJ = 4·2 MJ

The approximate values assigned to the constituents of food:-

1 gram of protein yields approx. 4 kcals = 17 kJ
1 gram of carbohydrate yields approx. 3·8 kcals = 16 kJ
1 gram of fat yields approx. 9 kcals = 38 kJ

Blood pressure

Sphygmomanometers in present use measure the blood pressure as the height of a column of mercury expressed in millimetres (mm/Hg). Sooner or later it will be in pascals (pa), or in practice, since this is a small unit, in kilopascals (kP). The delay is chiefly because of the large number of sphygmomanometers calibrated in mm/Hg, and it is proposed that these will remain in use.
Later they will show both mm/Hg and kP, and eventually only kP.
The kP gives a smaller range of figures than mm/Hg; for instance a blood pressure of $\frac{120}{80}$ mm/Hg would read in kP approximately $\frac{16}{10·8}$. The second figures are less discriminating than the first, and we must be alert to the importance of smaller numerical changes when we are working in kP.

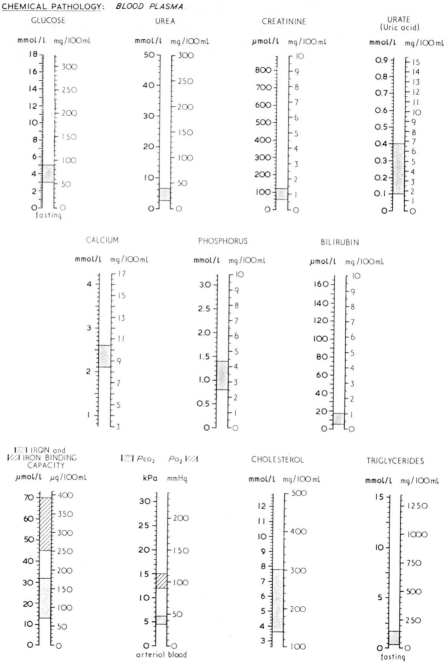

Fig. 133.

CONVERSION SCALES (2)
Traditional to SI units

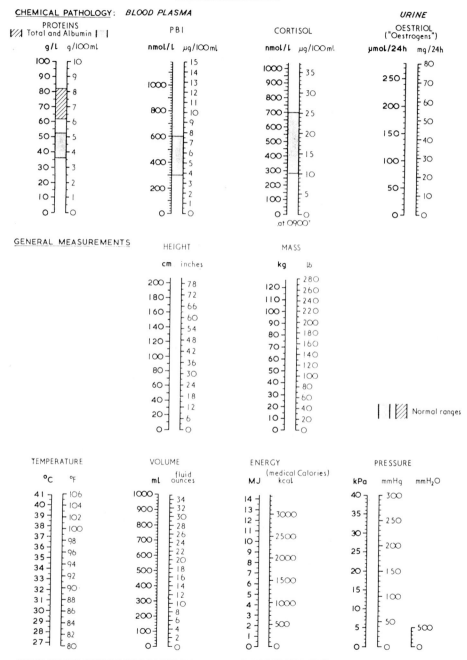

CHEMICAL PATHOLOGY: *BLOOD PLASMA*

GENERAL MEASUREMENTS

CHEMICAL PATHOLOGY CONVERSION SCALES ARE BASED ON THOSE PUBLISHED BY THE UNITED LEEDS HOSPITALS

Reproduced by kind permission of the Editor, *British Medical Journal*.

Clinical temperatures

The Fahrenheit thermometer scale has now largely been superseded by Centigrade. Celsius and Centigrade degrees are identical, so although the term Celsius has deen preferred to Centigrade, the nurse has no numerical adjustment to make.

Patient's height and weight

The metric system is in general use in this country for measuring patient's height and weight. A scale for conversion cm/inches and kg/lbs is given on p. 455.

Molar concentration is now to be used instead of the milliequivalent on laboratory reports. The chemical pathologist will for some time give the "normal" range of values on his report, and the nurse will notice that numerically these values are smaller than those returned in mg/100 ml or mEq. For instance, with reference to blood calcium, the mmol/1 figure is half that in mEq/1.

Chapter 18

Some Elements of Medical Statistics

Someone who reads the title of this chapter may well feel that this is a subject of rather marginal importance to a nurse. If, so consideration of a few questions might alter this opinion. How does she know what is the "normal" blood pressure, temperature and pulse rate? how did the pathologist arrive at the figures he sends to the ward on the normal range for haemoglobin, blood sugar, and all other electrolytes? how does one establish whether a new drug is an effective means of treating a disease, and how important are its side effects? how does the Department of Health and Social Service forecast how many geriatric institutions or maternity beds will be required in 1990? how effective is vaccination against poliomyelitis? has the nurse ever been asked to fill in a questionnaire by a researcher or by the General Nursing Council? A patient about to have a serious operation asks, "What chance have I got"? Probably what he wants to be told is, "Excellent, you'll be all right". In fact, figures will almost certainly be available that may show (for instance) that he has a 75% chance of being alive three years later.

All these situations are concerned with the collection and examination of facts and figures, and with their presentation in a meaningful and useful form; that is, with statistics. In the last paragraph it was asked how we knew what was the "normal" blood pressure; the answer is that a large number of observations will show that most of the figures are clustered around a central point. The word "normal" is widely used in everyday life, but technically it refers to this central group of characteristics which constitutes the norm. All forms of life show great variety in many of their characteristics, and this is one of the pleasures of social intercourse and of the study of natural history. Not all admit of variety; it is the norm in man to have two eyes, and five digits to each limb, but there is much diversity in such qualities as height, skin colour and intelligence, and in these there will be quite a range of people who belong to the norm. One of the tasks of medicine has been to establish what is the norm in physiological values like those quoted in the first paragraph, and how far departure from it is significant.

An observer might decide to record the systolic blood pressure of 100 people, and look at the figures obtained. It will at once be obvious that there are many variables that may make the raw figures valueless. The blood pressure varies with age, sex, emotion, and many diseases. Then there is observer error—one cannot make a critically accurate reading of a sphygmomanometer each time; different observers tend to record slightly higher or lower levels than others, while different instruments unless well maintained may give different results. Our observer decides to minimize these as far as possible by taking all readings himself, using the same instrument, on apparently healthy men aged 20 to 25 in a college. The figures obtained for the systolic pressure are as follows.

Mm Hg	Number of subjects	Mm Hg	No of subjects
110	1	126	10
112	3	128	9
114	6	130	7
116	9	132	5
118	11	134	2
120	12	136	1
122	12	138	1
124	11		

It can be seen at once that there is a very marked cluster around the 120–122 mm/Hg mark, but if these figures are expressed in a visual form, other facts will appear.

Along the bottom line in Fig. 154 is shown the attribute being investigated, that is the systolic pressure. This line is called the **abscissa**. The frequency with

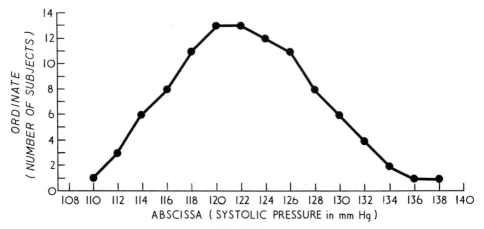

Fig. 134.

which each observation occurs is marked on the vertical line, the **ordinate**. By recording the number of observations for each figure, a **graph** is obtained, in exactly the same way as a nurse constructs a temperature chart.

Looking at the graph we can see that the greatest number of records is indeed at the 120–122 mark; this is the central location of the graph. Another prominent feature is that the graph is fairly symmetrical about this centre, falling rapidly in both directions so that only one observation occurs at the lower and higher extremes.

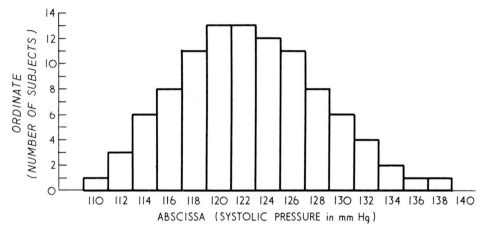

Fig. 135. A histogram is another way of presenting data.

So what is the "normal" systolic pressure in this group? The usual method of finding it is to add together the figures obtained, and divide by the number of observations. Thus the total of the 100 readings is 12,264, which divided by 100 gives 122·64 mm/Hg as the average or **mean**. Two other terms are used in finding the central point in data. The **median** is the value with an equal number of entries above and below it, and this falls in the 122 mm group also. The **mode** is the most frequently occurring figure, and in this group is also 120/122 mm.

It should not be thought that the mean, median and mode always coincide in this way. We might consider, to illustrate this fact, the incomes of a small hamlet of working country people in which also live a farm manager and a business man who is a commuter from the city. Their incomes are;-

| 1 of £10,000 | 1 of £2,500 | 9 of £2,000 |

The average or mean is

$$\frac{£10,000 + £2,500 + (9 \times £2,000)}{11} = \frac{£30,500}{11}$$

$$= £2,777$$

This figure is not very helpful as an expression of what is "normal" or average, since all but one of the group are below it. The most frequent figure in the group is £2,000, and this is the mode. The median would also fall in the £2,000 group, and so either the median or the mode would be more representative of the real financial state of the group than the mean or average. It can be seen that unless one looks carefully at how the data have been collected and presented misleading impressions can be gathered.

It has been noted that our blood pressure readings when charted produced a curve, highest in the centre where most records were grouped, and tailing away at each end. This shape is characteristic of many observations familiar in medicine, such as blood chemistry levels. If our sample were truly representative

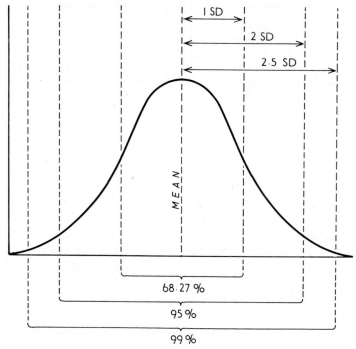

Fig. 136. Normal distribution curve.

of the group we were investigating, and if we made enough readings, we would obtain a smooth bell-shaped curve like the one in Fig. 136.

This curve is symmetrical about its mid point, which is the mean, and half our readings would be at one side of it, and half on the other. This is the **normal distribution curve**. A mathematical term useful in describing how close most of the observations are to the mean is the **standard deviation**. Nurses undertaking research will need to be familiar with the formula for obtaining this; some nurses may wish to know more about it, and should consult a book from the bibliography; most will only wish to note it as a way of expressing how close our observations lie to the mean, either above it (+) or below it (−). The diagram shows that 68·27% of our sample is within the range of one standard deviation of the mean, either above or below it (± 1SD); that 95% are within the range ± 1·96 SD, and that practically everyone (99%) is within the range ± 2·58 SD. So if our sample was a representative or truly random one, 99% of the population of 20–25 year old apparently healthy men would have a systolic blood pressure within ± 2·58 SD from the mean. The standard deviation of the mean in this case can be calculated as 5·989 or since we are working in whole numbers in this study, 6. This means that 68% of this group will have a systolic blood pressure of 123 ± 6, that is, 117 to 129 mm/Hg.

The data collected can be presented in another form, the bar chart. In our chart, the class width is the same all along the base line, and this form is called a **histogram.**

VITAL STATISTICS

In the first paragraph it was asked how the age of the population or the birth rate in the future could be foretold. The answer is that these are a projection into the future based on trends in the survival and birth rates at the present day. It must be admitted that these prophecies are not always correct. In forecasting the birth rate statisticians may know the number of women of marriageable age, and may take into account the impact of the Abortion Act and of contraception, but may fail to foresee rapid inflation or recession in the economy, which may make people postpone or limit their families for financial reasons.

Vital statistics are derived from the Registrar General's figures on the number of births, marriages, divorces, deaths, and notifiable disease. Census returns give the numbers of people in the community by age, sex and occupation, and any other information the Censor may require.

Plain figures derived from these sources are not very informative. The fact that more babies die in London than in Carlisle is due to the fact that London is the bigger city, and further treatment of these figures will be necessary. The

infant mortality rate is of great interest to all in the health service, because it measures the level of service provided during pregnancy and labour and of the social standards in a country. It is calculated thus-:

$$\frac{\text{Number of deaths of infants under 1 year of age}}{\text{Live births during the same period.}} \times 1000$$

The infant mortality rate in England and Wales in 1973 was 16·9. This rate can be subdivided to show the mortality rate for infants under 28 days old, and those from 28 days to a year. This separation is of importance because the causes of death in early days are connected with prenatal conditions e.g. prematurity and congenital deformities, while those occurring after the baby is a month old derive mostly from its environment and are acquired e.g. infections. Such figures show the health authorities where there is room for improvement, and allows them to compare our rates with those of other countries.

Mortality rates deal with the number of deaths in a community. Crude death rates are influenced by such factors as age and sex; more elderly people die than young ones, and men have a higher death rate than women at most ages, so in order to compare different areas or countries these rates have to be **standardized.** Government decisions about retirement ages, insurance contributions and pension levels may be linked to such rates.

Death rates can be calculated for different ages, different social classes, various occupations and diseases, and will give valuable information. For instance, the steady rise in the number of deaths from lung cancer prompted research into the cause, and this uncovered its connection with smoking. These rates will disclose such facts that death from myocardial infarction is occurring among men at an earlier age than formerly.

Morbidity rates refer to the amount of ill health or disease, and are rather more complicated to construct than mortality rates, since death only occurs once, but diseases come and go and recur, and a patient may suffer from more than one disease. There are two terms often used in connection with disease; these are **prevalence** and **incidence.** The prevalence rate refers to the cases of a disease in existence at some moment, or over a stated period, and the incidence rate indicates the number of new cases that arise in a stated time. For instance, in an epidemic of influenza, the weekly incidence rate will show whether the epidemic is still increasing or whether it is declining, and from this hospitals can plan what actions they should take, e.g. to suspend admissions from the waiting list. Prevalence rates will show the total number sick at any one time.

CLINICAL TRIALS

There is a constant need in medicine to establish the efficiency or otherwise of a new drug or a new procedure, and although this will in many cases involve research with animals, the time comes when a test must be made with human beings, and a **clinical trial** must be set up.

The principle involved is the comparison of two sets of observations; one comes from the patients receiving the new drug or treatment, and the other from a control group, who are either having standard treatment, or else some inactive substance or placebo. Two sets of problems present themselves in connection with trials. The first is how to ensure that any differences in results are not due to faulty techniques in the conduct of the trial, and the second problems are ethical. Since nurses are more likely to feel concern about the second than the first, we will begin with the latter.

Nurses sometimes feel revulsion at the idea that patients are used as guinea pigs, but this emotional expression should be avoided, and a more thoughtful attitude adopted. If we really do not know if a drug is effective, it is better to test it under controlled conditions, and decide whether it is to be recommended or not, than to let it drift on in use. Suppose a new drug is formulated which is said when given by a course of intramuscular injections to prevent venous thrombosis. Since this is such a common post-operative complication, an effective drug would be valuable. One may ask, is it ethical to do a trial and deprive the control group of the benefits of this treatment? The answer is that it is not ethical to use indiscriminately a series of injections which cannot be painless which may prove to be useless or even deleterious. Apart from this consideration it is not sensible to spend money on a drug of unproven merit when so many branches of the health service need more resources. In general, ethical and practical considerations would lead to the exclusion of pregnant women and of children from most clinical trials. All hospitals which undertake research have an Ethical Committee to which plans for clinical trials must be submitted for approval.

The first set of problems mentioned were in connection with the method of distinguishing real results, if there is a difference between the treated and untreated groups. This difference in a well planned and conducted trial is likely to be due to the real effects of the drug or treatment, but there are some obstacles to be overcome.

For instance, the results may not be statistically significant, i.e. no better than could be explained by chance. This is especially likely to occur if numbers in the trial are small, but correct analysis of the results will indicate if these are significant.

A second point of difficulty is that the treatment and control groups may differ in some important respects. The processes by which representative groups are assigned to one form of treatment or the other are not within our scope, but this is an aspect of setting up the trial that is fraught with difficulty, and the one most closely scrutinized by critics.

The third problem is how to ensure that patients are managed on identical lines, and the results evaluated without bias. For instance, a patient who knows he is receiving a new drug may feel hopeful about its effects, and report improvement. To avoid this, **blind trials** are commonly used, in which the patient is unaware what drug he is getting. Similarly, the physician may have an unconscious bias in favour of one treatment or the other, and may transmit this feeling to the patient, or may show his preferences in the way he evaluates the results. This bias can be nullified by adopting a system in which the doctor as well as the patient is unaware which drug he is giving. This is the much used **double-blind trial.**

The criteria for deciding what are the results of treatment are set beforehand, and the patients in the trial are if possible evaluated by an independent witness. One noticeable feature of most trials is that a proportion of patients show improvement on the placebo or inert substance sometimes used on control groups.

The hope of all those who conduct clinical trials is that there is a significant difference between the treatment and control groups, not attributable to chance or to faulty technique, and that the trial will offer clear guidance to colleagues on the effects of alternative treatments. A negative result, in which it appears that a new treatment is no advance on the old one, is of course valuable.

OBSERVATIONAL STUDIES

Surveys can be made of patients and the course of diseases in other ways than by clinical trials. **Retrospective studies** are those in which the investigator turns to the past for the source of his material. One of the best known of such studies, which illustrates well how work on the past may help practice in the future, was that of Gregg on congenital cataract in Sydney in 1941. Gregg was an ophthalmologist, who noticed in his practice a sudden increase in the number of cataracts in babies who also frequently had congenital heart defects. He felt that the number of cases suggested that there had been some toxic or infective cause, and investigated the history of the mothers of affected babies in the early months of pregnancy. He found that all had had german measles, and so established that this mild virus disease had severe consequences for the fetus if a woman contracted it in the early months of pregnancy.

Prospective studies are those in which the results will only be known in the future, maybe in some years' time. Studies are made of a group of people with some risk factor (e.g. a high blood cholesterol) and of a control group without this factor. The subsequent history of both groups is noted and compared.

The most famous work of this kind was the study of Doll and Hill, who in 1951 sent a questionnare to all doctors (about 60,000) in the United Kingdom on their smoking habits, and 41,000 answered. The first follow-up began four years later, when details of the cause of death of all respondents deceased during that time was determined. When age-adjusted rates were employed, the man-years of exposure to smoking indicated that smokers were thirteen times more likely to get lung cancer than non-smokers.

Sampling

If one wants to draw some conclusions about the physical or social characteristics or the opinions of a large group, it will not be possible to examine every member of this **target population** individually, and one uses instead a **sample** of this population. Unless this sample resembles the original group in essential characters and is adequate in numbers, the results will be misleading.

Supposing, for instance, an investigator wanted to forecast the result of a Parliamentary election, as many do. The target population is all voters in the constituency. If the investigator took the telephone directory, and asked every tenth subscriber which way he would vote, he would have a random sample of subscribers, but not of voters. He would not have sampled any of the under-privileged who do not have a telephone, and might vote in quite a different way from the better off.

Investigations frequently fail to give reliable data because of sampling errors such as this. In the world of advertising it is not unknown for a biased sample to be taken deliberately. For instance, one may read an advertisement that states, "Three out of five doctors recommend A's toothpaste", and it is often accompanied by a picture of a wise man in a white coat. What does this mean? It cannot be that 60% of all doctors recommend A's toothpaste, because there are scores of toothpastes on the market, but this is the general impression many receive. The advertiser used a very small sample, and probably had to do a series of surveys before he arrived at a run of five doctors of whom three out of five liked A's toothpaste.

In a similar way, we ourselves often make inferences from distorted samples of the population. For instance, a nurse in a medical ward in a teaching hospital may think a great deal about the patients with rheumatoid arthritis who are under her care, and about their disease as she sees it. She may decide that everyone who suffers from rheumatoid arthritis has a severe crippling disease with many problems. In fact, many people with rheumatoid arthritis are never admitted to hospital at all, and relatively few come to teaching hospitals, the admission lists of which are biased in favour of people who are the subject of research. Her sample is distorted, and no conclusions can be drawn from it, except about the kind of arthritics who are admitted to teaching hospitals.

If it is desired to discover the beliefs, tastes or intentions of a sample group, it will be necessary to question them, either by interview or by post. The schedule of questions must be carefully compiled to extract the required information. Each question must be simply phrased, and must be one that the respondent has the necessary knowledge to answer, and also one that he is willing to answer. Everyone is aware that when people are asked about their voting intentions before an election, there is a large number of "don't knows". These are dubbed floating voters, and all parties hope to capture the allegiance of this floating vote, but it is not very likely that many people who intend to vote have not really made up their minds, and "don't know" often means "shan't tell" or "don't care".

Questions about age and salary are seldom well received, and accurate answers cannot always be expected. Respondents tend to shade their answers according to whether they like the interviewer or not, and there is often a tendency to conform to what are thought to be the expectations of the interviewer. More reliable information is forthcoming if the interviewer does not know the exact purpose of the investigation, and so is an impartial collector of data. Questions must be framed to give a full selection of alternatives. For instance, if a sample of female staff nurses are asked:-

Which would you rather do:-
  a. make a career in nursing
  b. get married and quit nursing?

there may well be women who would like both to marry and to continue nursing, but their opinion will go unrecorded.

Postal Surveys

These may be thought more scientific and objective in that it is easier to identify a truly random sample, but there are drawbacks. Only about 5% of people refuse to give an interview, but about 80% fail to return a postal survey. The number who answer are those with a special interest in the topic. The genuine researcher when giving the results of a postal survey will always give the refusal rate.

People tend to take a rather ambivalent view of statistics. On the one hand, they may think of it as a dull subject, not relevant to real life, and it is hoped that this very slight allusion to some of the facts about medical statistics may show the nurse how important it is in her work. On the other hand, people may think that figures can be made to prove anything, and it is true that badly collected figures may give a misleading impression. Everyone presented with data should make an effort to see how reliable are the facts and the interpretation put on them, and should try in using technical terms to rise above the level of the politician who said the aim of his party was that all workers should receive an above average wage.

Chapter 19

Medical Terms

The terms used in describing medical conditions or surgical operations are often long and complex, but the majority are formed from a comparatively small group of Latin and Greek terms, and once these are known the meaning of many words can be recognized. No one has difficulty in grasping such compound words as waterfall, bookcase, workman, horsemanship. The study of some of the parts that make up scientific terms will enable their meaning to be understood.

For instance *pre*-operative and *post*-operative are words known to every nurse. The greater part of the word is the same, but the meaning has been altered by changing the front part. *Pre-* means "before"; a preface comes before the main part of a book, to prepare is to make ready beforehand, to predict is to foretell. *Post-* means "after"; a postscript comes after a letter, a post mortem examination takes place after death, a post-operative drug is given after operation. Such a part, which stands at the beginning of a word and can modify its meaning is called a *prefix*. Some of the commoner ones used in medicine are given below. A prefix is only part of a word, and is never used by itself.

PREFIXES

Pre- (before)
> e.g. *pre*dict, to foretell.

Ante- (before)
> e.g. *ante*natal, before birth.

Post- (after)
> e.g. *post*natal, after birth.

Ant(i) (against)
> e.g. *anti*dote, a remedy against poison, *ant*agonist, someone or some thing who is acting against another.

A, an (without)
> e.g. *a*moral, without ethical sense, *an*aemic, without blood. The an- form is used when the second part of the word begins with a vowel, e.g. *an*oxia, without oxygen, but *a*septic, without infection.

Sub (under)

    e.g. the *sub*clavian artery runs under the clavicle, the *sub*scapularis muscle is under the scapula.

Supra or super (above)

    e.g. the *supra* spinatus muscle is above the spine of the scapula; to *super*impose is to place above.

In (in or into)

    e.g. to *in*cise is to cut into.

Inter (between)

    e.g. the *inter*costal nerves run between the ribs.

Intra (within)

    e.g. *intra*cranial means within the skull.

Ex (out)

    e.g. to *ex*cise is to cut out.

Per (through)

    e.g. to *per*colate is to trickle through.

Peri (around)

    e.g. the *peri*cardium lies around the heart.

Circum (around)

    e.g. to *circum*cise is literally to cut around.

Iso (same)

    e.g. an *iso*tonic solution has the same strength (in salt) as the blood. Normal saline is *iso*tonic with the blood.

Hyper (excessive)

    e.g. *hyper*tonic saline is stronger than normal saline. *Hyper*thyroidism is excessive thyroid activity.

Hypo (weaker)

    e.g. *hypo*tonic saline is weaker than normal saline.

Olig(o) (few, scanty)

    e.g. *oligo*menorrhoea means few menstrual periods. *Olig*uria is diminished urinary output. The "o" is dropped before a following vowel.

Poly (many)

    e.g. *poly*menorrhoea, many or frequent periods.

Hemi, semi (half)

    e.g. the two cerebral *hemi*spheres are each half a sphere in shape. The *semi*circular canals of the ear are each half a circle.

Eryth (red)

    e.g. *eryth*ema is redness of the skin, an *eryth*rocyte is a red blood cell.

Leuk or leuc (white)
>   e.g. *leuco*plakia, white patches on tongue or vulva.

Cyan (blue)
>   e.g. *cyan*osis is blueness, erythrocyanosis is reddish-blueness.

Pyo (pus)
>   e.g. *pyo*derma means pus in the skin, *pyo*salpinx is pus in a Fallopian tube.

Dys (pain or difficulty)
>   e.g. *dys*entery is a condition in which there is pain in the intestine, *dys*uria is painful micturition.

Para (around)
>   e.g. a *para*-umbilical hernia occurs around the umbilicus.

Hydro (water)
>   e.g. *hydro*therapy is treatment by water, someone who is de*hydr*ated is short of water.

Micro (small)
>   e.g. a *micro*scope is for seeing small things.

Macro (large)
>   e.g. the *macro*scopic structure means something that can be seen with the naked eye.

Acro (an extremity)
>   e.g. *acro*cyanosis is blueness of the fingers and toes.

Just as a prefix stands at the beginning of a word, the suffix is at the end. One of the best known ones is -*itis*, meaning inflammation. Someone who has appendic*itis* usually undergoes appendic*ectomy*. The main part of each of these two words is the same, but the meaning has been completely altered by changing the suffix.

SUFFIXES

itis (inflammation)
>   e.g. tonsill*itis* is inflammation of the tonsil, periton*itis* is inflammation of the peritoneum, *otitis* media is inflammation of the middle ear.

-osis (a state or condition)
>   e.g. thyrotoxic*osis*, a toxic state of the thyroid gland. Carcinomat*osis* means a state in which malignant growths are present. Diverticul*osis* of the colon is a state in which small pouches, or diverticula are present. Should these become inflamed, the patient has diverticul*itis*.

-tome (an appliance for cutting)

> e.g. a micro*tome* cuts microscopic sections. An osteo*tome* is an instrument that cuts bone.

-ectomy (cutting out, or excision)

> e.g. appendic*ectomy* is the cutting out of the appendix.

-ostomy, -otomy (cutting an opening)

> e.g. a colo*stomy* is an opening into the colon. Phleb*otomy* is cutting open a vein.

-ology (knowledge or study)

> e.g. path*ology* is the study of disease. Cardi*ology* is the study of the heart.

-y (a suffix of nouns, or names of things)

> e.g. acromegal*y* is enlargement of the extremities, found in a pituitary disorder.

-ia (is another very common noun ending)

> e.g. in pneumon*ia*.

-phobia (fear or dislike)

> e.g. photo*phobia* is dislike of light. Claustro*phobia* is fear of enclosed places.

-algia (pain)

> e.g. neur*algia* is nerve pain.

-oma (a growth or tumour)

> e.g. fibr*oma*, a fibrous tissue tumour; carcin*oma*, a malignant glandular growth. There is no way in which the student can guess by looking at a name whether the growth is innocent or malignant, and study of the various names and their meaning is necessary.

-gen (producing or giving use to)

> e.g. fibrino*gen* gives rise to fibrin when acted on by thrombin during blood clotting. Hydro*gen* produces water when it combines with oxygen. An anti*gen* produces an immune reaction in the body. Urobilino*gen* gives rise to urobilin when the urine is exposed to air. An agglutino*gen* in the blood is concerned with clumping of sensitive blood cells. A patho*gen* is an organism that gives rise to disease.

-ase (the ending of the names of enzymes)

> e.g. lip*ase*, hyal*ase*.

-in (is another enzyme suffix)

> e.g. peps*in*, renn*in*.

-pnoea (breath or breathing)
>   e.g. dys*pnoea* means difficult breathing, a*pnoea* means without breath, or cessation of breathing.

-plegia (paralysis)
>   e.g. hemi*plegia*, a paralysis of one side of the body; para*plegia*, paralysis of the lower part (literally, paralysis going around).

-rrhoea (discharge or flow)
>   e.g. leuco*rrhoea* is a white vaginal discharge. Dia*rrhoea* is literally a running through.

-uria (urine)
>   e.g. poly*uria* is the frequent passage of urine; haemat*uria* is the presence of blood in the urine.

-scope (an instrument for viewing)
>   e.g. sigmoido*scope*, cysto*scope*. The process of using such an instrument is sigmoidoscopy, cystoscopy.

-gram (a picture)
>   e.g. electrocardio*gram*, a picture or chart of the heart's electrical activity.

The two sections above illustrate the variety of beginnings and endings that may be found in medical terms. Between them may come one or two or more portions of words, which can be termed word roots. Some of the more common are described here.

WORD ROOTS

Cyst (a bladder)
>   e.g. *cyst*itis is inflammation of the bladder. If the word is not qualified, it is taken to mean the urinary bladder.

Chole (bile organ)
>   e.g. *chole*cystogram, a picture (X-ray) of the gall bladder. *Chole*cystitis, inflammation of the gall bladder.

Aden (a gland)
>   e.g. the *aden*oids are glandular tissue (lymphatic) in the nasopharynx. An *aden*oma is a (benign) glandular growth.

Angio (a vessel or duct)
>   e.g. chol*angio*gram, an X-ray picture of the bile ducts. Lymph*angi*tis, inflammation of lymph vessels.

Haem (blood)
>	e.g. *haem*orrhage is a flow of blood. The "h" is omitted if the root is in the middle of a word, e.g. an*aem*ia, lack of blood; ur*aem*ia, a rise in the amount of urea in the blood.

Cyt (a cell)
>	e.g. *cyt*ology is the study of cells, an erythro*cyte* is a red cell.

Path (disease)
>	e.g. *path*ologist, a man who studies disease.

Therapy (treatment)
>	e.g. chemo*therapy*, treatment by drugs; physio*therapy*, treatment by physical means.

Thromb (a clot)
>	e.g. *thromb*osis, the process of blood clotting.

Phleb (a vein)
>	e.g. *phleb*itis, inflammation of a vein; *phleb*othrombosis, the formation of clot in a vein.

Derm (skin)
>	e.g. intra*derm*al injection is one made into the skin.

Gastr (stomach)
>	e.g. *gastr*oscope an instrument for inspecting the stomach.

Enter (the intestine)
>	e.g. gastro*enter*itis is inflammation of the stomach and intestine.

Proct (the rectum)
>	e.g. *proct*oscope, an instrument for looking into the rectum. A *proct*ologist is a specialist in diseases of the rectum.

Card (the heart)
>	e.g. the peri*card*ium is the serous outer covering of the heart.

My(o) (muscle)
>	e.g. *myo*cardium, the muscle of the heart; *my*algia, pain in muscle.

Hepat(o) (the liver)
>	e.g. *hepat*omegaly is enlargement of the liver.

Rhin (the nose)
>	e.g. *rhin*oplasty is an operation to refashion the nose; a *rhin*oceros is an animal with a horn on its nose.

Aur (the ear)
>	e.g. an *aur*iscope is an instrument for examining the ear.

Os, oris (the mouth)
>   e.g. an *or*al examination is a spoken one.

Cephal (the head)
>   e.g. the normal head-first position of the baby in the uterus is the *cephal*ic presentation.

Encephal (the brain) (literally, in the head)
>   e.g. *encephal*ogram, a picture of the brain.

Nephr or ren (the kidney, both the Greek and Latin roots being used)
>   e.g. a *nephr*ogram is a (radioactive) picture of the kidney; the kidney gets its blood from the *ren*al artery.

Oste (bone)
>   e.g. *oste*otomy means cutting into bone, *oste*ology is the study of the skeleton.

Arthr (a joint)
>   e.g. a pseud*arthr*osis is a false joint, usually formed by imperfect healing of a fracture.

Cost (rib)
>   e.g. the *cost*al margin means the border of the ribs.

Lysis (breaking down)
>   e.g. haemo*lysis*, the breaking down of blood cells.

Glyc(os) (sugar)
>   e.g. hyper*glyc*aemia is an excessive amount of sugar in the blood *Glycos*uria means sugar in the urine.

Scler (hard)
>   e.g. multiple *scler*osis is a disease in which (literally) there are patches of hardening in the nervous system.

Lith (stone)
>   e.g. *lith*otomy position in the theatre used to be the position for stone-cutting operations on the bladder, in those early days when it was dangerous to open the peritoneal cavity.

Melan (black)
>   e.g. a *melan*oma is a pigmented growth. *Mela*ena means black stools.

Morph (shape)
>   e.g. a meta*morph*osis is a change of shape.

Students who would like to test their ability to recognize medical terms should examine the following words, all of which are formed from term defined above. The answers may be found on the next page.

1. Leucocytosis	11. Dermatome
2. Lymphadenopathy	12. Encephalitis
3. Microcephalic	13. Orthopnoea
4. Thromboangiitis	14. Scleroderma
5. Cephalhaematoma	15. Nephrolithotomy
6. Hypoglycaemia	16. Rhinorrhoea
7. Hypernephroma	17. Macrocytic
8. Electroencephalogram	18. Polyarthritis
9. Cholecystgastrostomy	19. Anisocytosis
10. Hæmangioma	20. Polycythaemia

1. Leucocytosis   white/cell/condition
a rise in the number of white cells in the blood.

2. Lymphadenopathy   lymph/gland/disease
any pathological condition of lymph glands.

3. Microcephalic   small/headed
a congenital condition in which the head is abnormally small.

4. Thromboangiitis   clotting/vessel/inflammation
inflammation of blood vessels with clot formation

5. Cephalhaematoma   head/blood/swelling
a swelling on the head of the new born, due to bleeding under the periosteum of the skull.

6. Hypoglycaemia   lacking/sugar/blood
low blood sugar level.

7. Hypernephroma   excessive/kidney/swelling
a malignant kidney tumour.

8. Electroencephalogram   electric/brain/picture
a tracing of the electric activity of the brain.

9. Cholecystgastrostomy   gall/bladder/stomach/opening
an operation to make an opening between the gall bladder and the stomach.

10. Haemangioma   blood/vessel/swelling
a tumour formed of blood vessels.

11. Dermatome   skin/cutting instrument
This instrument is used to cut skin grafts.

12. Encephalitis   brain/inflammation.

13. Orthopnoea   upright/breathing
The patient can only breathe comfortably while sitting up.

14. Scleroderma   hard/skin
A rare condition in which the skin is thickened and hardened.

15. Nephrolithotomy   kidney/stone/incision
Removal of a stone from the kidney by operation.

16. Rhinorrhoea   nose/flow
Increased nasal discharge.

17. Macrocytic   large/celled
In some anaemias e.g. pernicious, the red cells are larger than normal.

18. Polyarthritis   many/joint/inflammation

19. Anisocytosis   without/similar/cell/condition
Red blood cells are not all of the same size or shape, e.g. in some varieties of anaemia.

20. Polycythaemia   many/cells/in the blood
a condition in which the number of red blood cells is higher than normal.

Index